Cover Image Credit/Copyright Attribution: IIIerlok_Xolms/Shutterstock

Michelle Kenyon · Aleksandra Babic
Editors

The European Blood and Marrow Transplantation Textbook for Nurses

Under the Auspices of EBMT

Editors
Michelle Kenyon
Department of Haematological Medicine
King's College Hospital NHS
Foundation Trust
London, UK

Aleksandra Babic
Istituto Oncologico della
Svizzera Italiana
Bellinzona, Switzerland

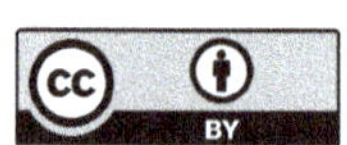

Foreword

Autologous and allogeneic haematopoietic stem cell transplantations (HSCT) are curative procedures for patients with haematological diseases and immune deficiencies.

This textbook is an easy-to-read primer for all those involved in the care of HSCT patients. It offers a solid and comprehensive overview of different nursing methods and requirements and their applications towards improving HSCT patients' outcome.

The book is divided into several chapters which allow reviewing the most important components of nursing and caring after HSCT both in the adult and paediatric patients. It also relies on real-life clinical situations to illustrate the scientific principles and concepts.

Cutting-edge and updated nursing techniques are presented, but the basic principles and general considerations are explained first.

This textbook developed under the auspices of the European Society for Blood and Marrow Transplantation (EBMT) by highly skilled and experienced colleagues in this field represents an invaluable resource that will be highly useful to all professionals involved in the modern management of HSCT patients.

EBMT is very proud of this unique achievement that has been long awaited because nursing science must be continually improved in order to provide the best patient care possible. It will contribute to better patient care and make it visible not only for nurses but also for all other stakeholders. Far from being all-inclusive, it will definitely serve as a catalyst for the interest of the readership.

Mohamad Mohty

Preface

The EBMT Nurses Group: promoting excellence in patient care through international collaboration, education, research and science

The EBMT Nurses Group (NG) plays an essential role in haematology and haematological stem cell transplantation nursing. The group was created 33 years ago and now has over 750 members in more than 60 countries worldwide with a principal nurse identified in almost each EBMT centre.

The EBMT NG's mission is to enhance and value the nurses' role all over the world, supporting and sharing knowledge through communication, advocacy, research, training and education. The group is dedicated to improving the care of patients receiving SCT and works towards promoting excellence in care through recognizing, building upon and providing evidence-based practice.

Over the last two decades, BMT nursing has grown rapidly and has acknowledged the need for care of the patients, their families and donors.

Advanced practice nurses have been taking a leading role in the care of patients, providing in holistic care; BMT nurses are involved in the decision-making process about treatment options for their patients, and they evidently contribute to an enhancement in their patients' quality of life. More and more, EBMT NG is conducting a research on topics based within clinical practice and is formulating their own research agenda.

The EBMT NG consists of a board and five committees (paediatric, research, global educational, scientific and communication and networking) and links with national groups/forums.

Recently, we enhanced our collaboration between EBMT and the Haematology Society of Australia and New Zealand (HSANZ) Nurses Group.

http://www.ebmt.org/Contents/Nursing/WhoWeAre/TheBoard/Pages/TheBoard.aspx

Bellinzona, Switzerland   Aleksandra Babic

Contents

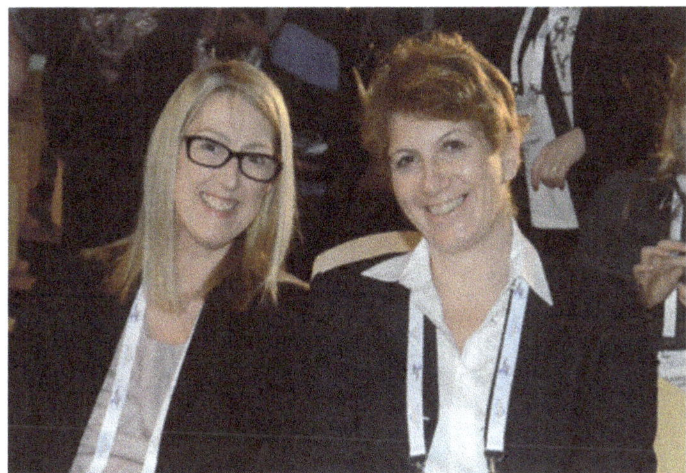

Michelle Kenyon works as Consultant Nurse (BMT Care and Survivorship) at King's College Hospital, London. She has worked for more than 25 years in the field of haemato-oncology and stem cell transplantation. Her interest in improving the patient experience of haematopoietic stem cell transplantation (HSCT) led her to write *The Seven Steps*, a patient information book (2002) and subsequently the *Next Steps* (2012). Around 50,000 copies of these titles have been distributed and are now used as the basis of informed consent for transplant recipients throughout the UK.

She studied her BSc in Cancer Nursing and MSc in Advancing Cancer Nursing Practice at King's College London, and undertook an empirical research study exploring the use of life-coaching in stem cell transplant survivors for her dissertation. She supports patients throughout their post-transplant recovery and has a particular interest in survivorship issues and the effects of treatment. She launched the HSCT long-term follow-up clinic at King's College Hospital in 2014 and has found the patient insights inspiring and the overall experience highly rewarding. She is the nurse representative on the BSBMT executive, Vice Chair EBMT (UK) NAP group and is Secretary of the EBMT NG.

Aleksandra Babic is a Nurse Manager, affiliate to Oncology Institute of Southern Switzerland (IOSI), in Bellinzona, as Transplant Unit Coordinator and Quality Manager. She received her nurse diploma from the College Center of Professional Formation in Dubrovnik, Croatia, in 1988, and was awarded a Master's degree in Nurse Management in 2006. Until 2016 she worked as a nurse manager in apheresis unit at IEO, European Institute of Oncology in Milan, and has published papers on peripheral blood stem cell collection and mobilisation (i.e. R-ESHAP Plus Pegfilgrastim as an Effective Peripheral Stem Cell Mobilization Regimen for Autologous Stem-Cell Transplantation in Patients with Relapsed/Refractory Diffuse Large B-Cell Lymphoma, Transfus Apher Sci. 2013; Successful Mobilisation of Peripheral Blood Stem Cells in Children Using Plerixafor: A Case Report and Review of the Literature, Blood Transfus. 2013; Who Should Be Really Considered as a Poor Mobilizer in the Plerixafor Era? Transfus Apher Sci. 2012) and photopheresis (i.e. Efficacy of Photopheresis Extracorporeal Procedure as Single Treatment for Severe Chronic GVHD: A Case Report, Transfus Apher Sci. 2013). In addition, Aleksandra has presented at a number of conferences worldwide, most recently including the GIIMA 3rd National Conference, GITMO and the EBMT 2015 conference: Validation of PBSC collection within JACIE program – A multicenter evaluation. From 2016 she is also a JACIE Quality Manager Inspector.

Aleksandra is the former EBMT NG President (European Blood and Marrow Transplant Society) Nurses Group, which includes more than 800 nurses in 64 countries worldwide. She is a former President of GIIMA, the Italian Nurses Group in Mobilisation and Aphaeresis, and the founder and a board member of the not-for-profit association, Nurses No Frontiers.

Brief History of HSCT Nursing: HSCT Nursing Through the Ages and Its Evolution

Since the beginning and progress of stem cell transplantations in the late 1950s/early 1960s, it was clear that nurses play a crucial role within the multiprofessional team caring for patients and their families undergoing this treatment. Nurses as core professionals along physicians and other healthcare workers care for patients and their families around the clock. Continuity of care is vital to patients' satisfaction as well as trust. In the beginning, care was considerably cumbersome with HSCT patients who needed to be treated in a sterile environment such as germ-free tents or bubbles. Being one of the nurses who still remembers how that had to be handled, it is clear that this work was very time consuming and specific material was needed because everything – from the linen and clothes of patients up to every single book, toy or newspaper – is all needed to be wrapped up and sterilized before given to the patient. Next to helping patients deal with the time in the germ-free environment, talking to their beloved ones through a plastic curtain or wearing a mask covering emotions on the face, nurses of course also needed to take care for the physical and psychological challenges patients faced.

- Nurses Field of Competences

To be able to care for patients and families, nurses need to perform duties and responsibilities that often comprise more tasks than the ones taught in nursing schools. Experience and long-term commitment to the care of HSCT patients can be a challenge but also very rewarding. Novices to the field will need to be supervised and supported by expert nurses from the beginning to be able to endure also burdensome situations in a very person-centred care.

– Coordinator, Communicator and Translator

Nurses play an important role as coordinator of all issues including coordinating procedures and care activities within the interprofessional context before, during and after transplantation. This includes organizing all necessary diagnostic tests and checkups prior to transplantation. Sometimes they are responsible also for the donor and his/her health including questions concerning the donation of stem cells and its consequences. The process of transplantation involves many professionals and specialties – therefore, all results need to come back to one single point of coordination. It is important to communicate all diagnostic tests, their results, and what they mean in the situation of the patient in a language that the patient understands. Often the medical language is difficult to understand by lay people, and therefore nurses play an important role in translating the meaning and consequences to patients and their families.

– Preparer and Educator of Patients for Transplantation and the Period After HSCT

Over the years, every centre developed modules, booklets or information brochures for patients which always supported the educational activities to prepare patients prior transplantation, help them through the phases of transplantation and make them ready for discharge and the time at home when no professional is around, and they have to make important decisions and cope with the situation in their own home environment. Specific attention has developed towards educating the long-term survivors and their next of kin in which nurses can play a prominent role because medical treatment activities are more in the background and day-to-day questions have to be dealt with. Some centres developed classes in which patients and families get together, gain the needed information and share concerns and discuss ways of coping. All this is often done under the auspice of nurses experienced not only in transplant nursing but also in principles of patient education.

– Carer, Administrator and Technician

The administration of chemotherapeutic, immunosuppressive and symptom-control drugs; blood products; and parenteral nutrition through a central venous access device has developed over the years. The accurate handling and care of the central venous catheter and infusion pump systems is vital in the process because the catheter is related to the highest risk of infections. In addition, nurses often need to make important decision when no physician is around to prescribe medication (such as during the night shift) to ease suffering such as pain, mucositis, diarrhoea or nausea.

– Social Supporter and Motivator

The distress during the time prior to undergoing HSCT, during isolation, in the recovery phase and the time after (long-term recovery) is not to be underestimated. Nurses play an important role as part of the interprofessional team in communicating, motivating and supporting patients throughout the entire process including the follow-up time. Connecting patients and family members with other professionals such as social worker, psychologist or spiritual carer whenever emotional distress is overwhelming, other questions arise and encouragement is needed is often considered very helpful.

Being culturally sensitive and meeting the spiritual needs of patients has become a recognized challenge in our often multicultural societies. Because of the 24/7 availability of nurses, they often detect these needs and are able to call for the necessary support that patients and families need.

Although over the years there were tremendous improvements in outcomes, namely, better survival rates, some patients and families need to face limited life expectancy. In this phase, the early support of palliative care in managing symptoms, helping patients in their often difficult and complex decision-making and discussing who of the family can be involved to take care and how to back up the family and look for additional offers to relieve and unburden family members is vital. Advance care planning should be integrated early into the care of stem cell recipients (Button et al. 2014), and nurses can address the above-mentioned topics and help patients and families to find a way in the often overwhelming and complex situation. An interprofessional palliative care service, supposedly even offered pre-transplantation (Loggers et al. 2016), could provide support in helping throughout often complex and instable situations which could lead to a better understanding of the situation, lessen distress and increase hope and quality of life (El-Jawahri et al. 2016) in the unit of care.

- Extended Practice Roles

In the late 1990s during the EBMT conference in Aix-les-Bain (France), nurses performing diagnostic and therapeutic interventions such as bone marrow or lumbar punctures – up to that time executed only by physicians – were strongly discussed and also criticized by the nursing audience. That can probably be considered as the beginning of the development of extended roles that nurses nowadays perform on a regular basis. Importantly, throughout the discussion, the core tasks of nurses remain in the hands of nurses and are not delegated to other professions.

Probably a suitable mix of skills and grades of nurses is the foundation of professional nursing within the interprofessional team. Nurses trained on an academic level and performing tasks as a nurse practitioner or clinical nurse specialist are considered as advanced practice nurses. Several role models exist throughout the European countries. Learning from the highly qualified nurses in the USA and their approach of nursing inspired many European nurses to go beyond what was up to then traditional in their own country. Being academically trained often enabled nurses to argue more based on evidence-reflected practice and led to being accepted by other academic professionals.

Being part of the interprofessional team with a strong shoulder-to-shoulder workforce together with physicians, physiotherapist, dietitians, social workers or chaplains, nurses found their unique role in being present with the patients 24/7 during the treatment but also in the time before and after the treatment. Nurses took over the responsibility to educate patients before the treatment about any aspects that are important to successfully undergo the procedure. Over the past decades, many nurses not only developed clinical skills but are also excellent researchers looking deeper into the phenomena of patients, family members and measuring outcomes based on a reflective way of practising nursing. The field of nursing research in HSCT has evolved from reflecting on symptom management and service development to quality of life and long-term survival topics.

Outcomes of research form the basis of standard operating procedures (SOPs) developed to support clinical practice, guarantee a high level of practice, and audit and accredit the transplant centres on evidence-based practice guidelines. The translation of evidence into clinical practice and taking into consideration the local circumstances is challenging. Still there are varieties among the nursing care in different transplant settings (Bevans et al. 2009). Therefore, networks of nurses in the field in which nurses discuss patient-centred outcomes are vital – not only to prevent the reinvention of the wheel but mainly to establish high-quality standards and data that are comparable in research. Nurses collaborate in local, national and international networks such as the EBMT Nurses Group, the American Society for Blood and Marrow Transplantation (ASBMT), the Special Interest Group of the American Oncology Nursing Society or the Haematology Nurses and Healthcare Allied Professionals Group (HNHCP). Also nurses reach out to cancer nursing organizations such as the European Oncology Nursing Society (EONS) because issues of haematological patients are not always specific to the stem cell transplant patient population but knowledge from the care for patients with other malignant diseases can be useful in the care.

The shift of the focus towards more educational tasks – especially since the emergence of oral drugs developed to cure haematological malignancies without the necessity of a stem cell transplantation such as tyrosine kinase inhibitors – changed the work of nurses tremendously. Unexpectedly – despite the anticipation that patients with cancer will always take their medication as prescribed by their physician – nurses needed to develop skills and knowledge of adherence. By collaborating together with the industry and patients, educational initiatives were developed to support patients in adhering to the prescribed regimen often over a very long disease and therefore symptom-free time.

- Importance of HSCT Nursing

The best compliment towards nursing was done by Prof. Edward Donnall Thomas (1920–2012), founding medical director of the Fred Hutchinson Cancer Research Center's Transplant Program who shared the 1990 Noble Prize in Physiology or Medicine with Dr. Joseph E. Murray: he stated that nurses and nursing was his secret weapon without whom he could not have achieved his goals. This acknowledges that nurses play a vital role as part of the interprofessional team in caring for the transplant recipients and their families. The statement of Prof. Thomas should be the basis on which nurses should develop the skills, knowledge and expertise to enhance a reflected care and be alert for any changes in treatments which might influence care. Picking up changes and supporting the developments will become a challenge in the often complex healthcare environment. Nurses will need to understand the challenges and shape the future care for any person trusting in what the interprofessional team has to offer – and maybe unravel the "secrets" of nursing and make it more visible of what nursing has to offer.

Bern, Switzerland   Monica C. Fliedner

Literature

Bevans M, Tierney DK, Bruch C, Burgunder M, Castro K, Ford R, et al. Hematopoietic stem cell transplantation nursing: a practice variation study. Oncol Nurs Forum. 2009; 36(6):E317–25. doi:10.1188/09.ONF.E317-E325.

Button EB, Gavin NC, Keogh SJ. Exploring palliative care provision for recipients of allogeneic hematopoietic stem cell transplantation who relapsed. Oncol Nurs Forum. 2014;41(4):370–81. doi:10.1188/14.ONF.370-381.

El-Jawahri A, LeBlanc T, VanDusen H, Traeger L, Greer JA, Pirl WF, et al. Effect of inpatient palliative care on quality of life 2 weeks after hematopoietic stem cell transplantation: a randomized clinical trial. JAMA. 2016;316(20):2094–103. doi:10.1001/jama.2016.16786.

Loggers ET, LeBlanc TW, El-Jawahri A, Fihn J, Bumpus M, David J, et al. Pretransplantation supportive and palliative care consultation for high-risk hematopoietic cell transplantation patients. Biol Blood Marrow Transplant. 2016;22(7):1299–305. doi:10.1016/j.bbmt.2016.03.006.

JACIE and Quality Management in HSCT: Implications for Nursing

Carole Charley, Aleksandra Babic,
Iris Bargalló Arraut, and Ivana Ferrero

Abstract

Laboratory medicine, along with the airline industry, has a long history of utilising quality management systems. It took until 1999 for The Joint Accreditation Committee of the International Society for Cellular Therapy (ISCT) and the European Group for Blood and Marrow Transplantation (EBMT), known as JACIE, to be established as an accreditation system in the field of haematopoietic stem cell transplantation (HSCT). The aim was to create a standardised system of accreditation to be officially recognised across Europe and was based on the accreditation standards established by the US-based Foundation for the Accreditation of Cellular Therapy (FACT).

Since the concept of JACIE was originally launched, many European centres have applied for initial accreditation with other centres gaining reaccreditation for the 2nd or 3rd time. Transplant units, outside of Europe, have accepted the importance of the JACIE Standards, with units in South Africa, Singapore and Saudi Arabia also gaining accreditation.

There is evidence that both donor and patient care have improved within the accredited centres (Passweg et al., Bone Marrow Transpl, 47:906–923, 2012; Demiriz IS, Tekgunduz E, Altuntas F (2012) What is the most appropriate source for hematopoietic stem cell transplantation?

C. Charley (✉) • I.B. Arraut
JACIE Accreditation Office, Barcelona, Spain
e-mail: carolecharley@gmail.com

A. Babic
Istituto Oncologico della Svizzera Italiana,
Bellinzona, Switzerland

I. Ferrero
Stem Cell Transplantation and Cellular Therapy
Laboratory, City of Health and Science of Turin,
University of Turin, Italy/JACIE Accreditation Office,
Barcelona, Spain

M. Kenyon, A. Babic (eds.), *The European Blood and Marrow Transplantation Textbook for Nurses*,
https://doi.org/10.1007/978-3-319-50026-3_1

Peripheral Stem Cell/Bone Marrow/Cord Blood Bone Marrow Res. (2012):Article ID 834040 (online)). However, there is a lack of published evidence demonstrating that this improvement directly results from better nursing care. Therefore, the authors conducted a survey of nursing members of the European Blood and Marrow Transplantation Nurses Group (EBMT (NG)) to identify how nurses working in the area of HSCT felt that JACIE impacted in the care they delivered and the general implications of JACIE for nurses.

Keywords

FACT-JACIE International Standards • Nurses implications • Quality management • Standard operating procedures

1.1 Background to JACIE

The 1990s saw an increase in the number of transplant teams performing haematopoietic stem cell transplantation (HSCT) (Passweg et al. 2012). The procedure that was initially considered experimental during the 1960s/1970s was becoming an established treatment for many blood cancers, solid tumours and acquired or congenital disorders of the haematopoietic system within adult and paediatric populations. Towards the end of the 1990s, the source of haematopoietic stem cells was collectable from the marrow, peripheral blood and cord blood and from autologous, sibling and unrelated donations (Demiriz et al. 2012).

In 1998 two leading European scientific organisations, The International Society for Cellular Therapy (ISCT) Europe and the European Group for Blood and Marrow Transplantation (EBMT), formed a joint committee to be known as the Joint Accreditation Committee for ISCT and EBMT (JACIE) (JACIE n.d.; Cornish 2008). The purpose of this new committee was to establish a system to allow transplant teams to self-assess against a group of standards (Cornish 2008), provide an inspection process and recognise compliance with the standards by awarding accreditation to those teams who worked within the field of HSCT. A pilot study of the JACIE inspection and accreditation process was carried out in Spain 2000–2002. This enabled JACIE to assess sections of the stan-

dards that gave rise to common difficulty experienced by the transplant teams and to assess what assistance, if any, would be required by the centres for them to obtain accreditation. The results of this pilot study underlined the need to implement national and international regulations (Pamphilon et al. 2008) within each European country. In January 2004, with the support from the European Union under the Public Health Programme (2003–2008), the JACIE accreditation process was launched (Pamphilon et al. 2008).

To enable a set of international standards for the provision of quality medical, nursing and laboratory practice in HSCT transplantation to be developed and recognised, JACIE collaborated with their American counterparts, the Foundation for the Accreditation of Cellular Therapy (*FACT*) (JACIE). The "FACT-JACIE International Standards for Hematopoietic Cellular Therapy Product Collection, Processing, and Administration" are revised on a regular basis.

JACIE remains a non-profit organisation with all members being an expert within their specialty: clinical, collection or processing procedures of HSCT. Clinicians, nurses and quality managers who are experts in their field can volunteer to become JACIE inspectors, if they meet the criteria set. Potential inspectors must attend a training programme, pass the inspector's exam and act as an observer within the inspection team as a trainee before their first official JACIE inspection. As the JACIE accreditation process has evolved, the inspection team membership has extended to include apheresis nurses and more recently experienced quality managers recognising the multi-professional components of our HSCT programmes. The accreditation process is continuous reflecting an established quality management system (QMS); therefore accredited centres are required to apply for reaccreditation every 4 years. In 2016, many transplant teams were achieving reaccreditation for the 2nd or 3rd time, whilst other centres are applying for their initial application. At the beginning of December 2016, the JACIE website (www.jacie.org) (2016) cited 334 successful initial accreditations; 197 successful reaccreditations from 26 countries had been granted since 2000. Although the initial aim of the accreditation scheme was a voluntary process, in many countries, health-care systems/commissioners or health insurance providers and tissue banking authorities increasingly view JACIE accreditation as important and demand accreditation to allow the procedure of HSCT to be performed.

Accreditation is the means by which a centre can demonstrate that it is performing to a required level of practice in accordance with agreed standards of excellence. Essentially it allows a centre to certify that it operates an effective QMS. Furthermore, due to the increased use of unrelated donors from different countries, interaction and collaboration between units are key elements for the success of stem cell transplantation. JACIE accreditation is a guarantee that the donor and the cellular product have been handled according to specific safety criteria.

A QMS is a mechanism to:

- Ensure that procedures are being performed in line with agreed standards, with full participation by all staff members. In a HSCT programme, this ensures that the clinical, collection and laboratory facilities are all working together to achieve excellent communication, effective common work practices, shared policies where appropriate and increases guarantees for improved patient outcomes and the use of international donor criteria for related donors (Gratwohl et al. 2014;

Anthias et al. 2015, 2016). Nurses have successfully taking on the role of improving communications for donor mobilisation, collections and liaising with the staff of the processing facility.

- Track and monitor collected cell products for safety and viability from the time of donation to the administration procedure. Patients' medical records must include not only the information of date and time of the collection but should include volume of collected product, type and volume of citrate and the product identification. A transport log will be required to ensure traceability of all products from collection to processing and then to clinical for administration.
- Identify errors and incidents that can be reviewed and corrective actions be implemented and allow a plan of action to be put into place to minimise the error reoccurring.
- Formalise training and competencies.
- Clearly identify the roles and responsibilities of all staff working within the transplant team or with outside agencies (clinical, collection, processing and support services; intensive care, radiotherapy, cleaning and transport services, laboratories and donor panels).
- Review documentation for evidence that standards have achieved compliance on a regular basis.

1.2 Preparing for JACIE Accreditation

1.2.1 Considerations

In the early stages of preparing for accreditation, extra resources may be required: a dedicated quality manager, data collection manager and support staff (pharmacist, dietician, social worker) to fulfil the standards and prepare for the inspection. Formalisation of the QMS and accreditation will depend on structures already in place.

There will be many processing facilities that are independent from the clinical transplant teams and may also be responsible for collections of apheresis products. In this situation, the processing facility and clinical facility have a choice of accreditation. They may decide to apply for separate or combined accreditation. However, in order to obtain JACIE accreditation, it is important that the QMS describes the communication processes between all facilities involved and provides the evidence that communications exist, e.g. minutes of weekly, monthly and annual meetings must include the names of the attendees, sharing evidence of engraftment and adverse events. It is important to remember a clinical facility must use an apheresis and processing facility that are JACIE accredited. Similarly, an apheresis facility must use a processing facility that is accredited before clinical and apheresis facilities can be awarded JACIE accreditation.

1.2.2 Implementing a Quality Management System

HSCT is a procedure with a high technological content, which requires extensive attention towards patients/donors who might introduce important problematic clinical factors and also towards sophisticated laboratory procedures related to the collection, manipulation, cryopreservation and transplantation of haematopoietic stem cells (HSCs). The continuous improvement of stem cell technology requires that all procedures regarding HSCT be guaranteed through the definition of qualitative standards recognised by scientific associations and international organisations. For the collection, processing and transplantation of HSCs, there are standardised procedures, which require specific clinical, haematological and laboratory knowledge and strict quality controls concerning all processes from cellular collection and manipulation to the administration of the collected product. Stem cell collection, processing, storage and transplantation must be carried out in a highly regulated manner to guarantee both safety and clinical efficacy. Therefore, quality assurance is a very important topic at all levels of HSCT, including robust nursing procedures, e.g. chemotherapy administration, use of stem cell mobilisation agents and collection of cellular material.

The implementation of a QMS arises from the need to develop an appropriate system to optimise the quality of the service offered by a stem cell transplantation unit, in a general context of health-care quality improvement. A QMS is a tool that can be used to rapidly identify errors or accidents and resolve them to minimise the risk of repetition. A QMS assists in training and clearly identifies the roles and responsibilities of all staff (Cornish 2008; Caunday et al. 2009).

In 1966, Avedis Donabedian wrote a paper entitled "Evaluating the Quality of Medical Care", where the concepts of structure, process and outcome in health care were introduced. The structure includes not only the physical aspects in which care is given but also the resources and tools available to the health-care team, the leadership and the staff. The process is how the health-care system and the patient interact. The outcome includes the effect of care on diseases and their prevention, such as the mortality rate, the error rate and the quality of life (Samson et al. 2007).

During the 1950s, Edwards Deming introduced the plan-do-check-act (PDCA) cycle, an iterative four-step management method used for the implementation and improvements of processes and products, also known as plan-do-study-act (PDSA). He also stressed the importance of viewing problems in the context of a system and that most mistakes were not the fault of the worker (Samson et al. 2007).

The major objective of the JACIE Standards is to promote quality medical and laboratory practice in HSCT and other therapies using cellular products; therefore dedicated quality management standards are found within the FACT-JACIE manual (clinical facility B04, marrow collection facility CM04, apheresis collection facility C04, processing facility D04).

Quality management is the management of activities involved in quality assessment, assurance and control that try to improve the quality of patient care, products and services in cellular therapy activities.

A QMS could be implemented applying the PDCA cycle for the management and continuous improvement of processes and products.

- **PLAN** means to establish the objectives and processes necessary to the centre. This means define the scope of the QMS and identify which processes within the scope are most important, those staff who are involved in the important processes and involve them in defining the targets to be used to measure the quality of the process. Ensure all staff knows how they can contribute to achieve the performance required.

One important aspect to consider when implementing a QMS is the organisation and interaction between the different facilities (clinical, collection and processing). The plan shall include an organisational chart of functions, considering clinical, collection and processing staff, in particular for those tasks that are critical to assuring product or service quality. Training plans should be defined and put in place. Documentation may be displayed in a variety of formats (job descriptions, training records, qualifications certificates, retraining).

A document system should be implemented serving multiple purposes for the QM programme. They provide instructions on:

- Activities, policies and processes controlling various steps within the activities
- Quality control and traceability of products, donor and patients

The Quality Management Plan (QMP) (or *Quality Management Manual*) should be one of the first documents developed when preparing for JACIE accreditation. The centre must have a standard operating procedure (SOP) outlining the method by which to create, approve, implement and update SOPs (known as the "SOP for SOPs"). Clinical and collection protocols or laboratory methods must be translated into written procedures, in paper form or an electronic version, and readily available to staff. The purpose of document control is to ensure the correct approved documents are in use.

In the 6th edition of the FACT-JACIE Standards, more specific requirements for validation and qualification studies have been delineated, and the concept of risk assessment has been implemented.

- Validation is documented evidence that the performance of a specific process meets the requirements for the intended application. For example, the procedure for thawing frozen cells should be evaluated, as there is a risk of contamination and loss of cells during the thawing process. A thawing control, on three procedures, could be performed to assess these criteria would validate the process.
- Qualification is documented evidence that the equipment/facility/utility is meeting the user requirement specification, working correctly and leading to the expected results. For example, "the dry shipper used for the transportation of frozen haematopoietic stem cells should be validated for temperature control".

During the implementation phase, risk management should be an ongoing part of the quality management process, to minimise hazards for processes, patients and staff. There are several methods for the assessment of the risk, such as Failure Mode and Effects Analysis (FMEA) or Failure Modes, Effects and Criticality Analysis (FMECA), methods of assessing potential failure mechanisms and their impact on system, identifying single failure points.

- *DO* means to implement the plan, execute the process and carry on the activities. Once the programme has been established and staff trained, the activities and the quality plan should be maintained, through the document system and the available resources. Policies and procedures could be revised, training programmes implemented and the outcome analysis of cellular therapy product efficacy reviewed to verify that the processes in use provide a safe and effective product.
- *CHECK* is to measure the results and compare them against the expected results or goals defined by the plan. Audits represent one of

the principal activities in this step and should be documented, independent inspection and retrospective review of activities to determine if they are performed according to written procedure and specified endpoints. They should be conducted to ensure that the QMS is operating effectively and to identify trends and recurring problems in all aspects of the programme. Moreover, the transplant programme should manage errors, accidents, deviations, adverse reactions and complaints and monitor activities, processes and products using measurable indicators (Harolds 2015).

- Finally, *ACT* is to improve the QMS based on the results of the previous steps. Investigation of errors and indicators and the implementation of corrective or improvement strategies are undertaken and monitored with follow-up assessment to determine the effectiveness of the change.

Data shown by Gratwohl and colleagues (Gratwohl et al. 2014) demonstrates the use of a clinical quality management system is associated with improved survival of patients undergoing allogeneic HSCT.

## 1.3	The JACIE Accreditation Process

### 1.3.1	Start Working with the Standards

The JACIE accreditation process begins when the transplant centre, with the support of the hospital management team (a key element in order to assure the required resources to successfully implement the JACIE accreditation process), agrees to start working according to the JACIE Standards.

It is important to gather all the necessary information before commencing the JACIE accreditation pathway. First read the JACIE Standards, access the guides, manuals and supporting documentation from the JACIE website (www.jacie. org). Then utilise the JACIE Inspection Checklist

as a self-evaluation tool. This document contains all the JACIE Standards and will help the centre establish their level of compliance against each standard and identify further work required to achieve accreditation. Furthermore, the checklist is the pivotal tool used continually throughout the JACIE accreditation process, until JACIE accreditation has been awarded.

### 1.3.2	Application for JACIE Accreditation

When the applicant has established a mature QMS, i.e. has been in place and operational for at least a year, a self-assessment of the standards has been performed and shows a high percentage of compliance the centre can formally apply for JACIE accreditation. The completed application form and inspection checklist should be submitted to the JACIE Office where the JACIE team will review and approve the application form, finalising this part of the process by signing the accreditation agreement with the centre.

Within 30 days of the application being approved, the applicant will be required to provide the preaudit documentation to the JACIE Office. The JACIE team and the inspectors will determine that all required documentation has been correctly submitted. The documents can be provided in the language of the centre/applicant; however in some exceptional cases, a translation in English of some key documents can be requested. The preaudit documentation should be submitted using the predefined folder structure described on the JACIE website, which includes relevant documentation for all areas of the Stem Cell Transplant Programme such as personnel documentation, donor consent information, labels and summary of QMS activities (Quality Management Plan, audit report, policies).

### 1.3.3	Arranging the Inspection Date

The JACIE Office will begin the process to assign an inspection date and the inspection team. However, this part of the process can take approximately 6 months from the approval of the application. The inspection team will consist of one inspector per facility to be inspected. For example, if the applicant has applied for adult clinical and bone marrow, apheresis and processing accreditation, the inspection team will consist of the following: clinical, apheresis and a processing inspector (The clinical inspector will be responsible for clinical and marrow collection facilities). The inspectors are selected according to their area of expertise: clinical, apheresis and processing. For instance, a clinician will inspect the clinical facility. If a paediatric unit is part of the inspection, a paediatrician will be assigned. When there is more than one facility per area, for instance, two apheresis units, an extra collection inspector will be included in the inspection team.

The applicant will be invited to view the list of JACIE inspectors, found on the JACIE website, and inform the JACIE Office if there are any inspectors that they prefer *not* to participate in their inspection, due to conflict of interest. The inspection will be performed in the language of the centre unless there are no JACIE inspectors that speak the language of the applicant centre; in these cases, the inspection will be performed in English with language support.

1.3.4 The Inspection

The inspection will take place over a period of 1–2 days and is a thorough examination of all aspects of the programme. The inspector will use the inspection checklist previously completed by the applicant to evaluate the centre's compliance with the standards.

The inspection is usually divided in the following parts:

- Introductory meeting by the programme director and the inspection team with all the programme personnel
- MEDA/B data audit and review of documentation
- Interviews with personnel
- Closing meeting with programme director

- Closing meeting summarising the inspection results with the transplant team

1.3.5 The Inspection Report

Following inspection, the inspectors submit their completed written report and inspection checklist to the JACIE Office. The inspection report is a fundamental part of the accreditation process. The report will be prepared and presented to the JACIE Accreditation Committee by the JACIE Report Assessors after their review and confirmation with the inspectors over any issues, if necessary.

The Accreditation Committee is a group of experts from all areas of Stem Cell Transplantation (Clinical, Collection and Processing) that discusses each individual report and determines corrective actions the centre is required to implement in order to achieve the JACIE accreditation. Please bear in mind that although the inspectors identify areas of non-compliance, it is the JACIE Accreditation Committee who decide the corrective actions, not the inspectors.

1.3.6 Corrections and Accreditation Award

A high percentage of all inspections reveal deficiencies and the degree of deficiency identified will vary in seriousness. In most cases, evidence of corrections can be submitted electronically. However, if the deficiencies are considered a risk for patients, donors or personnel, a focussed re-inspection will be required before JACIE accreditation can be finalised.

Centres are allowed a period between 6 and 9 months to implement and submit the corrections to the JACIE Office. The same team of inspectors will review and assess the adequacy of the corrections provided by the centre. Once the inspectors are satisfied that all points have been resolved and with the approval of the JACIE Accreditation Committee, the applicant will be awarded the JACIE accreditation for a 4-year period, subject to an interim audit at the end of the second year.

1.3.7 Post JACIE Accreditation

The inspection is the most visible part of the JACIE accreditation process. The most challenging part, once the JACIE accreditation has been awarded, is maintaining accreditation. At the second year of accreditation, the interim audit will be due, and if the system has not been maintained, the hard work invested in achieving accreditation will become void and centres return to the beginning of the process when applying for reaccreditation.

The JACIE Committee warns against failing to uphold standards or maintain the QMS between inspections. Those centres that fail to maintain their QMS due to lack of commitment or allow their system to devolve may discover standards that were compliant at the initial inspection may become partially or noncompliant during the inspection required for reaccreditation. Inspectors will identify failures to review documentation, perform audits and maintain competencies due to the lack of available evidence during the accreditation cycle.

1.4 JACIE Standards that Affect Nursing: Clinical and Collection

The JACIE Standards are divided into sections: clinical and donor (B), collection of marrow (CM), apheresis products(C) and laboratory (D). Many of these standards are shared across each facility as appropriate (Table 1.1).

It is not possible to describe, within this chapter, all the actions and evidence required to fulfil a full compliance for all the standards published in the latest edition of the JACIE Standards; therefore in Tables 1.2, 1.3 and 1.4, there are examples of appropriate standards, compliance and comments that have implications for nurses.

It is important that the nursing team takes ownership of the relevant standards and works towards achieving full compliance whilst being aware of the other standards that have implications on nurses or nursing (Table 1.5).

Table 1.1 FACT-JACIE Hematopoietic Cellular Therapy Accreditation Standards (6th edition)

QUALITY MANAGEMENT

CLINICAL PROGRAM STANDARDS PART B	COLLECTION FACILITY STANDARDS PART C	PROCESSING FACILITY STANDARDS PART D
B1 General	C1 General	D1 General
B2 Clinical Unit	C2 Apheresis Collection Facility	D2 Processing Facility
B3 Personnel	C3 Personnel	D3 Personnel
B4 Quality Management	C4 Quality Management	D4 Quality Management
B5 Policies and Procedures	C5 Policies and Procedures	D5 Policies and Procedures
B6 Allogeneic and Autologous Donor Selection, Evaluation, and Management	C6 Allogeneic and Autologous Donor Evaluation and Management	D6 Equipment, Supplies, and Reagents
B7 Recipient Care	C7 Coding and Labeling of Cellular Therapy Products	D7 Coding and Labeling of Cellular Therapy Products
B8 Clinical Research	C8 Process Controls	D8 Process Controls
B9 Data Management	C9 Cellular Therapy Product Storage	D9 Cellular Therapy Product Storage
B10 Records	C10 Cellular Therapy Product Transportation and Shipping	D10 Cellular Therapy Product Transportation and Shipping
	C11 Records	D11 Distribution and Receipt
	C12 Direct Distribution to Clinical Program	D12 Disposal
		D13 Records

Table 1.2 Examples of "non compliant" clinical standards (FACT-JACIE Hematopoietic Cellular Therapy Accreditation Standards: 6th edition)

B.03.07	NURSES		
B.03.07.01	The Clinical Program shall have nurses formally trained and experienced in the management of patients receiving cellular therapy.	Partially Compliant	No evidence of formal training in the transplant setting
B.03.07.02	Clinical Programs treating pediatric patients shall have nurses formally trained and experienced in the management of pediatric patients receiving cellular therapy.	Partially Compliant	Nurses are paediatric qualified but lack evidence of formal training in the transplant setting
B.03.07.03	Training and competency shall include:		
B.03.07.03.03	Administration of blood products, growth factors, cellular therapy products, and other supportive therapies.	Partially Compliant	Hospital policy does not include the administration of cellular products; therefore a policy for the administration of cellular products is required. This policy can then be used for training and competency testing
B.03.07.03.06	Palliative and end of life care.	Non Compliant	No training
B.03.07.04	There shall be written policies for all relevant nursing procedures, including, but not limited to:		
B.03.07.04.01	Care of immunocompromised patients.	Partially Compliant	Hospital policy used does not include the severely compromised transplant patient, therefore a policy or SOP required
B.03.07.04.03	Administration of cellular therapy products.	Partially compliant	Policy/SOP does not include administration of donor lymphocytes
B.03.07.06	There shall be a nurse/patient ratio satisfactory to manage the severity of the patients' clinical status.	Partially compliant	During the discussions with nursing staff there appears to be an informal policy in place to increase the number of nursing staff when required. A formal policy should be written

Table 1.3 Examples of "non compliant" quality management standards for clinical and apheresis facilties (FACTJACIE Hematopoietic Cellular Therapy Accreditation Standards: 6th edition)

B.04	QUALITY MANAGEMENT	COMPLIANCE	COMMENT
B.04.04	The Quality Management Plan shall include, or summarize and reference, policies and Standard Operating Procedures addressing personnel requirements for each key position in the Clinical Program. Personnel requirements shall include at a minimum:		
B.04.04.01 C.04.04.01	A current job description for all staff.	Partially Compliant	Job Description not available for all nursing grades/roles
B.04.04.02 C.04.04.02	A system to document the following for all staff:		
B.04.04.02.02 C.04.04.02.02	New employee orientation.	Partially Compliant	Orientation program in place but no evidence that nurse Smyth (only worked on the ward for 3 months) has participated in the orientation program
B.04.04.02.03 C.04.04.02.03	Initial training and retraining when appropriate for all procedures performed.	Partially compliant	No evidence of re-training for Nurse X who has returned from long-term absence.
B.04.04.02.05 C.04.04.02.05	Continued competency at least annually.	Partially compliant	Not all nursing staff have evidence that competencies are performed annually
B.04.04.02.06 C.04.04.02.06	Continuing education.	Partially Compliant	Education program in place but no attendance list for each education activity
B.04.08.03	Audits shall include, at a minimum:		
B.04.08.03.03	Annual audit of verification of chemotherapy drug and dose against the prescription ordering system and the protocol.	Non compliant	Not performed
B.04.11 C.04.11	The Quality Management Plan shall include, or summarize and reference, policies and procedures for cellular therapy product tracking and tracing that allow tracking from the donor to the recipient or final disposition and tracing from the recipient or final disposition to the donor.	Partially compliant	Policies and SOP are included with the QMP. Staffs do not complete the tracking forms.

Table 1.4 Examples of "non compliant" policy and procedure standards for clincial and apheresis facilties (FACTJACIE Hematopoietic Cellular Therapy Accreditation Standards: 6th edition)

B.05	POLICIES AND PROCEDURES	COMPLIANCE	COMMENT
B.05.01 C.05.01	The Clinical Program shall establish and maintain policies and/or procedures addressing critical aspects of operations and management in addition to those required in B4. These documents shall include all elements required by these Standards and shall address at a minimum:		
B.05.01.08	Administration of HPC and other cellular therapy products, including products under exceptional release	Partially Compliant	The policy has not been updated to include Cord blood
C06.01.07	Labeling (including associated forms and samples)	Partially Compliant	Labeling procedure should show more details regarding roles of physician and nurse involved in labeling operations
C.05.01.14	Equipment operation, maintenance, and monitoring including corrective actions in the event of failure.	Partially Compliant	No evidence of maintenance reports
B.07.04.04	Prior to administration of the preparative regimen, one (1) qualified person using a validated process or two (2) qualified people shall verify and document the drug and dose in the bag or pill against the orders and the protocol, and the identity of the patient to receive the therapy.	Non Compliant	No evidence of two persons verifying the drug.
B.07.06	There shall be a policy addressing safe administration of cellular therapy products.	Partially Compliant	The policy has not been updated to include Cord blood
B.07.06.04	Two (2) qualified persons shall verify the identity of the recipient and the product and the order for administration prior to the administration of the cellular therapy product.	Non Compliant	No evidence of two person verify the drug
B.07.06.06	There shall be documentation in the recipient's medical record of the administered cellular therapy product unique identifier, initiation and completion times of administration, and any adverse events related to administration.	Partially compliant	No evidence of start and completion times of the infused product written in the recipient's medical notes

Table 1.5 Examples of "non compliant" process control standards for apheresis facilities (FACT-JACIE Hematopoietic Cellular Therapy Accreditation Standards: 6th edition)

C.08	PROCESS CONTROLS	COMPLIANCE	COMMENT
C.08.10.01	Adequacy of central line placement shall be verified by the Apheresis Collection Facility prior to initiating the collection procedure.	Partially Complaint	No evidence that this standard is performed
C.08.11	Administration of mobilization agents shall be under the supervision of a licensed health care professional experienced in their administration and management of complications in persons receiving these agents.	Partially Compliant	The responsibilities of administration of growth factors should be clearly defined in the appropriate policies especially for those donors where shared care is in place
C.08.12.01	Methods for collection shall include a process for controlling and monitoring the collection of cellular therapy products to confirm products meet predetermined release specifications.	Partially Compliant	Criteria for HPC-A collection should be defined together with ranges of expected results concerning HPC product characteristics

1.4.1 Staffing and Nursing
(Table 1.2)

Senior staff should be aware that the patient's pathway, during the transplant process, can be unpredictable. There are episodes when the patient will experience complications of the treatment required for HSCT that will require a higher intensity of nursing care. During such episodes, the nursing management should have an established contingency plan to provide adequate nursing care for these patients. Possible options could be:

- Nursing staff within the team allowed to work extra shifts
- The employment of additional nursing staff with relevant experience from the hospital pool of nurses or from nursing agencies
- Transfer of the patient to a high dependency or intensive care setting

Whatever the contingency plan, there should be evidence in place, such as a written policy for staffing. This policy should describe the plan of action to be taken for small teams, apheresis, quality management and data collection teams, in case of planned or unplanned long-term absence from work, therefore allowing the patient's or donor's pathway to continue without affecting the nursing or medical care given.

Not only should there be adequate nursing staff, the nurses should be qualified, trained and competent in the roles they perform.

JACIE can be a challenge and an opportunity for nurses in:

- Reviewing existing procedures
  - Especially those that have been performed automatically in the same way despite being inefficient
- In adopting measures for clinical risk management
  - Paying more attention to long-term planning for continuing education of personnel, procedures and tools for monitoring, verifying and in achieving competence maintenance
- Development and implementation of internal audits and quality indicators

Furthermore, JACIE is an opportunity for nurse recognition within the organisation they work, in terms of contribution to the overall results achieved.

1.4.2   Training and Competencies (Tables 1.2 and 1.3)

All hospitals should have their own programme for training, annual review/appraisal and competencies. The structure already in place for recording the individual staff members training can also be used to record the JACIE Standards' requirements. A new system for training records for JACIE is not required if the following is undertaken.

- Basic training:
  - A route that leads to the skills acquisition in order to obtain new or improved "performance"
- Educational training:
  - The set of activities, including basic training, aimed to develop and enrich the staff on the technical, special, managerial and cultural side aspects of their role
- Competence:
  - The proven ability to use knowledge and skills
- Competency maintenance:
  - The minimum activity that is required to be performed by each operator in order to retain the assessments defined in the specific job description.
- Competency matrix:
  - The activities performed must be recorded in order to perform an annual assessment (quantitative and qualitative) for the activities that can be recognised.

It is important that training and competency programmes are structured and ongoing, with documented evidence of training topics and dates. Most importantly, an attendance register for training and competency sessions is required. Whilst initial supervised training is more easily documented, annual competency maintenance

can be difficult to show (Table 1.3). Ongoing training for clinical personnel should reflect:

- Their experience
- Individual competencies and proficiencies
- Orientation for new staff
- Preceptorship

Training needs to be flexible to reflect staff requirements and should be performed in a timely manner to demonstrate annual updating.

When staff cannot attend a particular training session due to staffing issues, holidays or sickness, a self-teaching system, e.g. an electronic system that includes the presentation and self-assessment tool, may be an option to consider.

For those centres that apply for a combined adult and paediatric JACIE accreditation, it is important that training sessions should include relevant age-specific issues for each topic, especially if the two age group populations are nursed within the same ward environment. Where adult and paediatric patients are nursed on separate wards, training sessions may be separate for certain topics, but it is also important to share sessions, where appropriate, to provide evidence that both population groups are an integrated part of a combined transplant facility.

The FACT-JACIE International Standards Accreditation requires that the clinical programme have access to personnel who are formally trained, experienced and competent in the management of patients receiving cellular therapy. Core competencies are specified within the standards, and evidence of training in these competencies must be documented. This may be achieved by evidence of in-service training, attendance at conferences, etc.

During September 2016, the EBMT (NG) in collaboration with JACIE and the EOC (Ente Ospedaliero Cantonale - multicentre Swiss hospital name, www.eoc.ch) launched the first video recorded course, aimed at physicians, nurses and technicians working within JACIE-accredited centres. The course focused on competency maintenance and could be accessed in person, on the day, or through online conferencing and is now a source of video recorded e-sessions, lectures and questionnaires, available online free of charge. Upon correct answering of questionnaires on every topic, participants to the in-site or online conference are able to obtain a Certificate of Competence that is validated by EBMT and JACIE that can be used as evidence towards the JACIE inspection. In addition, the activities were granted a CME certification by EBMT/EBAH and Swiss CME credits (The course is available at http://www.dsit.it/prj/ebmt2016/inex2.php). This initiative was based on an online test system using a SharePoint internal hospital standard operating procedures compliant with FACT-JACIE standards, developed by the Bellinzona transplant centre (Babic et. al. 2015).

1.4.3 Benefits of Quality Management (Table 1.3)

The key aim of the JACIE process is to implement a QMS into clinical practice. Despite the difficulties that maybe encountered, the process can be useful for integration of staff from all disciplines and professional collaboration. Staff education plays a key role in the implementation of the whole system and in particular for the quality management system (Piras and Aresi 2015). The majority of the quality standards are aimed at providing evidence that there are systematic processes in place. Furthermore, several of the standards relate to having systems in place to record initial qualification, training and competencies and minimal qualifications for the trainer. The hospital system can be utilised for these standards, and this evidence can be shown to the inspectors. However, not all hospital record systems register the training qualification required by a member of staff who has a training role.

1.4.4 Audits (Table 1.3)

Some nurses may be unfamiliar with this area. One approach is to view audits as assessing the care you give, reviewing the evidence and making changes to improve the patient's or donor's experience and/or nursing care given. After a predeter-

mined period of time, it is necessary to reassess the changes made to measure any improvements resulting from those changes. This is referred to as "closing the audit loop". A nursing audit schedule works best when the nursing teams initiate the audit topics. It is important to include the audits required by JACIE, e.g. (1) the verification of the chemotherapy drug and dose against the prescription and the protocol and (2) the verification of the haematopoietic stem cell infusion.

It is important that the audit is performed by personnel that are not directly involved within the activity to be audited.

1.4.5 Reporting Adverse Events (Table 1.3)

To enable adverse events to be fully reported, it is important that a culture of "no blame" is present. The hospital should have an established reporting system in place, and it is important that the adverse events for transplantation and collection of cellular products including apheresis and marrow can be coded separately to other departmental adverse events. This allows for clarity and a true record of the number of events recorded for the transplant programme. Each episode is reviewed and changes made if required. This is then followed by an audit of the changes made to minimise a reoccurrence. Nurses working with patients and donors have a very important role in reporting adverse events.

It is important that all adverse events are recorded in the quality meeting minutes, quarterly and annual reports and most importantly shared with all the sections involved in delivery of the transplant programme (clinical, collection and processing), as appropriate. For example, if a recipient has a reaction to a stem cell infusion or there is a deviation from the time specified for each infusion of thawed cells, these events should be reported and shared with the processing facility.

Where adverse events have been shared across departments, the inspector will require evidence that the events were discussed, and if any changes were made to practice that this was recorded, policies were updated and the episode monitored.

1.4.6   Tracking of Collected Products (Table 1.3)

To enable the safe collection, storage and distribution of collected products, it is important that each stage of the process is recorded. Therefore, collection, laboratory, transport and clinical staff should be involved in signing a transport log to accept the product and in some cases recording the temperature of the product. Policies should be in place to include what to do if there is a deviation in practice, e.g. temperature of the product falls outside the range of temperature agreed within the transport policy. It is important that policies and standard operating procedures that include responsibilities of more than one facility are shared and members of staff have ready access.

The donor and recipient's medical notes must be completed, as part of the tracking system, to record the collection or transfusion of the collected product. The cellular product identification, time and date should also be included in the medical notes

1.4.7   Common Deficiencies: 5th Edition of the JACIE Standards

During the annual meeting of the EBMT (2015), the results of a review of JACIE inspection reports against the 5th ed. of the JACIE Standards were presented (JACIE Quality Management 2015). The aim of the review was to identify common deficiencies within the standards. Of reports issued against the 5th ed. of the JACIE Standards, 95% (145/152) had been reviewed.

Standards relating to clinical personnel were rated as the group of standards with the highest number of deficiencies. This was due to the lack of evidence:

- In training and competencies for physicians
- Relating to donor and recipient informed consent
- Of diagnosis and management of graft versus host disease, both acute and chronic

Other clinical standards that highlighted lack of evidence were related to the administration of the preparative chemotherapy regimen and the administration of the transplanted product. The inspectors could not find evidence that two personnel had checked the identity of the recipient against the dose of the material to be infused.

There were issues with quality management standards for clinical, collection and processing. Third-party agreements/service-level agreements failed to state the responsibilities of each facility involved within the process, e.g. who was responsible for transportation of the collected cellular product either from the collection facility to processing or transportation from processing to the clinical facility. For those clinical facilities that provide shared care for donors prior to collection of cellular material, it is important that third-party agreements/service-level agreements also include the responsibilities for the administration of mobilisation products. These responsibilities should be described within the appropriate standard operating procedure/policy (SOP), and it is important that all parties involved with the shared care have access to the SOP.

Labelling of collected products was a common issue, either non-compliance with the International Society of Blood Transfusion (ISBT128) standards for labelling or personnel failed to complete all the data fields on the label. Often the volume and name of the citrate used and start and completion time of the collection were missing.

1.5   JACIE: Implications on Nursing – The Nurse's Perspective

Research demonstrates that patient outcomes and donor care are improved (Anthias et al. 2016; Gratwohl et al. 2011) when treatment is delivered within a JACIE-accredited centre. Therefore, it could be assumed that the JACIE accreditation process has had implications on nursing practice. A literature search was performed (using PubMed and Google search engine with the following parameters: quality management, standard operating procedures, nurse education, JACIE accreditation and audit), but no results were found reflecting the dearth of nursing research on implications of JACIE for nursing. Therefore, a simple survey was sent to the members of the European Group for Blood and Marrow Transplantation Nurses Group (EBMT (NG)) via email. The aim of the survey was to establish what implications the JACIE process had for nurses in their daily practice.

1.5.1 Results of the Survey

The survey (in the form of a word document) was distributed via email to 322 nurse members of the EBMT nurses group (EBMT (NG)). 135/322 (41%) nurses opened the email received and the response rate was 31/322 (9.62%). One reply was rejected due to the transplant centre not working towards JACIE accreditation; therefore 30/322 (9.3%) replies from 11 countries were evaluated:

Nurses who responded to the survey performed a variety of roles within the area of HSCT, worked in 11 different countries, and their replies varied from "no implications on daily routine" to "nurses obtaining new skills in areas such as developing standard operating procedures and risk management".

1.6 Results

A total of 322 EBMT (NG) members were contacted via email with a response rate of 9.62% (31 replies) from 12 countries. One reply was rejected due to the transplant centre not working towards JACIE accreditation therefore 30 replies from 11 countries were evaluated:

The role, seniority and the involvement of the nurse, in the JACIE process, could have an influence on how each respondent responded.

97% (29/30) of respondents were classified as senior nurses:

Seven ward managers
Fourteen* clinical nurse specialists (CNS)
Five quality managers
Three nurse coordinators
One nurse consultant responsible for SOPs in clinical and processing facility

3% (1/30) of respondents were classified as a staff nurse/junior nurse.

*One CNS role includes data manager and one CNS is responsible for JACIE

The majority of nurses, 93.3% (28/30), worked within the clinical area**, 3.3% (1/30) worked in the apheresis facility and 3.3% (1/30) within the processing facility.

**Two clinical nurses worked in a second area (one in apheresis and one in processing)

1.7 Does the JACIE Process Have Any Implications for Nurses?

The survey showed an overwhelming response (90% (27/30)) that the JACIE process has implications for nurses with 10% (3/30) stating JACIE had no implications for nurses.

The respondents offered either none or several examples of their experiences:

26/27 (96%) offered one or more citations
15/26 (58%) offered two citations
10/26 (38%) offered three citations
1/26 (3.8%) offered four citations
4/27 (15%) offered no citations

1.7.1 Implications: Staff Nurse's/ Junior Nurse's Point of View

The only staff nurse/junior nurse to respond to the questionnaire described their role, instead of describing any implications that had occurred in working towards their first JACIE accreditation: "Nurses were involved in checking procedures, therefore providing documented evidence in education and patient care". This is a good demonstration that all staff within the transplant programme should be involved in the accreditation process.

1.7.2   Implications: Ward Manager's Point of View Can Be Summarised as Follows

JACIE has provided an improved structure to produce written procedures, which are reviewed regularly.

This uniform working allows procedures to be described precisely, enabling all staff performing the procedure to perform the task in the same way and can be used an educational tool especially for new members of staff. The experience of JACIE has improved patient care, improved communication between all members of the team and has allowed for a closer working relationship. Nurses were able to learn new skills especially in understanding risk management.

1.7.3   Implications: Clinical Nurse Specialist's Point of View Can Be Summarised as Follows

Initially the documentation and developing the JACIE programme took many years and was hard work. Extra work had to be incorporated into a busy schedule, and time had to be allocated to attend the many meetings relating to JACIE. Now accreditation has been achieved, and the team works within an established programme. All the effort was worthwhile because everyone feels confident with the quality standards and programme. Quality is always a priority.

Additional management hours were required to administer/manage the increased numbers of protocols and procedures. New presentation skills were learnt in presenting audit results to the transplant team, and new opportunities arose to develop a donor care programme to conform to the JACIE Standards.

There was only one negative feedback: "Unfortunately no impact on daily practice".

1.7.4   Implications: Quality Manager's Point of View Can Be Summarised as Follows

The transplant team now has a greater awareness and importance of standard operating procedures (SOPs) by working within a document controlled system and being included in the multidisciplinary team meetings. Within the paediatric setting, there has been an improvement in medical SOPs for the care of the HSCT paediatric patients as well as an improvement in collaboration with the adult clinic, apheresis and stem cell laboratory teams. Patient outcome reviews have been valuable in improving care.

The JACIE audit programme has encouraged the transplant team to perform internal audits, which has led to improvements in quality assurance.

1.7.5   Implications: Nurse Coordinator's Point of View Can Be Summarised as Follows

JACIE has highlighted more attention is required for nurse training, evaluation of competencies, document control and the registration process. The standards relating to donors has emphasised to the team the importance of the role of a "donor advocate", to prevent a conflict of interest of the transplant physician, and JACIE is a very useful working tool, especially for new colleagues.

1.8   Conclusion of the Survey

Although there was a very low response to the survey (9.62%), the results represent the views of senior nurses (97% of respondents). After reviewing the 45* comments from the 30 respondents, the authors of this survey would like to suggest that the JACIE accreditation process has had a positive impact on nurses. Only 9% of comments could be classified as having a negative impact on the nurse due to extra workload.

* See Appendix 1.1 for a full list of citations written by the respondents to the survey.

A further study is required within the BMT nursing community to fully understand the implications for nurses during the initial JACIE accreditation phase and post JACIE accreditation whilst maintaining and improving the quality system that is now embedded into daily practice. The study could be based on the Donabedian model looking at structure, process and outcomes.

The JACIE Standards are reviewed every 3 years, allowing them to be adapted to the rapidly developing field of HSCT. Nurses are required to maintain compliance with the QMS and JACIE Standards and must familiarise themselves with the changes that occur in each edition of the JACIE Standards. Each edition will present fresh challenges to achieve the standards especially given the present day competing pressures on resource and finance. It is noteworthy that none of the surveyed nurses mentioned this aspect as a concern for nurses in their practice. As nurses working within JACIE-accredited centres, it is important to provide evidence of our continued monitoring of practice and processes through the QMS and not regard the JACIE accreditation process as a tick box exercise.

1.9 Discussion Points

Since the introduction of JACIE accreditation, nurses have submitted oral and poster presentations at the annual EBMT (NG) conference on the topic "Preparing for JACIE". The small response to our EBMT (NG) survey and a literature search that could not identify published articles on the topic of "JACIE and implications for nurses" could suggest the JACIE accreditation process has not impacted greatly on nurses.

One of the five Deming principles (Health Catalyst 2014) that help health-care process improvements:

"Quality improvement is a science of process management. If you cannot measure it you cannot prove it, therefore quality improvement must be data driven".

As specialised nurses, working in the field of HSCT, we should be asking ourselves why are we not publishing our data or audit findings. Using the development of the apheresis collection services across Europe as an example, many teams will be nurse led. When the collection of HSCs became an established practice, the number of nursing teams increased, training became more formalised and apheresis nurse forums were established to try and reinforce policies and procedures. A QMS was introduced in the form of JACIE accreditation with risk management and audit became integral to the apheresis nurse role.

Deming also states:" If nurses are going to manage care, they require the right data delivered in the right format at the right time and in the right place". Therefore, nurses with the HSCT programme should take ownership, perform audits, assess the results, make changes to patient care and reassess. These experiences and findings should be shared and published.

If the reluctance to publish is a lack of ownership of quality management, or nurses perceive quality management as the responsibility of the quality manager, then they must be reminded that JACIE has a significant impact upon each and every role and that they must be aware and fully participate in the process. Audit, review of policies and procedures, competencies and risk assessment will become a key part of the nursing routine for the QMS to be maintained and to evolve.

Key Readings
- JACIE 6th Ed. Manual
- JACIE 6th Ed. Standards
- www.jacie.org
- JACIE Quality Manual
- Smith J, Jones M Jr, Houghton et al (1999) Future of health insurance. N Engl J Med 965:325-329

Acknowledgements The authors would like to thank the JACIE Office for the use of materials and Tuula Rintala Apheresis Nurse JACIE Inspector and member of the JACIE Accreditation Committee for her help and advice.

Appendix 1.1. Citations Classified in the Role of the Nurse

1. 1. Staff nurse/junior nurse: citation classed as positive (only one citation)
   - As nurses, we have checked procedures to enable the team to demonstrate our work on education and patient care.
2. Ward manager's citations

Citations classed as positive:
   - Improved structure to create procedures.
   - A more uniformed way of working.
   - (Almost) everything we do is now described in the policies, and everybody performs the procedure the same way, which is better for the patient.
   - Communication processes have improved between the different professionals (e.g. nurses, physicians) improving the way we are working together.
   - We now have the knowledge to implement the method and the instruments of risk management.
   - There have been improvements on patient care, central venous catheter management, team work and communication and safety of the patients.
   - A tool that can be used to helped introduce new staff to the daily routine of transplant care.

Citations classed as neither negative nor positive:
   - Started to use many procedures.
   - We regularly update the quality documentation.
   - Description of working processes.
   - It's an Issue of quality management.

3. Clinical nurse specialist's citations

Citations classed as positive:
   - Now we are JACIE accredited and working within an established programme, it was well worth it and, we feel confident about our quality standards and programme.
   - Quality is always a priority in every aspect of the transplant process.
   - Maintain patient records more accurately.
   - We have started the donor care programme according the JACIE.

Citations classed as neither negative nor positive
   - Preparation of QMS and developing SOPs x four citations.
   - Increased number of protocols and procedures to follow and manage, requiring additional management hours to administrate.
   - We had to prepare and update all SOP documents from the nursing field.
   - As a centre preparing for our 1st accreditation, we are preparing documents, SOP and the nurses' education programme.
   - Perhaps not implications, many checklists and SOPs have been revised or developed which has developed our work.
   - I personally worked on the SOPs and routines in HSCT.
   - I was required to present results at the clinical audit meetings and answer questions.

Citations classed as negative:
   - Initially the documentation and developing the programme took many years and was hard work.
   - As our quality manager is from a laboratory background, I have had to incorporate clinical quality lead into my CNS role, and this has added to my workload.
   - Finding time for many meetings related to quality and JACIE was difficult due to other demands.
   - Unfortunately no impact on daily practice.

4. Quality manager's citations

Citations classed as positive:
   - There is a greater awareness of the routines.
   - An improved structure.

- Patient safety is highlighted.
- All nurses are working in a more quality assured way, by only using adequate and current documents and working procedures.
- The internal audits, which we have performed for several years, whilst working with JACIE, have led to improvements in quality assurance.
- Before JACIE accreditation, we actually did not have strict medical SOPs for treatment of our paediatric transplant patients.
- Since first accreditation as a separate paediatric centre, we have broadened our corporation with the adult clinic, apheresis and stem cell lab. Since then SOPs are more in common. "Nurses are now involved and appreciate being involved in the review meeting for patient outcome".

Citations classed as neither negative nor positive:
- More SOPs to write
- Increased audits
- Working with documents and internal audits
- Updating SOPS, ensuring staff, including the multidisciplinary team, understand the importance of following the SOP

5. Nurse coordinator's and nurse consultant citations

Citations classed as positive:
- Separate donor and recipient management.
- JACIE is a good working tool, especially for new colleagues.

Citations classed as neither negative nor positive:
- More attention in the control of the working activities.
- More attention in the registration of processes.
- More attention in the nurse training and evaluation of competency.
- My mission is to work for the HSCT programme of quality programme improvement process as required by the accreditation body JACIE.

References

Anthias C, Ethell ME, Potter MN, Madrigal A, Shaw BE. The impact of improved JACIE standards on the care of related BM and PBSC donors. Bone Marrow Transpl. 2015;50:244–7. https://doi.org/10.1038/bmt.2014.260; published online 10 November 2014

Anthias C, O'Donnell PV, Kiefer DM, et al. European Group for Blood and Marrow Transplantation Centres with FACT-JACIE Accreditation Have Significantly Better Compliance with Related Donor Care Standards. Biol Blood Marrow Transpl. 2016;22(3):514–9.

Babic A, Wannesson L, Trobia M, Lazzaro M. Transplant unit personnel competency maintanance: online testing by sharepoint application. EBMT. 2015; oral presentation N003.

Caunday O, Bensoussan D, Decot V, Bordigoni P, Stoltz JF. Regulatory aspects of cellular therapy product in Europe: JACIE accreditation in a processing facility. Biomed Mater Eng. 2009;19:373–9.

Cornish JM. JACIE accreditation in paediatric haemopoietic SCT. Bone Marrow Transpl. 2008;42:S82–6. https://doi.org/10.1038/bmt.2008.290.

Demiriz IS, Tekgunduz E, Altuntas F. What is the most appropriate source for hematopoietic stem cell transplantation? Peripheral Stem Cell/Bone Marrow/Cord Blood Bone Marrow Res. 2012; (2012):Article ID 834040 (online).

Gratwohl A, Brand R, Niederwieser D. Introduction of a quality management system and outcome after hematopoietic stem-cell transplantation. J Clin Oncol. 2011;11. https://doi.org/10.1200/JCO.2010.30.4121.

Gratwohl A, Brand R, McGrath E, van Biezen A, Sureda A, Ljungman P, Baldomero H, Chabannon C, Apperley J. Joint Accreditation Committee (JACIE) of the International Society for Cellular Therapy and the European Group for Blood and Marrow Transplantation, and the European Leukemia Net. Use of the quality management system "JACIE" and outcome after hematopoietic stem cell transplantation. Haematologica. 2014;99(5):908–15.

Harolds J. Quality and Safety in Health Care, Part I. Five Pioneers in Quality. Clin Nucl Med. 2015;40(8):660–2.

Health Catalyst. www.healthcatalyst.com Proprietary.© 2014. Five deming principles that help healthcare process improvement by John Haughom, MD).

https://www.ebmt.org/Contents/Resources/Library/Slidebank/Pages/JACIE2015. 24 Mar 2015 – JACIE Quality Management Day 2015. Common deficiencies, Carole Charley.

Pamphilon D, Apperley JF, Samson D, Slaper-Cortenbach I, McGrath E. JACIE Accreditation in 2008: demonstrating excellence in stem cell transplantation. Hematol Oncol Stem Cell. 2008;2(2):311–9 (online).

Passweg JR, Baldomero H, Gratwohl H, et al. The EBMT activity survey: 1990-2010. Bone Marrow Transpl. 2012;47:906–23; pubilised online 30th April 2012.

Piras A, Aresi P, Angelucci E. Analysis of the accreditation process. JACIE Transplant Program Businco. Prof Infern. 2015;68(2):167–73. https://doi.org/10.7429/pi.2015.6822167.

Samson D, Slaper-Cortenbach I, Pamphilon D, McGrath E, McDonald F, Urbano Ispizua A. Current status of JACIE accreditation in Europe: a special report from the Joint Accreditation Committee of the ISCT and the EBMT (JACIE). Bone Marrow Transpl. 2007;39:133–41.

www.Ebmt.org home/quality Management/about JACIE www.jacie.org. Accessed 15 Dec 2016.

HSCT: How Does It Work?

2

Letizia Galgano and Daphna Hutt

Abstract

The HSCT (haematopoietic stem cell transplant) is a particular treatment for many haematological and non-haematological diseases. Broadly, there are three different categories of transplantation, autologous, allogeneic and syngeneic, which can be applied to most disease scenarios. Haematopoietic stem cells can be derived from the bone marrow, peripheral blood and umbilical cord blood. HSCT treatment can be divided into separate phases that start with the harvest of the stem cells and passing through the conditioning, aplasia and engraftment until the recovery of the haematopoietic functions. HSCT is indicated in many diseases, and these indications depend on numerous factors such as the disease type, stage and response to previous treatment. Among non-malignant diseases, aplastic anaemia, sickle cell disease and, more recently, autoimmune diseases can also be effectively treated with HSCT. One third of the transplants in children are performed for rare indications such as severe combined immunodeficiencies. Allogeneic HSCT can also cure a number of non-malignant diseases in children, such as Wiskott-Aldrich syndrome and chronic granulomatous disease (CGD). This chapter will include transplant in primary immunodeficiency in children as well as inherited bone marrow failure and inborn errors of metabolism.

Keywords

HSCT • Indications • Autoimmune diseases • Haemoglobinopathies
Paediatric • Immunodeficiencies

L. Galgano (✉)
Department of Transfusion Service and Cell Therapy
BMT Unit, AOUCareggi Hospital, Florence, Italy
e-mail: lgalga@tin.it

D. Hutt
Department of Pediatric Hematology-Oncology and
BMTs, Edmond and Lily Safra Children Hospital,
Sheba Medical Center, Tel-Hashomer, Israel
e-mail: dhutt@sheba.health.gov.il

© EBMT and the Author(s) 2018
M. Kenyon, A. Babic (eds.), *The European Blood and Marrow Transplantation Textbook for Nurses*,
https://doi.org/10.1007/978-3-319-50026-3_2

2.1 What Nurses Need to Know

2.1.1 Introduction

Haematopoietic stem cell transplantation (HSCT) is a therapeutic option for several haematological diseases including acute and chronic leukaemia, lymphoma and multiple myeloma, some of inherited disorders such as severe combined immunodeficiency and thalassemia and other inborn errors of metabolism (Maziarz 2015).

HSCT involves the use of autologous haematopoietic stem cells (HSC) obtained from the patient's own bone marrow (BM) or peripheral blood (PBSC) or allogeneic HSC where the donor cells come from a family-related or an unrelated donor, from the bone marrow, peripheral blood or cord blood.

The collected HSC are infused into a recipient (Gratwohl et al. 2010). Before the infusion, the recipient is treated with a conditioning regimen (see Chap. 6), involving the use of different types and dosages of chemo and/or radiotherapy and/or immunosuppressant drugs (such as antithymocyte globulin) (Copelan 2006).

2.1.2 Aims of HSCT

- In the autologous setting, patients with chemosensitive malignant diseases are offered high-dose chemotherapy in order to destroy or further reduce the malignant disease, ablating the marrow with this aggressive therapy. In this case, the stem cell infusion is intended to treat the prolonged chemotherapy-induced hypoplasia and not the disease itself (Maziarz 2015; Michel and Berry 2016).
- In the allogeneic setting (see below Sect. 2.2):
  - In malignant haematological disease, donor HSCs replace the immune system and help to eradicate malignancy (Maziarz 2015; Michel and Berry 2016).
  - In non-malignant diseases, where the cause is dysfunction of the haematopoietic stem cell (HSC), the HSCT procedure replaces the inefficient patient immune system with the donor one (Michel and Berry 2016; Hatzimichael and Tuthill 2010).

2.1.3 Outcomes

Outcomes vary according to:

- The stage of the disease
- The age of the patients
- The lapse of time from diagnosis to transplant
- The histocompatibility between donor and recipient
- The donor/recipient sex combination (the overall survival decreases for male recipients having a female donor) (Sureda et al. 2015a)
- Advances in immunogenetics and immunobiology
- Conditioning regimens
- Disease characterization and risk stratification
- Immunosuppression
- Antimicrobials
- Other types of supportive care

All these factors contribute to improvements in disease control and overall survival (Maziarz 2015).

Patient selection influences outcomes. Patients with better overall functional performance status, limited comorbidities and underlying organ damage have more favourable outcomes (Maziarz 2015).

2.1.4 Nursing Considerations

Patients require specific care to overcome the physical and emotional problems resulting from this treatment. Usually after myeloablative conditioning, HSCT recipients typically experience a period of profound pancytopenia lasting days to weeks depending on the donor source. The rapidity of neutrophil recovery varies with the type of graft: approximate recovery time is 2 weeks with G-CSF-mobilized peripheral blood stem cells, 3 weeks with marrow stem cells and can be as long as 4 weeks with umbilical cord blood stem cells.

However, re-establishment of immune system takes at least several months due to prolonged lymphocyte recovery process, and some patients continue to show immune deficits for several years after HSCT (Mackall et al. 2009). During this period, the patient has a high risk of developing complications; thus, HSCT units require multidisciplinary teams of physicians, nurses, pharmacists, social workers, nurse practitioners, physician assistants, nutrition experts and occupational and physical therapists, in addition to a specialized facility and technical resources (Maziarz 2015).

Nurses who work in HSCT units have a key role in treatment management and require specific training to:

- Understand, prevent and manage the early and late effects of HSCT.
- Care for multiply treated patients.
- Inform and educate patients and their caregivers.
- Administer drugs and blood products safely.
- Manage the central venous catheter (cvc).
- Give emotional support.

These topics will be covered in later chapters.

2.2 Different Types of HSCT

HSCs may be obtained from autologous (BM or PBSC) or allogeneic (HLA-matched related (MRD), HLA-matched unrelated (MUD) or HLA-mismatched related or unrelated donors and UCB) sources (Table 2.1).

Table 2.1 Summary of HSCT types and HSC sources

Type of transplantation	Cell source	Donor
Autologous	Bone marrow Peripheral blood	Recipient
Allogeneic	Bone marrow Peripheral blood Umbilical cord blood	Related Unrelated
Syngenic	Bone marrow Peripheral blood	Monochorionic twin

Adapted from Tura (2003)

2.2.1 Autologous Haematopoietic Stem Cell Transplantation

Autologous HSCT is defined as "a high dose chemotherapy followed by the reinfusion of the patient's own HSC" (cit. NCI Dictionary). After mobilization (see Chap. 5), the patient's HSCs are collected and cryopreserved. Auto-HSCT facilitates the prompt reconstitution of a significantly depleted or ablated marrow following very aggressive chemotherapy and sometimes radiotherapy intended to eradicate haematologic and non-haematologic malignancies (Michel and Berry 2016).

There is no risk of rejection or graft versus host disease (GvHD) and no GvT (graft versus tumour) effect (see Chaps. 11 and 12). Graft failure can occur rarely, and some trials demonstrate how relapse remains an issue for the majority of patients with multiple myeloma (Michel and Berry 2016; Mackall et al. 2009).

2.2.2 Allogeneic Stem Cell Transplantation

In allogeneic transplantation, the recipient receives HSCs from a *related* or *unrelated* donor who can be fully or partially human leukocyte antigen (HLA)-matched (Fig. 2.1); related donors are family members; unrelated donors are identified through a donor registry or from a cord blood bank. In allogeneic HSCT, the major histocompatibility complex (MHC) HLA class I and II molecules located on chromosome 6 play an important role (Maziarz 2015). (Please refer to Chap. 3 for HLA typing and donor selection.)

In allogeneic HSCT, the aim of conditioning is to:

- Kill tumour cells (in malignant diseases).
- Eradicate existing bone marrow tissue (in order to provide space for engraftment of transplanted donor stem cells).
- Suppress the patient's immune response and minimize the risk of graft rejection of the donor HSC (Maziarz 2015).

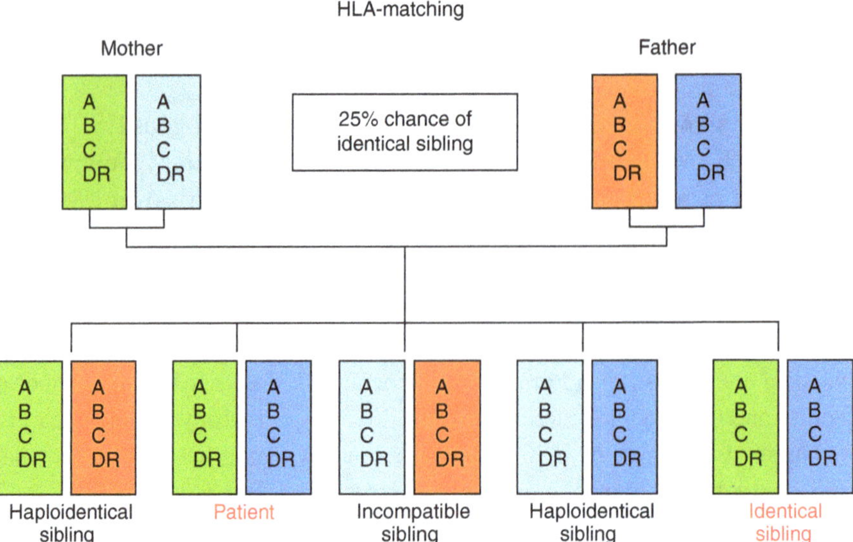

Fig. 2.1 Scheme of HLA compatibility (Adapted from: Soiffer 2008)

Allogeneic HSCT has been subject to several improvements during recent years.

Reduced intensity conditioning regimen, alternative donor transplants and new stem cell sources have increased the accessibility and availability, especially for older patients who have poor tolerance of the high toxicity of the treatment. These improvements have resulted in reduced transplant-related mortality, although relapse remains an issue (Michel and Berry 2016).

2.2.2.1 Allogeneic Transplantation from HLA-Matched Related Donor (MRD)

The ideal donor is an HLA-identical sibling. Patients have a 25% chance of each sibling being fully HLA-matched, because siblings inherit 50% haplotype from each parent (Fig. 2.1).

If donor is an identical twin, they are referred to as syngeneic (see Sect. 2.3).

2.2.2.2 Allogeneic from Unrelated Donor (MUD, MMUD)

If recipient has no sibling or the blood tests confirm that there is no HLA compatibility with the sibling, then a search of "Bone Marrow Donors Worldwide" registry database (BMDW) is activated (Apperley et al. 2012).

If the donor histocompatibility is fully matched with the recipient, the donor is called a matched unrelated donor (MUD); if there is a partial incompatibility, the donor is called a mismatched unrelated donor (MMUD).

The time between the activation of the unrelated donor research and the beginning of transplantation procedure is fundamental. The more time spent in the search phase, the greater is the risk that the patient's disease will worsen or die (Hatzimichael and Tuthill 2010).

2.2.2.3 Cord Blood Transplantation

Unrelated donor umbilical cord blood unit transplantation (UCBT) provides an alternative donor option in patients who lack a conventional MRD and MUD. Advantages of UCBT include the capacity to tolerate greater degrees of HLA mismatch than is possible using MUD (Bashey and Solomon 2014).

UCBT have the advantage that the cryopreserved units at the cord blood banks are readily available, with results comparable to those from an unrelated donor or only partially compatible units (also HLA 5/8 loci). UCBT shows a lower incidence of GvHD, without losing the GvL effect (Copelan 2006) (see Chap. 12). However, delayed haematopoietic recovery and slow immune reconstitution and acquisition cost remain important challenges (Bashey and Solomon 2014).

2.2.2.4 Haploidentical Transplantation

In case of unavailability of a conventional HLA identical sibling, MUD or CB unit, it is possible to transplant with an available haploidentical donor. The donor may be a parent, child, brother, sister or other relative that matches for one haplotype (HLA-mismatched related donors with compatibility >6/8 loci).

The most important criterion for a haploidentical transplant is the urgency of the transplant in order to avoid early relapse or progression of the disease (Aversa 2015).

The advantages of the haploidentical transplantation are:

- The donor can be changed in case of a poor stem cell mobilizer or if optimal graft composition was not achieved.
- Easy family donor availability (if patients are not fostered or orphans without other relatives).
- The benefit of natural killer (NK) cell alloreactivity.
- Easy access to donor-derived cellular therapies after transplantation (Aversa 2015).

There are two haploidentical procedures:

- Haploidentical transplantation with haematopoietic stem cells T-replete with cyclophosphamide in immediate post-transplant phase that involves the induction of transplantation tolerance; it appears to have overcome many of the obstacles historically associated with haploidentical donor transplantation, such as too high rates of graft rejection and post-transplant infections (Bashey and Solomon 2014), and promotes a graft versus leukaemia (GVL) therapeutic benefit with improved survival (Maziarz 2015).
- Haploidentical transplantation with depletion of T-lymphocytes exists in aggressive and severe immune depleting conditioning regimen followed by infusion of mega-doses of highly purified peripheral stem cells (Bashey and Solomon 2014).

2.2.2.5 Syngeneic Transplantation

Syngeneic is a type of transplantation where the donor is the recipient's monochorial twin and who is genetically identical to the patient. There is no immunological conflict such as GvHD (graft versus host disease) (see Chap. 11) but at the same time no beneficial GVL (graft versus Leukaemia) effect (Mackall et al. 2009).

(see Chaps. 9 and 11 for HSCT complications)

2.3 The Stem Cell Sources

HSC can be isolated from the bone marrow (BM), peripheral blood after mobilization (PBSC) and umbilical cord blood (UCB) (Maziarz 2015).

"Bone marrow cells are capable of repopulating all hematopoietic and lymphocytic populations while maintaining capacity for self-regeneration, assuring long -term immunologic and hematopoietic viability" (Maziarz 2015).

Until the early 1990s, the bone marrow (BM) represented the only source of stem cells. However, this practice has almost been replaced by peripheral blood stem cells (PBSC). More recently, cord blood (CB) has been shown to be a good alternative source of haematopoietic stem cells. All three types of HSCs regardless of source are capable of regeneration after a high-dose chemoradiotherapy treatment (Richard 2000).

2.3.1 Peripheral Blood Stem Cells

PBSCs have been increasingly used in both auto- and allo-HSCT. Mobilization of haematopoietic stem cells to the peripheral blood can be achieved by the administration of growth factors such as G-CSF (allo-HSCT) and/or myelosuppressive chemotherapy (auto-HSCT) (Apperley et al. 2012).

An advantage HSCT performed with PBSC is a relatively rapid recovery of haematopoiesis compared to BM and increases the disease-free survival and overall survival in high-risk haematological malignancies. The disadvantage is an increased risk of chronic GvHD in the allogenic HSCT because of an increased number of T cells circulating (Maziarz 2015).

2.3.2 Bone Marrow

BM is traditionally harvested from the posterior iliac crests under general or epidural anaesthesia in a surgical room where trained haematologists or surgeons collect stem cells and blood directly from the bone marrow cavity in the bilateral posterior iliac crest region using aspiration needles.

HSCT performed with BM leads to less GvHD compared to PBSC source, but has the disadvantage of a slower neutrophil and platelet engraftment (Maziarz 2015).

2.3.3 Umbilical Cord Blood

Cord blood cells are collected and cryopreserved from the umbilical cord immediately after birth, but generally before the placenta has been delivered in order to avoid clots (Demiriz et al. 2012). UCB cells have been used both in related and unrelated HLA-matched and HLA-mismatched allogeneic transplants in children and in adults (Demiriz et al. 2012; Apperley et al. 2012). The advantage is a low criteria for a match (4/6 match is acceptable) increasing the chance of identifying a suitable cord unit or cord units in a matter of days. Less GvHD is often observed. A key disadvantage is often slower engraftment compared to BM and PBSC and increased infection complications due to slow rate of haematopoietic recovery (Maziarz 2015).

(see Chaps. 3 and 5).

2.3.4 HSCT Phases

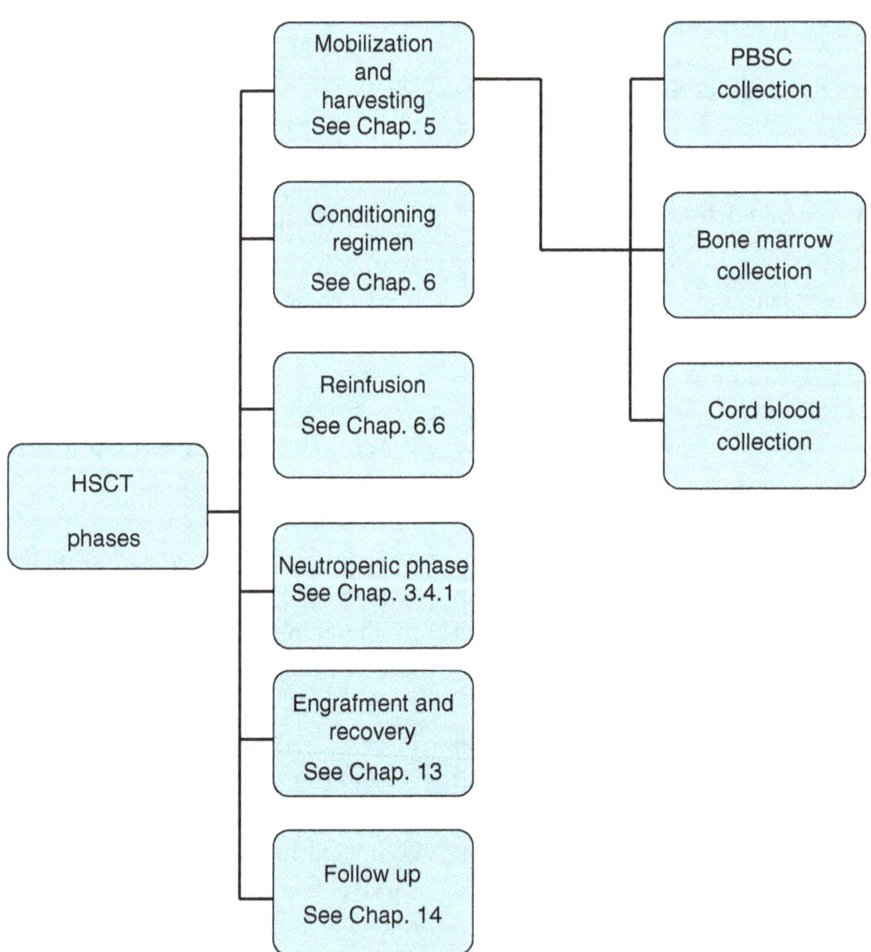

2.3.4.1 Neutropenic Phase

After the chemotherapy, the blood count decreases for about 7–14 days in autologous HSCT and until 20–30 days in allogeneic HSCT. The neutropenia occurs when the absolute neutrophil count is <500 cells/mm^3 (Maziarz 2015).

During this period, several complications may occur:

- Increased risk of infections due to a not effective immune system. Infection following HSCT is associated with significant morbidity and mortality, so prevention is critical to improve outcomes. The risk of infection is based on multiple variables including the type of transplantation (autologous or allogeneic), source of haematopoietic cells (related or unrelated donor, peripheral blood, bone marrow, or cord blood), underlying disease, disease status (remission or relapse), intensity of the preparative regimen (ablative or non-myeloablative), prior infections, endogenous microflora and environmental exposure to microorganisms. In addition, risk may vary based on infection control measures used by transplantation centres. Practices in infection control such as type of isolation, dietary restrictions and antimicrobial prophylaxis vary widely among transplantation centres. Nurses are pivotal in implementing practices to prevent and manage infections and associated effects following HSCT (Sureda et al. 2015a).
- Bleedings because of thrombocytopenia (platelets have a slow recovery after transplantation).
- Tiredness caused by the decreasing of haemoglobin levels.
- Pain because of mucositis.
- Reduced nutrition. Oral intake is usually severely reduced because of, on one side, the oral mucositis that many patients develop and, on the other side, the prolonged post conditioning nausea. When oral intake is reduced and the body mass index decrease, total enteral/parenteral nutrition may be provided especially for children.

2.4 Indications for Transplant in Malignant Disease

The patient assessment for a transplant procedure is complex and includes several factors such as the patient's overall health and performance status, comorbidities, disease risk/status (e.g. remission state and responsiveness to treatment) and graft and donor source. For example, autologous transplantation is not useful for diseases in which normal HSCs cannot be collected as in CML or myelodysplasia (Rowley 2013).

The indications for transplant are based on best available evidence from clinical trials or, where clinical trials are not available, registry, multicentre or single centre observational studies (Majhail et al. 2015). The HSCT specialist determines if transplant should be considered as an option for disease consolidation, but the final decision will be made in conjunction with the patient (Maziarz 2015).

There have been major changes in indications, such as the rise and fall of autologous HSCT for breast cancer or of allogeneic HSCT for chronic myeloid leukaemia (CML), and in technology, as illustrated by the change from the bone marrow to peripheral blood, the rapid increase in use of unrelated donors and the introduction of reduced intensity conditioning. It is clear how some guidance is warranted, for transplant teams, hospital administrators, health-care providers and also patients (Apperley et al. 2012).

The HSCT indications are not the same in children and in adults (Table 2.1).

The Table 2.2 is a scheme of the main indications for autologous and allogeneic transplantation. It includes the standard of care.

2.4.1 Indications for Allogeneic HSCT

Adult patients with acute myeloid leukaemia (AML) should always be considered for allo- or auto-HSCT, while allo-HSCT cannot be recommended as first-line treatment for chronic myeloid leukaemia (CML) because of the efficacy of the first-line therapy with imatinib for

Table 2.2 Indication for transplant: Recommendation categories (see text for definition): Standard of care (S); Standard of care, clinical evidence available (C); Standard of care, Rare indication (R)

	Adult		Paediatric	
Disease	Auto	Allo	Auto	Allo
Acute myeloid leukaemia				
CR1, intermediate risk/not in remission		C		C
CR1, high risk/CR2+		S		S
Acute promyelocytic leukaemia, relapse	R	R	R	R
Acute lymphoblastic leukaemia				
CR1, high risk/CR2		S		S
CR3+/not in remission		C		C
Chronic myeloid leukaemia		C		C
Myelodysplastic syndromes				
Low risk		C		C
High risk/juvenile myelomonocytic leukaemia/ therapy related		C		S
T-cell non-Hodgkin lymphoma				
CR1, high risk/CR2		S		S
CR3+/not in remission		C		C
Lymphoblastic B-cell non-Hodgkin lymphoma (non-Burkitt)				
CR1, high risk/CR2		S		S
CR3+/not in remission		C		C
Burkitt's lymphoma				
First remission/first or greater relapse, sensitive	C	C	C	C
First or greater relapse, resistant		C		C
Hodgkin lymphoma				
Primary refractory, sensitive/first relapse, sensitive/ second or greater relapse	C	C	C	C
Primary refractory, resistant/first relapse, resistant		C		C
Multiple myeloma	S	C		
Anaplastic large cell lymphoma				
Primary refractory, sensitive/first relapse, sensitive/ second or greater relapse	C	C	C	C
Primary refractory, resistant/first relapse, resistant		C		C
Solid tumours				
Germ cell tumour/Wilm's tumour, relapse/ osteosarcoma, high risk/medulloblastoma, high risk/ other malignant brain tumours	C		C	
Ewing's sarcoma, high risk or relapse	S		S	
Non-malignant diseases				
Severe aplastic anaemia, new diagnosis, relapse/ refractory		S		S
Sickle cell disease		C		C
Thalassemia		S		S

Table 2.2 (continued)

Disease	Adult		Paediatric	
	Auto	Allo	Auto	Allo
Fanconi's anaemia/dyskeratosis congenita/Blackfan-diamond anaemia/congenital amegakaryocytic thrombocytopenia/severe combined immunodeficiency/T-cell immunodeficiency, SCID variants/Wiskott-Aldrich syndrome/haemophagocytic disorders/lymphoproliferative disorders/severe congenital neutropenia/chronic granulomatous disease/other phagocytic cell disorders/IPEX syndrome/other autoimmune and immune dysregulation disorders/mucopolysaccharoidoses (MPS-I and MPS-VI)/other metabolic diseases/osteopetrosis/globoid cell leukodystrophy (Krabbe)/metachromatic leukodystrophy/cerebral X-linked adrenoleukodystrophy		R		R
Juvenile rheumatoid arthritis/systemic sclerosis	R		R	

Adapted from: Majhail et al. (2015)

chronic patients, even if HSCT remains the only curative treatment. Allo-HSCT at the moment is the only curative option for patients with myeloproliferative disorders such as primary myelofibrosis and is considered the treatment of choice for adult patients with myelodysplastic syndromes (MDS). Allo-HSCT from an HLA-identical sibling or MUD is a treatment option for young patients previously treated with fludarabine-containing regimens and poor-risk disease. Patients with acquired severe aplastic anaemia (SAA) are considered for a first-line HLA-identical sibling HSCT (if available) or in case a haploidentical donor or a mismatch 9/10 donor. Allo-HSCT is the only treatment for Fanconi anaemia. More than 20% of allo-HSCT are performed in patients under 20 years, and at least one third are performed for rare indications. Clinical trials are limited because of small numbers, and chronic GvHD is still major limitation for the procedure. Well-matched donors must be considered as the primary cell source (Sureda et al. 2015a; Majhail et al. 2015; Rowley 2013).

2.4.2 Indications for Autologous HSCT

Auto-HSCT remains the standard of care for patients with Hodgkin lymphoma in first chemosensitive relapse or refractory to the first-line therapy and in chemosensitive relapse of DLBCL (diffuse large B-cell lymphoma), while in relapsed patients, allo-HSCT should be considered. Auto-HSCT is clearly indicated for patients with multiple myeloma (MM) who respond to first-line treatment, but age and general health should be considered; in MM all-HSCT has a curative potential, but the risk of mortality needs to be considered; autologous is also a standard of care for follicular lymphoma in first or subsequent relapse, while the auto-HSCT consolidation is considered a standard part of first-line treatment of younger(<60–65 yrs) patients with mantle cell lymphoma and for peripheral T-cell lymphomas and represent a reasonable treatment option. Patients with amyloidosis and without severe heart failure benefit from high dose-therapy and auto-HSCT, while allo-HSCT should be considered in relapsed younger patients after at least one new drug such as lenalidomide or bortezomib (Sureda et al. 2015a).

HSCT in solid tumours needs further prospective trials (Sureda et al. 2015a).

For further information on HSCT in non-malignant paediatric indication, see below.

2.5 Indications for Transplant in Non-malignant Diseases in Children

More than 20% of allogeneic haematopoietic stem cell transplants (HSCT) are performed in patients below 20 years. However, at least one third of HSCTs in children are performed for rare indications (Sureda et al. 2015b). Allogeneic HSCT can cure several non-malignant disorders in children.

2.5.1 Transplant in Primary Immunodeficiencies

Primary immunodeficiencies are genetic disorders characterized by defective or impaired innate or adaptive immunity. Of these, severe combined immunodeficiencies (SCIDs) are the most severe, leading to death in infancy or early childhood unless treated appropriately (Sureda et al 2015b).

2.5.2 Severe Combined Immunodeficiencies

Severe combined immunodeficiencies (SCIDs) are a genetically heterogeneous group of rare inherited defects characterized by severe abnormalities of immune system development and function (Gaspar et al. 2013; Gennery 2015). Most of the genetic defects responsible for SCID are inherited in an autosomal recessive fashion and therefor are more common in infants born to

consanguineous parents (Rivers and Gaspar 2015). The incidence of SCID varies according to ethnicity (Booth et al. 2016). The different forms of SCID can have different patterns of lymphocyte development. Nearly all SCIDs have absent T cells but are then further divided by the presence or absence of B and NK cells (Fig. 2.2; Rivers and Gaspar 2015; Booth et al. 2016). Patients with SCID usually present in early infancy with recurrent, severe or opportunistic infections. Multiple pathogens may coexist, and opportunistic infection, for example, with *Pneumocystis jiroveci*, is common (Gennery 2015). This can also be accompanied by failure to thrive with persistent diarrhoea and persistent oral thrush. Infants that present with lymphopenia should be further evaluated (Rivers and Gaspar 2015).

The severity of the clinical and immunologic situation requires prompt intervention, and for most patients, the only curative treatment is allogeneic HSCT (Gaspar et al. 2013; Gennery 2015). Gene therapy and enzyme replacement therapy are available for some specific genetic subtypes (Gennery 2015). The objective of HSCT in patients with SCID is to provide normal haematopoiesis, facilitating correction of the immune defect. Therefore, it is critical to minimize potential long-term effects of treatment but to establish effective long-term immune function (Gennery 2015). Once the diagnosis of SCID is made, there is an urgency of finding a suitable donor (Gaspar et al. 2013) and proceeding to transplant. Factors

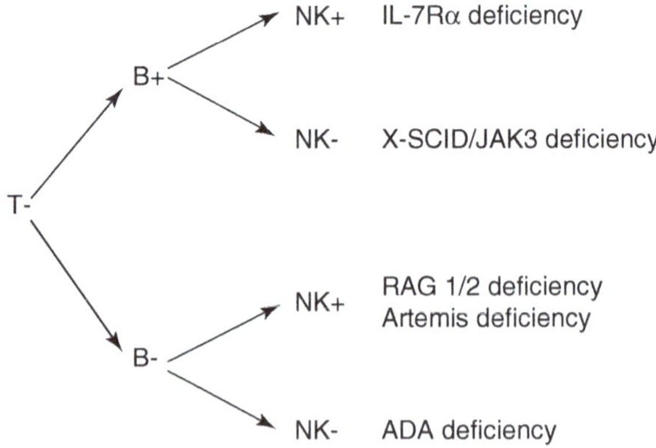

Fig. 2.2 Some of the more common immunophenotypes in SCID (Reproduced from Rivers and Gaspar 2015)

that influence the prognosis include the age, the type of SCID and the clinical state at the time of diagnosis, in particular the presence of infection and the degree of HLA matching with the donor (Sureda et al. 2015b).

2.5.3 Non-SCID Primary Immunodeficiencies

The three of the more common non-SCID primary immunodeficiency (PID) disorders are as follows: 1. Chronic granulomatous disease (CGD) patients with CGD have a reduced ability of phagocytes (particularly neutrophils) to kill bacterial and fungal pathogens. 2. Wiskott-Aldrich syndrome (WAS) is an X-linked immunodeficiency caused by mutations in the WAS gene, presenting with thrombocytopenia, eczema and immunodeficiency. 3. Haemophagocytic lymphohistiocytosis (HLH) is a life-threatening disease of severe hyper inflammation caused by uncontrolled proliferation of activated lymphocytes and macrophages (Booth et al. 2016).

Conditioning There is a debate about the best approach of treatment. Different centres are using a wide variety of conditioning regimes (Booth et al. 2016). In the presence of an HLA-identical family donor, HSCT can be performed in certain types of SCID (particularly those with an absence of NK cells) without any conditioning regimen. These patients can have donor T-cell (and occasionally B-cell) reconstitution, thereby potentially sparing short- and long-term toxicities (Dvorak et al. 2014; Gennery 2015; Sureda et al. 2015b). Dvorak et al. (2014) compared the outcome of transplants in SCID patients' undergoing unrelated donors or unrelated cord blood transplants with matched sibling transplants both with no conditioning. They concluded that patients lacking a matched sibling donor can proceed to an unrelated transplant without the use of conditioning chemotherapy in the same manner as with a matched sibling donor but with careful GvHD prophylaxis.

In contrast to SCID disorders, HSCT in non-SCID PID always requires conditioning therapy.

Over the last 15 years, the use of reduced intensity conditioning approaches has been explored in order to reduce acute and late effects (Booth et al. 2016). The EBMT and ESID (European Society for Immunodeficiencies) have published in 2011 guidelines for stem cell transplantation for primary immunodeficiencies (EBMT and ESID 2011).

Outcome In recent years, the outcome of HSCT has improved considerably with overall survival rates now approaching 90% in optimal circumstances (Gennery 2015). This is most likely due to earlier diagnosis; improved supportive care, including the initiation of bacterial and fungal prophylaxis; and early referral for HSCT (Booth et al. 2016). For many patients with PID, partial donor chimaerism is sufficient to induce cure if the affected recipient cell lineage is replaced completely or partially by donor cells, although complete donor chimaerism is best in some diseases (Gennery 2015). Pai et al. (2014) reported the results of 240 infants who received a transplant for SCID, at 25 centres in the USA between January 2000 and December 2009. The overall survival rate at 5 years was 74%; most deaths were within the first year after transplant and were due to infections (39%) or pulmonary complications (37%). Mortality was increased for patients who had active infection at the time of transplantation.

2.5.4 Newborn Screening

Over the past decade, the concept of newborn screening for SCID has moved into reality in a number of countries around the world. Early diagnosis of these conditions will significantly improve the outcome for SCID patients, allowing a rapid move to curative therapy before symptoms and infections accrue (Gaspar et al. 2013; Booth et al. 2016). Detection of SCID at birth allows immediate protection with prophylactic Immunoglobulin substitution and antibiotics, thus keeping children free from infection until a definitive procedure can be undertaken (Gaspar et al. 2013). Screening is based on a qPCR assay for T-cell receptor excision circles (TRECs) which can be performed on the dried blood spot tests—Guthrie already taken as part of universal newborn screening for other inherited conditions. TRECs are essentially a marker of thymic output and their levels are severely reduced in SCID and in a number of other conditions. If low TREC levels are detected, then assay is repeated before the patient is called for further immunological evaluation (Booth et al. 2016).

The optimal way to approach transplant in those infants identified through newborn screening programs has yet to be determined (Booth et al. 2016). It generated considerable debate among many members of the SCID transplant community (Gaspar et al. 2013). The use of chemotherapy in pre-symptomatic children with SCID is difficult for physicians and families to accept (Booth et al. 2016).

2.5.5 Inherited Bone Marrow Failure

The inherited bone marrow failure (BMF) syndromes are a rare group of syndromes that are characterized by impaired haematopoiesis and cancer predisposition. Most inherited BMF syndromes are also associated with a range of congenital anomalies (Mehta et al. 2010).

Fanconi anaemia (FA) is the most common inherited BMF syndrome (Mehta et al. 2010). It is an autosomal recessive disorder that is characterized by a wide variety of congenital abnormalities, defective haematopoiesis and a high risk of developing acute myeloid leukaemia and certain solid tumours. The indication for HSCT in FA is the development of bone marrow failure (Tischkow and Hodgson 2003). Virtually all patients with FA will require treatment with allogeneic HSCT (Mehta et al. 2010).

Diamond-Blackfan anaemia (DBA) is characterized by red cell failure, the presence of congenital anomalies and cancer predisposition. The classic presentation of DBA usually includes anaemia with essentially normal neutrophil and platelet counts, in a child younger than 1 year (Vlachos and Muir 2010).

Dyskeratosis congenita (DC) is a multisystem disorder, with a disruption in telomere biology leading to very short telomeres underpinning its pathophysiology. Bone marrow failure is a key feature in DC and is the leading cause of mortality (Barbaro and Vedi 2016). DC is genetically heterogeneous with X-linked, autosomal dominant and autosomal recessive subtypes. The clinical features include cutaneous manifestations of abnormal skin pigmentation, nail dystrophy, mucosal leukoplakia and BMF, pulmonary fibrosis and predisposition to malignancy. Allogeneic HSCT remains the only curative approach for the BMF (Mehta et al. 2010).

Congenital amegakaryocytic thrombocytopenia (CAMT) is a rare autosomal recessive disorder characterized by isolated thrombocytopenia at birth due to ineffective megakaryocytopoiesis and progression to pancytopenia in later childhood. HSCT remains the only known curative treatment for CAMT (Mehta et al. 2010).

2.5.6 Inherited Diseases: Inborn Errors of Metabolism

Most of the metabolic diseases considered for HSCT are lysosomal storage diseases that rely on transfer of enzyme from donor-derived blood cells to the reticuloendothelial system and solid organs (Sureda et al. 2015b). This group of rare diseases includes mucopolysaccharidosis (MPS) as Hurler's syndrome and leukodystrophy as X-linked adrenoleukodystrophy (X-ALD) and infantile Krabbe disease. The success of SCT in metabolic diseases is determined particularly by the degree of tissue damage present by the time of transplantation and the rate of progression of the disease (Steward and Jarisch 2005). If damage to the central nervous system is present, it is irreversible and therefore a contraindication for transplant (Boelens et al. 2008).

References

Apperley J, Carreras E, Gluckman E, Masszi T. editors. ESH-EBMT handbook. 2012, [Online] pp. 111, 309, 311.

Aversa F. T-cell depletion: from positive selection to negative depletion in adult patients. Bone Marrow Transplant. 2015;50:S11–3.

Bashey A, Solomon SR. T-cell replete haploidentical donor transplantation using post-transplant CY: an emerging standard-of-care option for patients who lack an HLA-identical sibling donor. Bone Marrow Transplant. 2014;49:999–1008.

Champlin RE. Blood stem cells compared with bone marrow as a source of hematopoietic cells for allogeneic transplantation. Blood. 2000;95:3702–9.

Copelan EA. Hematopoietic stem-cell transplantation. N Engl J Med. 2006;354:1813–26.

Demiriz IS, Tekgunduz E, Altuntas F. What is the most appropriate source for hematopoietic stem cell transplantation? Peripheral stem cell/bone marrow/cord blood. Bone Marrow Res. 2012.; [online]

Gratwohl A, Baldomero H, Aljurf M, Pasquini MC, Bouzas LF, Yoshimi A, Szer J, Lipton J, Schwendener A, Gratwohl M, Frauendorfer K, Niederwieser D, Horowitz M, Kodera Y. Hematopoietic stem cell transplantation a global perspective, worldwide network of blood and marrow transplantation. JAMA. 2010;303(16):1617–24.

Hatzimichael E, Tuthill M. Hematopoietic stem cell transplantation. Stem Cells Cloning. 2010;3:105–17. Published online 2010

Mackall, et al. Background to hematopoietic cell transplantation, including post transplant immune recovery. Bone Marrow Transplant. 2009;44:457–62. https://doi.org/10.1038/bmt.2009.255. p.458

Majhail NS, Farnia SH, Carpenter PA, Champlin RE, Crawford S, Marks DI, Omel JL, Orchard PJ, Palmer J, Saber W, Savani BN, Veys PA, Bredeson CN, Giralt SA, LeMaistre CF. Indications for autologous and allogeneic hematopoietic cell transplantation: guidelines from the American Society for Blood and Marrow Transplantation. Biol Blood Marrow Transplant. 2015;21(11):1863–9.

Maziarz RT. Blood and marrow transplant handbook. 2nd ed. Cham: Springer; 2015. p. 3–11, 29–33

Michel RP, Berry GJ, editors. Pathology of transplantation. Cham: Springer; 2016. p. 401–40.

Mohty M, Harousseau JL. Treatment of autologous stem cell transplant-eligible multiple myeloma patients: ten questions and answers. Haematologica. 2014;99(3):408–16.

Pai S-Y, Logan BR, Griffith LM, et al. Transplantation Outcomes for Severe Combined Immunodeficiency, 2000–2009. N Engl J Med. 2014;371:434–46.

Passweg JR, Baldomero H, Bader P, Bonini C, Cesaro S, Dreger P, Duarte RF, Dufour C, Kuball J, Farge-Bancel D, Kröger N, Lanza F, Nagler A, Sureda A, M Mohty for the European Society for Blood and Marrow Transplantation (EBMT). Hematopoietic stem cell transplantation in Europe 2014. Bone Marrow Transplant. 2016;51:786–92.

Rowley S. Hematopoietic stem cell transplantation for malignant diseases. New York: Elsevier; 2013. p. 1020–1.

Sureda A, Bader P, Cesaro S, Dreger P, Duarte RF, Dufour C, Falkenburg JHF, Farge-Bancel D, Gennery A, Kröger N, Lanza F, Marsh JC, Nagler A, Peters C, Velardi A, Mohty M, A Madrigal for the European Society for Blood and Marrow Transplantation. Indications for allo- and auto-SCT for haematological diseases, solid tumours and immune disorders: current practice in Europe, 2015. Bone Marrow Transplant. 2015a;50:1037–56. https://doi.org/10.1038/bmt.2015.6, published online 23 March 2015

References for Indications for Transplant in Non-malignant Diseases in Children

Barbaro P, Vedi A. Survival after hematopoietic stem cell transplant in patients with dyskeratosis congenita: systematic review of the literature. Biol Blood Marrow Transplant. 2016;22:1152–8.

Boelens JJ, Wynn RF, Bierings M. HSCT for inborn errors of metabolism. In: Carreras E, Gluckman E, Gratwohl A, Masszi T, Apperley J, editors. Haematopoietic stem cell transplantation, 5th. s.l. France, Paris: ESH EBMT; 2008. p. 544–53.

Booth C, Silva J, Veys P. Stem cell transplantation for the treatment of immunodeficiency in children: current status and hopes for the future. Expert Rev Clin Immunol. 2016;12:713–23. https://doi.org/10.1586/1744666X.2016.1150177.

Dvorak CC, Hassan A, Slatter MA, Hönig M, Lankester AC, Buckley RH, Pulsipher MA, Davis JH, Güngör T, Gabriel M, Bleesing JH, Bunin N, Sedlacek P, Connelly JA, Crawford DF, Notarangelo LD, Pai SY, Hassid J, Veys P, Gennery AR, Cowan MJ. Comparison of outcomes of hematopoietic stem cell transplantation without chemotherapy conditioning by using matched sibling and unrelated donors for treatment of severe combined immunodeficiency. J Allergy Clin Immunol. 2014;134:935–43.

EBMT & ESID- European Society for Immunodeficiencies have published in 2011 guidelines for stem cell transplantation for primary immunodeficiencies. [Online].

Gaspar HB, Qasim W, Davies EG, Rao K, Amrolia PJ, Veys P. How I treat severe combined immunodeficiency. Blood. 2013;122:3749–58.

Gennery A. Recent advances in treatment of severe primary immunodeficiencies [version 1; referees: 2]. F1000Research. 2015;4:1–10. 10.12688/f1000research.7013.

Mehta P, Locatelli F, Stary J. Bone marrow transplantation for inherited bone marrow failure syndromes. Pediatr Clin N Am. 2010;57:147–70.

Rivers L, Gaspar HB. Severe combined immunodeficiency: recent developments and guidance on clinical management. Arch Dis Child. 2015;100:667–72.

Soiffer RJ, editor. Haematopoietic stem cell transplantation. 2nd ed: Humana Press; 2008. p. 19–23.

Steward CG, Jarisch A. Haemopoietic stem cell transplantation for genetic disorders. Arch Dis Child. 2005;90:1259–63.

Sureda A, Bader P, Cesaro S, Dreger P, Duarte RF, Dufour C, Falkenburg JHF, Farge-Bancel D, Gennery A, Kröger N, Lanza F, Marsh JC, Nagler A, Peters C, Velardi A, Mohty M, Madrigal. Indications for allo- and auto-SCT for haematological diseases, solid tumours and immune disorders: current practice. Bone Marrow Transplant. 2015b;50:1037–56.

Tischkowitz MD, Hodgson SV. Fanconi anaemia. J Med Genet. 2003;40:1–10.

Tura S, editor. lezioni di ematologia. Bologna: Esculapio; 2003. p. 272–85.

Vlachos A, Muir E. How I treat diamond-blackfan anemia. Blood. 2010;116:3715–23.

Donor Selection

Mairéad Níchonghaile

Abstract

Allogeneic haematopoietic stem cell transplant (HSCT) is the treatment of choice for a variety of malignant and non-malignant disorders. The aim of HSCT is to replace the patient's haematopoiesis with that taken from a donor, and a prerequisite is the identification of a suitable donor. It is an intense and demanding process and puts considerable strain on both recipients and donors. The choice of donor has an impact on the transplantation process from scheduling to outcome. There are several common donor issues whether the donor is related or unrelated including eligibility, confidentiality, informed consent and right to refuse consent.

Keywords

Eligibility • Confidentiality • Informed consent • Donation • HLA match • Donor selection

3.1 Introduction

Allogeneic haematopoietic stem cell transplant (HSCT) is the treatment of choice for a variety of malignant and non-malignant conditions. The aim of HSCT is to replace the patient's haematopoiesis with that taken from a donor, and a prerequisite is the identification of a suitable donor. There are three conditions which have to be met for a donor to be considered suitable – the donor needs to be suitably matched, healthy and willing to donate (Kisch 2015). Allogeneic HSCT is an intense and demanding process and puts considerable strain on both recipients and donors.

Donors can be related or unrelated (Fig. 3.1), and the primary consideration is the degree of HLA compatibility of the donor to the recipient and this is considered the most important factor to determining overall success and the transplant-related mortality (Kulkarm and Treleaven 2009).

M. Níchonghaile
St James's Hospital, Dublin 8, Ireland
e-mail: maireadnichonghaile@eircom.net

© EBMT and the Author(s) 2018
M. Kenyon, A. Babic (eds.), *The European Blood and Marrow Transplantation Textbook for Nurses*,
https://doi.org/10.1007/978-3-319-50026-3_3

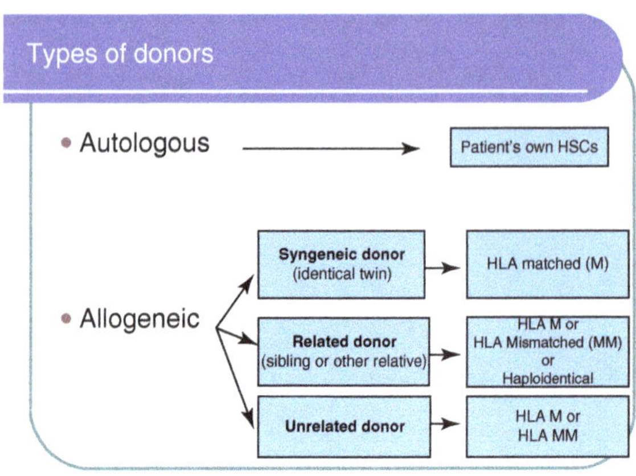

Fig. 3.1 Types of donors

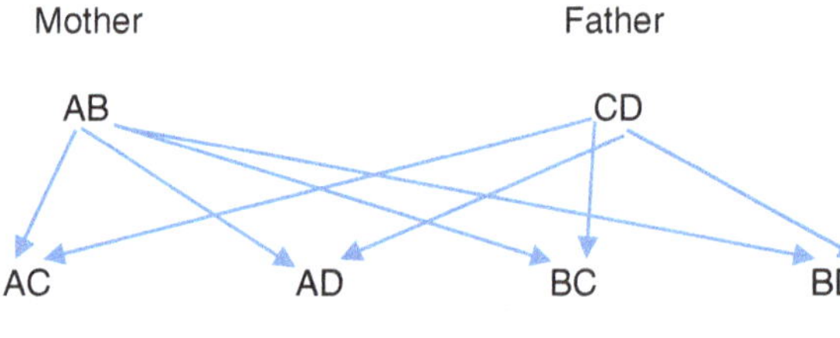

Fig. 3.2 HLA typing

3.2 Human Leukocyte Antigens

Human leukocyte antigens (HLA) are part of the major histocompatibility complex and is highly polymorphic, meaning that there are a lot of variations of the HLA type with humans, and they are found on the short arm of chromosome 6. The primary role of HLA molecules is to preserve peptide to T cells, enabling them to recognise and eliminate "foreign" particles present in an individual and also to prevent the recognition of self as foreign. Due to the Mendelian[1] inheritance of HLA types, the first place to look for a potential donor is within the immediate family (Fig. 3.2). Our HLA type is inherited from our parents – one haplotype from each parent giving rise to a one in four chance that sibling may match another.

Table 3.1 shows the wide variety and number of HLA alleles (the variant forms of the gene)

that have been identified. HLA typing can be serological or DNA based though currently the majority of HLA typing is DNA based.

Table 3.2 shows an example of the nomenclature used for HLA typing. HLA typing looks at matching recipients and donors at HLAs A, B and C (class I typing) and HLAs DR, DQ and DP (class II typing). The nomenclature used is the gene name followed by an asterisk with a four-digit allele name; the first two digits indicated the serological groups and the last two digits the number of the allele within the group.

When we speak of matching, we describe the potential donors as being fully matched (6/6 within the related setting or 10/10 when referring to unrelated donor), a one- or two-antigen mismatch or a haplotype match (i.e. 3/6 or 5/10). The example below shows a patent and his potential sibling donors.

Below is a list of examples when describing degrees of HLA matching between recipient and potential donor.

Table 3.1 The number of HLA alleles currently named at each locus (April 2011)

HLA locus	Number of class I alleles	HLA locus	Number of class II alleles
HLA–A	1601	HLA–DRB	1027
HLA–B	2125	HLA–DQA1	44
HLA–C	1102	HLA–DQB1	153
		HLA–DPA1	32
		HLA–DPB1	149

EBMT Handbook 6th Edition (2012) page 76

Table 3.2 An example of HLA nomenclature and its relation to HLA typing techniques

Typing method	Nomenclature
Serological	A1
DNA based: Low resolution	A*01
DNA based: Low resolution	A*01:01/01:4 N
DNA based: Low resolution	A*01:01

EBMT Handbook 6th Edition (2012) page 77

---

[1] Mendelian inheritance is where a person inherits two alleles, one from each parent. These alleles may be the same or different.

	Patient	Donor
Full/Complete	A*1, B*8, DRB1*03, DRB3*01 A*31, B*35, DRB*04, DRB4*01:02N	A*1, B*8, DRB1*03, DRB3*01 A*31, B*35, DRB*04, DRB4*01:02N
HLA Mismatched	A*1, B*8, DRB1*03, DRB3*01 A*31, B*35, DRB*04, DRB4*01:02N	A*3, B*7, DRB1*01 A*24, DRB1*15, DRB5*01/02/03N
Haplotype Match	A*1, B*8, DRB1*03, DRB3*01 A*31, B*35, DRB*04, DRB4*01:02N	A*1, B*8, DRB1*03, DRB3*01 A*3, B*7, DRB1*01
Single Antigen Mismatch	A*01, B*8, DRB1*03, DRB3*01 A*31 , B*35, DRB*04, DRB4*01:02N	A*01, B*8, DRB1*03, DRB3*01 A*28, B*35, DRB*04, DRB4*01:02N
Single Allelic Mismatch	A*01:01, B*8, DRB1*03, DRB3*01 A*31, B*35, DRB*04, DRB4*01:02N	A*01:0 2, B*8, DRB1*03, DRB3*01 A*31, B*35, DRB*04, DRB4*01:02N

The differences leading to the mismatch are highlighted in red

The possibility of having a suitably matched sibling donor varies depending on ethnicity as distinct HLA types that occur differ among ethnic groups and family size. If a suitable matched sibling donor is not available, a search can be undertaken of the volunteer unrelated donor panels that are part of BM Donors Worldwide. There are now in excess of 18 million volunteer unrelated donors registered on these panels.

Gragert et al. (2014) published the chances of identifying a suitable matched donor for a recipient requiring allogeneic HSCT. While a person of Caucasian background has a relatively good chance of identifying a potential donor, some ethnic groups have a much lower probability of finding a match through unrelated donor searching. This has led to an increase in the use of alternate donors, e.g. a haploidentical donors or alternative cell sources, e.g. cord blood stem cells. The use of haploidentical transplantation with improved conditioning and GVHD prophylaxis means that nearly all patients will gave the potential of a haploidentical donor (Table 3.3).

3.3   Eligibility for HLA Typing of Potential Related Donors

Every institution will have their own requirements regarding eligibility to be HLA typed, and there should be a policy available locally. The main eligibility criteria is willingness to be tested – this does not imply consent to donation – and that the potential donor is not suffering from any conditions that may be a threat or a risk to the recipient or that may be aggravated in themselves by the donation process. As a result potential donors who have had a malignancy previously or have an autoimmune condition should be excluded or given special consideration. Relevant guidance can be found at http://www.worldmarrow.org/donorsuitability/index.php/Main_Page#Related_donors

Sibling donors actively participate in the quest for a cure for their sibling, but this exposes them to an invasive medical procedure that can lead to stress and anxiety and places them in a complex situation. While it can have a beneficial effect for the donor and the family unit as a whole, donors often feel responsible for the recipient outcome.

With respect to unrelated donors, each registry will have their own inclusion/exclusion criteria, but they usually follow the advice of the WMDA (World Marrow Donor Association) on whose website there is comprehensive guidance with respect to donor eligibility. To be listed as a volunteer donor on a blood stem cell registry, you must be:

- Between 18 and 60 years old (age limits may vary per country)
- In good health
- Ready to donate stem cells to *any* patient in need

Table 3.3 Likelihood of identifying HLA-matched adult donors and cord blood units

U.S. Racial and Ethnic Group	Likelihood of identifying an adult donor[a]		Likelihood of identifying a cord-blood unit for patients ≥20 Yr of age[b]			Likelihood of identifying a cord-blood unit for patients <20 Yr of age?		
	8/8 HLA match	≥7.8 HLA match	6/6 HLA match	≥5/6 HLA match	≥4/6 HLA match	6/6 HLA match	≥5/6 HLA match	≥4/6 HLA match
				Percent				
White European	75	97	17	66	96	38	87	99
Middle Eastern or North African	46	90	6	46	91	18	75	98
African American	19	76	2	24	81	6	58	95
African	18	71	1	23	81	5	56	95
Black South or Central American	16	66	2	27	82	7	58	96
Black Caribbean	19	74	1	24	81	6	58	95
Chinese	41	88	6	44	91	19	77	98
Korean	40	87	5	39	89	17	73	98
South Asian	33	84	4	41	90	14	73	98
Japanese	37	87	4	37	88	16	72	97
Filipino	40	83	5	42	89	19	76	98
Southeast Asian	27	76	3	37	89	12	70	98
Vietnarnese	42	84	6	44	89	20	76	98
Hawaiian or Pacific Islander	27	72	3	32	84	10	64	96
Mexican	37	87	6	45	91	19	75	98
Hispanic South or Central American	34	80	5	43	90	17	73	98
Hispanic Caribbean	40	83	5	40	89	17	71	98
Native North American	52	91	10	54	93	25	80	99
Native South or Central American	49	87	11	53	93	26	79	98
Native Caribbean	32	77	4	35	86	14	66	97
Native Alaskan	36	83	7	47	91	18	75	98

Gragert et al. 2014
[a]Data are the probabilities of identifying an adult donor who is available
[b]Data are the probabilities of identifying a unit with an adequate cell dose

To donate umbilical cord blood, a future mother must generally be:

- Over 18 years of age
- In good health
- Pregnant without complications
- Registered well before the onset of labour

3.4 Algorithm of Donor Choice and Selection

Many factors affect the choice of donor, and with the selection of donor sources now available, the possibility of offering HSCT has extended to almost all patients who require it (Apperley et al. 2012).

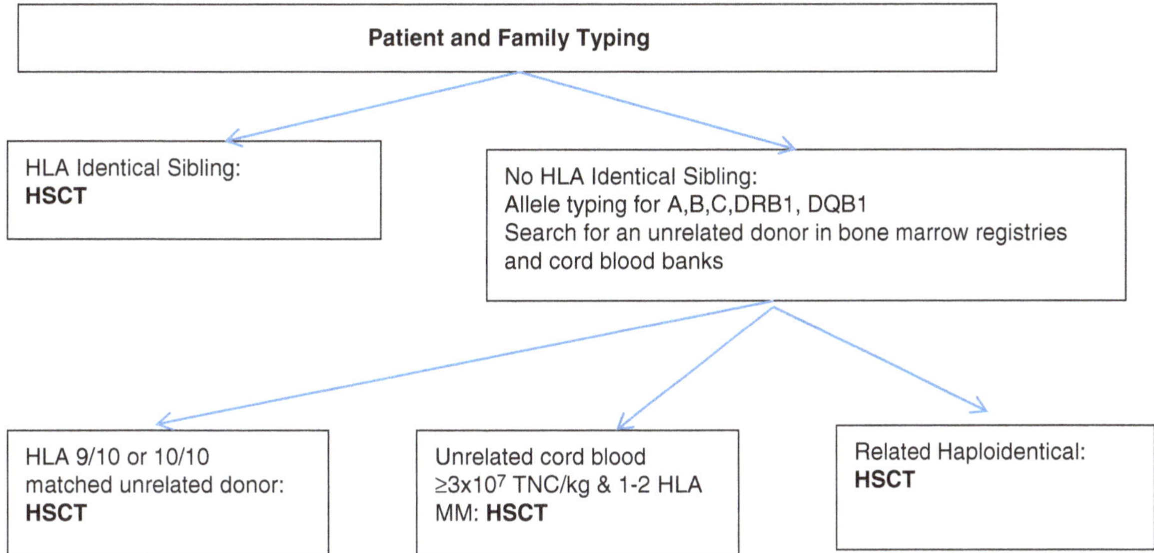

EBMT 2012 Handbook page 102

3.4.1 Donor Selection

The main determinants when selecting a donor whether related or unrelated are as follows:

The "perfect" donor does not exist – no current algorithm will guarantee a positive outcome will always occur.

3.4.2 HLA Match

The most significant factor in success and overall outcome is the degree of match between the donor and recipient.

1. Most data suggest a 10/10 match is the best choice.
2. In many circumstance a 9/10 match can be considered as good as a 10/10 but where the mismatch occurs is important. A mismatch at HLA DQB1 has been shown to have the least likely adverse outcome. Worse outcomes have been seen where the mismatch is at class I. Choosing a HLA A, B or C mismatch should be based on local studies and experience as it can be population or ethnically dependent.

3. Two or more mismatches are associated with a poorer outcome (Shaw 2009).

3.4.3 Cytomegalovirus (CMV) Status

Cytomegalovirus (CMV) is a common virus that can infect almost anyone. Most people don't know they have CMV because it rarely causes symptoms. However, if you're pregnant or have a weakened immune system, CMV is cause for concern. Once infected with CMV, your body retains the virus for life.

Where possible the donor-recipient pairing should be CMV matched with preference given to a CMV compatible donor, i.e. negative donor in a CMV-negative recipient. The CMV status of the donor is less important in a CMV-positive recipient, but there is some evidence that a CMV-positive donor is preferable in a CMV-positive recipient as it may protect the patient from CMV infection (Rovira et al. 2012). Analysis has shown that prior donor CMV exposure significantly reduces the risk of CMV reactivation in CMV-positive recipients as immunity against CMV seems to be transferred with the donor cells and protects CMV-positive recipients from reactivation.

3.4.4 Blood Group

Blood group mismatch is not a contraindication to HSCT, and there is conflicting data about the role of blood group mismatch in relation to post HSCT relapse, but the majority of research suggest that is does not influence HSCT outcome (Kulkarni and Treleaven 2009).

Matching donor and recipient blood group may benefit the recipient as it may reduce the number of transfusions and the period of transfusion dependency post HSCT. Blood group matching is an important consideration in transplants where BM stem cells are the product of choice as it removes the requirement for the product to be red cell depleted to reduce the risk of intravascular haemolysis in the recipient.

3.4.5 Sex Match

Donor-recipient sex match is an important predictor of transplant-related mortality (TRM) with the combination of a male recipient with a female donor known to have an increased risk of chronic GVHD and a higher TRM but not necessarily a reduced relapse risk in all diseases.

3.4.6 Parity

If only female donors are available, it is recommended where possible to use a nonparous female donor as -parous females have a higher chance of having HLA-specific antibodies due to exposure to foetal antigens in utero. It is accepted that recipients (either male or female) who have a HSCT from parous donors have a higher risk of chronic GVHD (Kollman et al. 2001).

3.4.7 Age

The younger the donor at the time of HSCT donation has a favourable outcome after HSCT. It appears that the risk of acute GVHD (Grade 3 or above) and chronic GVHD is higher, and overall survival can be lower with increased donor age (Kollman et al. 2001).

3.4.8 Donor Evaluation

All donors should be medically assessed and consented independently from the recipient medical team. The maxim of "Do No Harm" to the donor is paramount, and no donor should be selected where there is a risk of aggravating or exacerbating a potential medical issue in the donor.

Table 3.4 lists the investigations that should be undertaken for all donors. There is a concern that related donors may not always be as forthcoming about their health as they do not wish to jeopardise their relative's transplant. The table lists the mandatory virology screening that is required on all donors – specific or additional testing may

Table 3.4 Pre-transplant investigations of the donor

Blood group and antibody screening
Coagulation studies
Complete blood count
Full/confirmatory HLA typing
Liver function tests
Urea and creatinine
Pregnancy test
Viral serology – Cytomegalovirus
Epstein-Barr virus
Hepatitis B surface antigen and core antibody
Hepatitis C antigen
HIV
HTLV
Treponemel screen
Herpes simplex virus
Varicella zoster virus
Toxoplasma
Chest X-ray
Electrocardiogram
Under certain circumstances
Cytogenetic studies (chromosome fragility) if family history
Bone marrow examination
Echocardiogram or MUGA scan
Haemoglobin electrophoresis
Lung function tests
Haemoglobinopathy screen

be required in certain countries, e.g. screening for West Nile virus if donor resides in an at risk area, or if the countries' regulations require it, e.g. Tri-NAT assay.

3.5 Special Considerations

3.5.1 Screening of Elderly Donors

With more than 25% of HSCT now being performed in recipients >55 years of age, the chance of a higher age in matched sibling donors is also greater. This group of donors are more likely to have age-related medical conditions, and additional testing may be required to reduce the risk of donor-derived disease, e.g. transmission of an immune-mediated condition, e.g. asthma or psoriasis to the recipient, and reduce the risk to the donor. This includes PSA (prostate-specific antigen) in males, occult blood in stools, possible BM aspirate if results are abnormal, protein electrophoresis and CT chest if there is a history of smoking.

3.5.2 Screening of Paediatric Donors

Paediatric sibling donors are a unique underreported group with special challenges for the HSCT team and the family. Parents of the paediatric donor are in the difficult position of having to consent to both the donation and the transplant. JACIE and other professional bodies suggest the use of independent assessor and donor advocates in the case of paediatric donors to ensure the needs of the paediatric donors are met and that they are protected. Hutt et al. (2015) state that the intense experience of HSCT has a long-term impact on the whole family indicating the need for follow-up and psychological support. There can be a striking difference between the donors' and parents' view of the situation with the donor feeling a closer relationship with the recipient and also feeling responsible for them as well as the fact that the recipient owes them a debt of gratitude. Parents are concerned with two chil-

dren and often feel that the donation process has a positive effect on family life not understanding any negative effect it may have on the donor feeling a pressure to donate or having that feeling of responsibility.

The needs of paediatric donor are sometimes left unmet since parents and healthcare professionals cannot always see the effect of the donation process on them. This can also be said to be the case in adult donors although they at least have life experience and knowledge which enables them to process and deal with their feelings in a way that a child often cannot.

3.5.3 Confidentiality

Information and care of the HSCT patients and their donor should be kept separate. Healthcare professionals must minimise their influence and that of the recipient and other family members which could complicate the potential donors' decision to donate or not. Families are complex entities, and potential donors and recipients can be estranged or influenced, and donors can feel pressured to donate. A model of care which is independent to the recipient (i.e. independent medical assessment and counselling of the potential donor) increases the potential donors' sense of security and allows for informed consent or refusal of donation. It is essential to separate the care of the donor from that of the recipient so that each individual can be focussed upon. The privacy of the donor must be respected and protected, and all potential donors should be given information at the time of the HLA typing about the potential process.

3.5.4 Donor Consent and Clearance

All donors should be reviewed and consented prior to the recipient commencing conditioning chemotherapy. They should be medically cleared and understand the implications if they withdraw their consent or participation once the recipient's conditioning has commenced.

3.5.5 Stem Cell Source

While this is primarily dictated by the transplant medical assessment and the type of HSCT that the recipient is undergoing, the donor will also influence that decision. The donor has a choice in which type of donation method that they prefer, and both should be discussed. The donor may also have medical issues which influence the cell source, e.g. donors with significant back injuries or issues may not be suitable for bone marrow harvest, and unrelated donors who do not have adequate peripheral venous access may not be considered for apheresis due to the reluctance to insert a central access device in an unrelated donor.

Conclusion

Allogenic HSCT is a standard therapy in a number of malignant and non-malignant conditions. The choice of donor is a complex issue with far-reaching consequences both for the recipient and the donor.

References

Apperley J, Carreras E, Gluckman E, Masszi T. Haematopoeitic stem cell transplantation. 6th revised ed. 2012.

Gragert L, et al. HLA match likelihoods for hematopoietic stem-cell grafts in the U.S. registry. N Engl J Med. 2014;371(4):339–48.

Hutt D, Nehari M, Munits-Shenkar D, Akalay Y, Toren A, Bielorai B. Haematopoietic stem cell donation: psychological perspectives of paediatric sibling donors and their parents. Bone Marrow Transplant. 2015;50:1–6.

Kisch, AM. Allogeneic stem cell transplant. Patient and sibling donors perspective. Malmo University. 2015.

Kollman C, Howe CW, Ansetti C, et al. Donor characteristics as risk factors in recipients after transplantation of bone marrow from unrelated donors. Blood. 2001;98:2043–51.

Kulkarm S, Treleaven J. Patient selections: preliminary interview and screening of patient and donor. In: Treleaven J, Barrett AJ, editors. Haematopoietic stem cell transplantation in clinical practice. Churchill Livingstone: Elsevier; 2009.

Rovira M, Mensa J, Carreras E, Infections in HSCT In: Apperley J, Carreras E, Gluckman E, Masszi T. The EBMT Handbook: Haematopoeitic stem cell transplantation. 6th revised ed. 2012.

Shaw B. Human leukocyte antigen matching, compatibility testing and donor selection. In: Treleaven J, Barrett AJ, editors. Haematopoietic stem cell transplantation in clinical practice. Churchill Livingstone: Elsevier; Edinburgh 2009.

Transplant Preparation

4

Caroline Bompoint, Alberto Castagna,
Daphna Hutt, Angela Leather, Merja Stenvall,
Teija Schröder, Eugenia Trigoso Arjona,
and Ton Van Boxtel

Abstract

HSCT is a complex procedure, which involves a long and complicated pathway for the patient and the intervention of many health professionals. Within this multidisciplinary team, the transplant coordinator, usually a nurse, is the 'essential marrow', the heart and the vital backbone of this procedure; they are an essential transplant ingredient facilitating a fluidity of the pathway and a good transmission of information. Written information about the procedure is beneficial for patients either prior to clinic visit or during clinic to allow the patients and relatives to reflect on conversations. Transplantation carries a significant risk of morbidity and mortality, and these should be considered regarding the 'need' to transplant, based upon risk of disease, versus risk of the transplant. Pre-transplant assess-

C. Bompoint (✉)
HSCT Unit, Saint Eloi hospital, Montpellier, France
e-mail: c-bompoint@chu-montpellier.fr

A. Castagna
Pediatric Hemato-Oncology and HSCT Unit, AOUI
Verona, Verona, Italy

D. Hutt
Department of Paediatric Hematology-Oncology and
BMT, Edmond and lily Safra Children Hospital,
Sheba Medical Center, Tel-Hashomer, Israel

A. Leather
The Christie NHS Foundation Trust, Manchester, UK

M. Stenvall • T. Schröder
Pediatric Hematology, Oncology and Stem Cell
Transplantation Unit, University Hospital,
Helsinki, Finland

E.T. Arjona
Hospital U y Polytechnic "LA FE", Valencia, Spain

T. Van Boxtel
UMC Utrecht, Utrecht, The Netherlands

© EBMT and the Author(s) 2018
M. Kenyon, A. Babic (eds.), *The European Blood and Marrow Transplantation Textbook for Nurses*,
https://doi.org/10.1007/978-3-319-50026-3_4

ments must also be undertaken, and the results of these along with suitable donor medical clearance and cell availability are essential to ascertain that transplant is a valid option and can proceed safely. Dealing with fertility preservation upon diagnosis of cancer is often challenging; this issue is even more complex for paediatric patients. PDWP recommends that counselling about fertility preservation opportunities should be offered to each patient receiving HSCT.

This chapter will also focus on vascular access for optimal treatment of haematology patients because stem cell treatment cannot be performed without it. Constant advances in haematology have raised challenging ethical dilemmas concerning end of life, palliative care, patient information, donor concerns and impartiality and issues related to the risk we run to our patients. Nurses provide a key role in patient education, providing pre- and post-transplant advocacy and counselling, plan hospitalisations and consultations. They also act as educators and role models to nursing students and share knowledge in accordance with local policies and JACIE guidelines.

Keywords

Transplant coordinator • Nurse • Multidisciplinary team (MDT) • Ethics • Complex procedure • Venous access

4.1 The Role of Transplant Coordinator

The role of the transplant coordinator (TC) is to ensure that timely events occur for each patient and their families undergoing haematopoietic stem cell transplant (HSCT), ensuring that patients are physically and psychologically prepared for the treatment. Many transplant coordinators are nurse specialists who focus their role on the individual needs of the patient and families; however, some centres have medical staff that organise transplants. TC provide a high level of care and management, inform and educate the patient, have holistic knowledge of the patient, participate in specific or advanced nursing practices (bone marrow sampling, HLA typing, transplant recipient care) and coordinate all the transplant logistics.

The transplant coordinator ensures that a suitable source of cells is available following the high-dose chemotherapy or immunosuppressive treatment that the patient will receive.

The TC supports the patient education and coordination of all care and embodies a clinical nursing function where emphasis is placed on specialisation in a clearly defined area of care.

The TC also takes cares of the donor, to welcome and accompany the donor in his procedures: information, assessment, reimbursement of expenses and psychological follow-up.

They are involved in the creation of information tools for the patient and the donor which are evaluated in order to have an accurate knowledge of patients' needs. A TC actively participates in the JACIE process of accreditation of transplant centres by writing and evaluating SOPs.

Within the last decade, transplant centres across Europe have invested in new nursing roles allowing quality, continuity and coordination of care, providing a link between all members of the transplant team (physicians, nurses, cell therapy, immunologist, radiotherapists to name a few) and actively participating in the accreditation process.

4.2 Information and Consent

Written information is considered to be beneficial for patients either prior to clinic visit or during clinic to allow the patients and relatives to reflect on conversations (Patient Information Forum 2010). It is good practice to have had in-depth discussions with patients on at least two occasions prior to transplant consent and admission. There are many good information leaflets available for patients and their relatives to gain an overview of the procedure, some generic and others disease specific. Information should be offered to the patient early in their transplant journey where appropriate. Consent for transplant should be taken prior to admission and before the donor in allogeneic transplants starts any mobilisation therapy. Each country will have different legislation to follow, and guidelines for this will be available within your centre. Consent should be obtained by medical personnel who have received the appropriate, documented training in consenting to medical treatment and examination. Usually, for transplant consent due to its complexity and significant mortality risk, it would be considered as reasonable that this will be taken by the patient's consultant or designated deputy, to ensure all known factors and concerns are addressed appropriately.

Consent and information given to the patient should be balanced against the risk of disease. Indications and suitability of potential transplant candidates are identified, as indicated by EBMT guidelines and local policy. Yet decisions are the responsibility of medical teams with input from other members of the multidisciplinary team (MDT) based around EBMT guidelines; however, the patient needs to be in agreement and fully informed of the process, and the final decision should be with the patient, with appropriate support and guidance.

During the consent process, patients should be informed of the reason for transplantation and the risks and potential benefits associated with the procedure; this will vary depending upon conditioning, individual risk factors and the donor chosen. Information should include (but not be exclusive to) the risk of graft versus host disease (GVHD), infection, bleeding, multi-organ damage/failure, infertility, hair loss, pain and possibility of death.

Consent for data collection is also important and is in line with the data protection act since 1998 and allows EBMT to collect anonymous information about the transplant, disease groups and outcomes, enabling future developments, trends and research opportunities. Patients should provide consent for their centre to send this information.

4.3 Information and Consents in the Paediatric Population

Informed consent is an essential part of healthcare practice. Parental permission and childhood assent is an active process that engages both adults and children, in their health care. Paediatric practice is unique in that developmental maturation allows, over time, for increasing inclusion of the child's and adolescent's opinion in medical decision-making in clinical practice and research (Katz et al. 2016).

A paediatric patient or a minor can be defined as a patient who has not reached the legal age of majority (in most countries, 18 years of age), a patient younger than 18 years. An adolescent refers to a person in the transition between childhood and adulthood, classically defined as 13–18 years of age. A child refers to a person from the ages of 1 through 12 years, and an infant refers to a person in the first year of life (Katz et al. 2016).

Children and parents have the right to informed participation in all decisions involving their health care so that they can make informed consent. Participation in decision-making requires advance information about all measures that need to be taken. The right of children to participate in their health care requires that staff members shall create an environment based on trust. Staff members shall have the capacity to listen, share information and give sound guidance. They have to respect the right of children to express their view in all matters affecting them, give due weight to their opinion in accordance with their competence and render a culturally appropriate interpretation of the child's view and accept that children have the right to not express an opinion or to express their views through their parents (European Association for Children in Hospital 2016).

EACH Charter points out that the rights of the children and parents to informed consent require that staff members respect the child's and the parents' ability and competence. The staff need to provide adequate and timely information to the child and the parents regarding their child's health condition, the purpose and value of treatment, the process and the risks. They have to offer adequate, reliable information on alternative forms of treatment. They have to advise and support the child and the parents to evaluate the proposed course of action and acknowledge and take seriously the child's and parents' knowledge and experience relating to their child's general health condition or present condition (European Association for Children in Hospital 2016).

Children have the right to express their views and may disagree with their parents. Providing they are mature enough to make decisions in their own best interests, staff should respect the child's opinion, depending on the stipulations of national laws. Staffs are required to proceed with the utmost care to properly evaluate the situation. Hospital staff should also ensure that the necessary counselling and support is given to the parents (European Association for Children in Hospital 2016).

4.4 Role of Risk Assessment and Co-morbidity Scores

Transplantation carries a significant risk of morbidity and mortality, and these should be considered regarding the 'need' to transplant, based upon risk of disease, versus risk of the transplant; often this can be finely balanced. Suitability must be individualised to each patient need and requirements and discussed in detail with the patient with regard to the decisions.

Some patients are not solely living with the haematological disease or disorder and may have other factors that need to be taken into account. The presence of one or more diseases or disorders along with a primary diagnosis is called co-morbidity. This may be psychological or physical and may include illnesses such as diabetes and cardiac, respiratory or renal disease. Sometimes social and practical considerations may exclude a patient from undergoing stem cell transplant, yet as nurses we must aim to support where possible to ensure the best treatment options can be delivered.

Co-morbidity index tools have been used to predict outcomes in patients with cancer for several years, and some validated index tools such as Charlson co-morbidity index (CCI) consider medical history to estimate a prognosis or one-year mortality. Each factor is assigned to a point number of 1, 2, 3 or 6. Patients may have more than one disorder in each group, clearly increasing risk; however, the CCI was felt not necessarily relevant to patients undergoing HSCT because the factors within the groups would often already be considered an exclusion to transplant and did not reflect frequent morbidities experienced by haematology patients (Sorror et al. 2005). Subsequently the HCTI, which is considered more relevant to HSCT, was designed. This tool reflects the conditions that some of the patients face prior to transplant, which may be as a result of previous therapies used to treat the disease or indeed the disease itself and can be used to risk assess potential co-morbidity prior to allogeneic transplant.

Karnofsky Performance Status, also known as KPS, has scores ranging from 0 to 100 (0 being deceased and 100 being normal with no problems with activities of living or disease present).

KPS can be used to infer a patient prognosis and ability to perform activities of normal living. Dependent on the indication for transplant and patient wellbeing prior to commencing conditioning, a KPS may limit options and be suggestive of outcome (Karnofsky et al. 1948).

100	Normal; no complaints; no evidence of disease
90	Able to carry on normal activity; minor signs or symptoms of disease
80	Normal activity with effort; some signs or symptoms of disease
70	Cares for self; unable to carry on normal activity or to do active work
60	Requires occasional assistance, but is able to care for most of their personal needs
50	Requires considerable assistance and frequent medical care
40	Disabled; requires special care and assistance
30	Severely disabled; hospital admission is indicated although death not imminent
20	Very sick; hospital admission necessary; active supportive treatment necessary
10	Moribund; fatal processes progressing rapidly
0	Dead

Post-transplant performance scores can be used to determine ongoing treatment. Similar to the KPS, the Lansky score is specific to children and activities that they will encounter (Lansky et al. 1987) and may be the preferred tool in the paediatric setting.

100	Fully active, normal
90	Minor restrictions in strenuous physical activity
80	Active, but gets tired more quickly
70	Greater restriction of play *and* less time spent in play activity
60	Up and around, but active play minimal; keeps busy by being involved in quieter activities
50	Lying around much of the day, but gets dressed; no active playing participates in all quiet play and activities
40	Mainly in bed; participates in quiet activities
30	Bedbound; needing assistance even for quiet play
20	Sleeping often; play entirely limited to very passive activities
10	Doesn't play; does not get out of bed
0	Unresponsive

4.5 Fertility Preservation

With advancing treatments more and more women and children are cured of a cancer or haematological disease but may subsequently be deprived of their ovarian function or exposed to premature menopause due to the ovarian toxicity of treatments. Any patient undergoing therapy likely to impair fertility should be referred according to local referral pathway.

Fertility is a well-known and significant concern for patients receiving high-dose chemotherapy +/− radiotherapy. However, the risk to fertility depends on the treatment received and the age of the individual at transplant. Evidence suggests that some young patients under the age of 16 at transplant may recover some gonadal function in later life (Suhag et al. 2015); however, this is dependent upon conditioning therapy, although the majority of the patients treated will be rendered infertile as a consequence of treatment. In male patients, there is some evidence that following induction therapy spermatogenesis may recover after 5–10 years of treatment, but this is very much variable (Tal et al. 2000, Viviani et al. 1999). Azoospermia rates range from 10% to 70% in males following stem cell transplant; again, this is often dependent on conditioning agents employed (Anserini et al. 2002, Jacob et al. 1998).

Fertility options must be discussed prior to initiation of ANY chemotherapy regime, and consequently many patients should have already had a discussion regarding fertility preservation well before transplant discussions are undertaken particularly if they have had induction therapy for their diagnosis. However, it is also essential for this to be clarified and discussed in detail prior to transplant conditioning.

Although ovarian function is more affected by chemotherapy and certainly high-dose regimes, female fertility preservation remains challenging. Egg harvests are not often viable for later fertilisation. IVF followed by embryo storage can be more effective but takes 2–3 weeks revolving around the menstrual cycle and is not always feasible, especially in newly diagnosed patients with aggressive disease. Post-transplant, donor eggs may be a possibility for some women who may have limited options and should be explored in a full discussion with a fertility specialist.

Male patients should be offered sperm storage before initiation of any treatment. Radiotherapy and Alkylating agents amongst others have a severe impact on spermatozoa. Assuming that masturbation is possible, this is much simpler to organise than for female patients. It can usually be arranged and performed quickly in an andrology department. Once collected, the semen is analysed for sperm number, motility and quality. Quality of the sperm may be affected by several factors, including disease and current wellbeing of the patient.

4.6 Fertility Preservation in the Paediatric Population

The numbers of long-term survivors following haematopoietic stem cell transplantation (HSCT) have been noticeably increasing in recent years. Preparative regimens are associated with a high risk of infertility. Infertility is considered a major late effect in patients receiving haematopoietic stem cell transplantation (HSCT) (Borgmann-Staudt et al. 2012).

The infertility induced by cytostatic drugs is dependent on type and dosage of the drug used and also on the patients' age at the time of treatment.

More than two-thirds of former paediatric patients who had received allogeneic HSCT showed signs of impaired fertility. Significant risk factors were total body irradiation (TBI) for males and busulfan (Bu) for females (Borgmann-Staudt et al. 2012).

For radiation therapy, variables for infertility risk also include the:

- Age and developmental maturity of the patient
- Dose and fractionation of therapy
- Site of radiation therapy

The oocyte median lethal dose for radiation therapy is less than 2 Gy and sperm production is susceptible to damage at doses of more than 1.2 Gy; testicular Leydig cell function seems to be present at radiation doses up to 20 Gy (Fallat et al. 2008).

The alkylating agents, such as cyclophosphamide and busulfan, which have frequently been used in the treatment of childhood cancer, are far more gonadotoxic than other chemotherapeutic agents (Schmidt et al. 2010).

Hypogonadism is common after HCT (Sklar et al. 2001; Smith et al. 2014). In both boys and girls, hypergonadotropic hypogonadism (primary gonadal failure) is more common than hypogonadotropic hypogonadism (due to hypothalamic pituitary dysfunction) (Baker et al. 2009).

Children with hypogonadotropic hypogonadism have an absence of sex hormone production, delayed puberty, delayed pubertal growth spurt and a decrease in final adult height (Bourguignon 1988).

The type of presentation depends on the pubertal status at the time of HCT (Dvorak et al. 2011; Sanders et al. 2011). Puberty status is defined in two categories: 'Pre-puberty' for children aged up to 12 years and 'puberty' for children aged 13 years and older at the time of HSCT (Borgmann et al. 2011).

The earliest manifestation of impaired sex hormone production is delayed puberty in prepubertal patients, but older patients may show asynchronous or incomplete pubertal development, primary or secondary amenorrhea and infertility due to azoospermia or premature menopause. Sex steroids are also required for the growth spurt during adolescence. Delayed or incomplete puberty occurs in about 57% of females and 53% of males (Dvorak et al. 2011; Sanders et al. 2011).

In prepubertal males, the only option here is testicular tissue freezing. Options for use are autologous transplantation, xenografting or in vitro maturation. No children have been born from the use of prepubertal test tissue. In post-pubertal males, the most common option here is freezing of ejaculated sperm, but storage of testicular tissue is also a possibility (Shenfield et al. 2004).

4.6.1 Fertility Counselling

Studies emphasise the need for comprehensive counselling for patients undergoing HSCT, particularly those receiving TBI- or busulfan-based preparative regimens and their parents regarding fertility-preserving measures (Borgmann-Staudt et al. 2012).

Counselling patients of child-bearing age or their parents regarding future fertility when faced with a life-threatening cancer diagnosis is difficult but extremely important. Therefore, the health-care team has a responsibility to provide screening to identify these patients, provide education so that an informed decision can be made as rapidly as possible and have a team ready to preserve fertility once a decision has been made.

4.6.2 When?

Counselling at the primary diagnosis would be ideal.

In the current treatment era, optimal care for paediatric patients with cancer would include fertility preservation options at diagnosis prior to therapeutic exposures that can cause azoospermia. Sperm banking can be offered to even early pubertal patients, while development of methods to preserve spermatogonia from prepubertal patients represents an area of active research (Dilley 2007).

4.6.3 Issues

Fertility preservation is often possible, but to preserve the full range of options, fertility preservation approaches should be discussed as early as possible, before treatment starts. The discussion can ultimately reduce distress and improve quality of life. The discussions should be documented in the medical record (Loren 2013).

In 2015, the *Nordic Network for Gonadal Preservation after Cancer Treatment in Children and Young Adults* revised its Recommendations on Fertility Preservation (RTP) for girls and young women with childhood cancer:

> 'All girls should be examined regarding pubertal development (Tanner stage and menstrual history) at diagnosis and should be informed of the risk for impaired fertility following the planned treatment'.

4.6.4 Who?

Regarding this, in 2013 the original language used by the American Society of Clinical Oncology (ASCO) has been revised: The word 'oncologist' was replaced with 'health-care provider' to include medical oncologists, radiation oncologists, gynaecologic oncologists, urologists, haematologists, paediatric oncologists and surgeons, as well as nurses, social workers, psychologists and other no physician providers.

Regarding the role of health-care providers in advising patients about fertility preservation options, ASCO recommends:

All oncologic health care providers should be prepared to discuss infertility as a potential risk of therapy. This discussion should take place as soon as possible once a cancer diagnosis is made and before a treatment plan is formulated. (Loren et al. 2013 Recommendations for Fertility Preservation for Patients with Cancer).

However, what remains unclear is how these discussions are initiated, whether these discussions occur with all patients and which members of the oncology team are responsible for communicating with patients about these risks and available options (Nobel Murray et al. 2015).

In 2008, the bioethics committee, 2006–2007, from the American Academy of Paediatrics (AAP) published in this technical report reviews the Guidance for Counselling of Parents and Patients about Preservation of Fertility Options in Children and Adolescents with Cancer.

'Evaluation of candidacy for fertility preservation should involve a team of specialists, including a paediatric oncologist and/or radiation oncologist, a fertility specialist, anesthetist, and a mental health professional.

1. Cryopreservation of sperm should be offered whenever possible to male patients or families of male adolescents.
2. Current fertility-preservation options for female children and adolescents should be considered experimental and are offered only in selected institutions in the setting of a research protocol
3. In considering actions to preserve a child's fertility, parents should consider a child's assent, the details of the procedure involved, and whether such procedures are of proven utility or experimental in nature.

   In some cases, after such consideration, acting to preserve a child's fertility may be appropriate.
4. Despite it's not an options for children, instructions concerning disposition of stored gametes, embryos, or gonadal tissue in the event of the patient's death, unavailability, or other contingency should be legally outlined and understood by all parties, including the patient if possible.
5. Concerns about the welfare of a resultant offspring with respect to future cancer risk should not be a cause for denying reproductive assistance to a patient' (Fallat et al. 2008).

However, in 2015, the Nordic Network and Nordic Society of Paediatric Haematology and Oncology (NOPHO) revised the recommendation provided in 2012.

4.6.5 Recommendations on Fertility Preservation for Girls and Young Women with Childhood Cancer

After treatment All girls who have received alkylating agents or abdominal irradiation should after sexual maturation be offered referral to a gynaecologist or fertility specialist for evaluation, counselling and considering the possibility for ovarian hyper-stimulation and cryopreservation of oocytes.

4.6.5.1 Menstruating Girls

If the girl is menstruating, mature enough to give informed consent and is facing cancer therapy with very high risk of infertility, therapy can be delayed 1–2 weeks, and ovarian hyper-stimulation and cryopreservation of oocytes may be considered. The responsible oncologist must be consulted to make sure that no contraindications, such as bleeding disorders or too long delay of cancer therapy, to such procedures are present. The girl should get information adjusted to her age.

4.6.5.2 All Girls Regardless of Maturational Stage

All efforts should be done to minimise the radiation exposure to the ovary, such as optimal dose planning and irradiation modality, shielding and oophoropexy. Present knowledge indicates that a radiation dose lower than 10 Gy may preserve some ovarian function.

Girls, who are facing or receiving oncological treatments associated with a very high risk of infertility, could be offered the experimental procedure of ovarian cortical tissue cryopreservation.

In menstruating girls, cryopreservation of ovarian tissue can precede controlled ovarian hyper-stimulation (see above). The responsible oncologist must be consulted to make sure that no contraindications to such procedures are present.

4.6.6 Recommendations on Fertility Preservation for Boys and Young Men with Childhood Cancer

4.6.6.1 Pubertal and Post-pubertal Males

All males who are physically mature enough to produce sperm should be offered cryopreservation of sperm before oncological treatment with potentially gonadotoxic effect (i.e. all chemotherapy and radiotherapy with the gonads in the radiation field) is started.

All boys should be examined regarding pubertal development (Tanner stage and testicular volume). If the volume of testes is between 6 and 8 ml, there is a reasonable probability of sperm in an ejaculate.

The boy should be informed by a professional, specially assigned for this purpose, e.g. an andrologist, paediatric endocrinologist or fertility specialist, according to local availability and routines. It is important that the autonomy of the boy is respected and that he is offered the opportunity of individual consultation.

If the boy is unable to produce an ejaculate, alternative methods like vibrator stimulation or electro stimulation during anaesthesia could be offered.

If the boy is unable to produce an ejaculate or has azoospermia, an invasive procedure to retrieve testicular sperm may be considered, provided that the boy is motivated himself. The responsible paediatric oncologist must first be consulted to make sure that no contraindications (such as risk of tumour spread (e.g. in ALL) or bleeding disorder) to such procedures are present.

The boy, as well as his parents, should get verbal and written information about the procedures and the legal implications. The information should be adjusted to the boy's age, and he must give his informed consent to the cryopreservation.

4.6.6.2 Prepubertal Boys

Boys, who are facing oncological treatments associated with a very high risk of infertility, could be offered the experimental procedure of testicular biopsy cryopreservation. At present, there are no methods to ensure fertility after such procedures; thus, further research is warranted. Since the patient number is limited, the cryopreservation and research should be centralised.

The parents and, if old enough, the boy should get verbal and written information about the research project and give informed consent to the cryopreservation and to participate in the research.

4.6.7 Techniques

The objective of ovarian tissues' cryopreservation is to maintain viability of tissue after long-term storage. It is the basis for all forms of fertility preservation for cancer sufferers. Cryopreservation requires cooling tissue from 37 °C to the temperature of liquid nitrogen (−196 °C), storing at this temperature and then rewarming to 37 °C at some later date.

Freezed ovarian cortex segments can be used for later thawing and transplanting either back to the ovarian site (orthotopically) or to some other location (heterotopically). The ovarian cortex is used because it is this part of the ovary that is particularly rich in primordial follicles. In order for cryoprotectants to penetrate the tissue, the cortical strips need to be no more than 2 mm thick. Tissue samples from cancer patients need to be evaluated by a pathologist to detect the presence of any metastatic cancer cells (Agarwal and Chang 2007).

Spermarche occurs over a wide age range and is associated with a highly variable testicular volume, including in individuals with testicular volumes of less than 5 mL, pubic hair stage I or both. As a result, intraoperative assessment of the biopsy sample at the time of tissue retrieval has been suggested to be useful for allocation of tissue to a specific freezing protocol (Anderson et al. 2015).

For pubertal patients in whom complete spermatogenesis has occurred, semen cryopreservation is a well-established option. Recommendations are that all men and teenage boys should be offered semen cryopreservation for prepubertal patients and pubertal patients who are not able to produce a semen sample; approaches for fertility preservation are experimental (Anderson et al. 2015).

Sperm cryopreservation after masturbation is the most established and effective method of fertility preservation in males. Sperm should be collected before initiation of cancer therapy because of the risk that sperm DNA integrity or sample quality will be compromised.

Nevertheless, recent progress in andrology laboratories and with assisted reproductive techniques allows successful freezing and future use of a very limited amount of sperm; collection of semen through masturbation in adolescents may be compromised by embarrassment and issues of informed consent. Alternative methods of obtaining sperm besides masturbation include testicular aspiration or extraction, electro ejaculation under sedation or anaesthesia or from post masturbation urine sample. Testicular aspirates do not freeze well and cannot be used as a method of preserving sperm (Fallat et al. 2008).

4.6.8 Fertility Preservation Options for Children and Young Adults with Distinction Between Established and Experimental Options

- In prepubertal boys, before onset of spermatogenesis, testicular biopsy and cryopreservation are options (experimental). In pubertal and post-pubertal male patients, the ability to produce a sperm-containing ejaculate enables sperm cryopreservation (established); if this is not possible, testicular biopsy with cryopreservation of sperm or tissue is needed.
- In prepubertal girls, ovarian stimulation is inappropriate, so ovarian tissue cryopreservation can be offered (experimental). After puberty, cryopreservation is an option, but ovarian stimulation enables recovery of mature oocytes for cryopreservation or of embryos after fertilisation (established) (Anderson et al. 2015).
- *Safety of tissue with regard to contamination with tumour/leukaemia cells.* Cancer contamination in the cryopreserved tissue is a contraindication for re-transplantation. Experimental studies are ongoing regarding the in vitro maturation of oocytes for fertilisation from such tissue. Further research is warranted. The parents and, if old enough, the girl should get verbal and written information about the experimental procedure, its associated risks and legal implications and give informed consent to the cryopreservation (NOPHO).
- In the interest of the child, the PDWP recommends that counselling about fertility preservation (FP) opportunities should be offered to each patient receiving SCT, as part of the pre stem cell transplant (SCT) workup. The PDWP recommends that should be offered by a dedicated and trained task force that may include medical staff from the stem cell transplant unit as well as fertility preservation specialists. The presence of dedicated nurse staff and psychologists in the counselling task force should be considered to create a broader communication opportunity for the patient, who may be more at ease with non-medical staff (PDWP, EBMT 2017).

4.6.9 Sexuality in Adolescents and Young Adults

Children at risk for impaired growth as a result of cancer therapy should be examined regularly, with their growth plotted on the appropriate growth chart.

Monitoring should be more frequent from the time of expected onset of puberty through the fusion of growth plates at full sexual maturation (Nobel Murray 2015).

Although we know that, after the transplant, some adults process experience psychological and social issues, there is an absence in the literature about the 'adolescents and young adult' (AYA) HCT population (Cooke et al. 2011).

The AYA cancer population is a vulnerable group due to variety of social, psychological and developmental reasons. AYA patients also can have disturbed endocrine function, body image disruptions and sexual problems (Cooke et al. 2011).

Who should be in charge of talking with children? It is impossible to consider parent–child interactions on the topic of fertility without framing the issue within the larger, complicated topic of parent–child discussions about sex, given that the two are inextricably linked. Discomfort in the general area of discussing sexuality will impact the parental willingness and perception of competence in discussing fertility, especially at a moment of high stress (Clayman 2007). The growing literature on parent–child discussions of sex reflects the tendency of mothers to discuss this topic more frequently with their children, particularly daughters; even when both parents are involved, they are more likely to talk about sex with daughters rather than sons (Clayman 2007).

In 2006, Sloper's study concludes that there was an emphasis on the need for professionals to raise the subject sooner, more frequently, in a low-key way and without ambiguity. Respondents wished professionals would treat them as partners, therefore prioritising their input over their parents.

4.6.10 Conclusion

Dealing with fertility preservation upon diagnosis of cancer is challenging even for a young adult patient. This issue is even more complex for paediatric patients where decision-making generally falls to the parents but where high cancer survival rates increase the possibility of survivors needing to confront infertility later in life. Parents and adolescent patients report that achieving a healthy state is most important and that while they are interested in fertility preservation options, they may not be willing to delay treatment for pursuit of those options. Optimal care of paediatric cancer patients undergoing gonadotoxic therapy should include enrolment in available trials that will continue to refine knowledge of the effects of therapy on fertility for both male and female patients. Patients and families need information at diagnosis regarding the potential impact of therapy on fertility as well as referral to appropriate specialists for fertility preservation when desired. Studies and resources that allow potentially fertility-sparing interventions such as ovarian cryopreservation will not only need to be expanded, but adequate education and support for oncology providers who screen for patients at risk will be key. For patients that did not undergo fertility-sparing procedures prior to treatment, careful monitoring of reproductive function is warranted, and current technologies will still allow many of those patients to parent their own biological children (Dilley 2007).

4.7 Transplant Workup

HSCT is often considered as part of a therapeutic pathway, dependent on disease response and initial presentation. It is often proposed as a consolidation treatment to avoid a relapse. Prior to discussions regarding transplantation, it must be considered that the recipient can withstand the procedure without excessive risk and that there is no contraindication and the disease status is suitable to undergo the procedure. Transplanting patients with relapsed or relapsing disease may not provide sufficient benefit for the patient given the risks of the procedure and is often considered as futile. Pre-transplant assessments (disease status, bloods with virology status, radiology, cardiac, pulmonary and renal examinations) must be undertaken, and the results of these along with suitable donor medical clearance and cell availability are essential to ascertain that transplant is a valid option.

The results of this pre-transplant assessment will help to inform and adapt the transplant modality: conditioning regimen, type of graft, stem cell source and post-transplant strategy (immunomodulation, DLI). It also allows doctors to detect any abnormalities that could lead to post-transplant complications. This complete review serves as a reference and facilitates comparison of results of the examinations carried out before and after the transplant. In some cases the pre-transplant workup/assessment may mean that the risk of transplant is considered too great and therefore is no longer a suitable option due to higher-than-acceptable rates of morbidity and mortality and should be discussed with the patient. The previously mentioned morbidity indexes are useful in helping to determine this.

During transplant workup, the patient should be offered to meet other members of the multidisciplinary team such as social worker, dietician, physiotherapist, psychologist, etc. where possible.

Transplant workup may vary from centre to centre and will be dependent on clinical indication. The list below is not exclusive but gives indication of workup required prior to transplant admission. The transplant coordinator would usually organise and collate this information and results.

- Full blood count.
- U & E and liver function profile.
- Virology transplant assessment including HIV; Hep B, C, and E; CMV; and EBV status.
- Group and save sample.
- HLA antibody screen.
- Coagulation.
- Tissue typing and verification typing of patient and donor for allogeneic transplants.
- Patients who have been heavily transfused prior to transplant should have serum ferritin levels taken to identify iron overload, >1000 ng/ml.
- Cardiac function is assessed by echocardiography (ECHO) or MUGA scan (ECHO is favourable). Healthy individuals typically have left ventricle ejection fractions (LVEF) between 50% and 65%.
- Calculated creatinine clearance or eGFR to estimate renal function.
- Pulmonary function tests
- Bone marrow aspirate and trephine +/− cytogenetics, dependent on disease and cytogenetics at diagnosis.
- Lumbar puncture +/− IT chemotherapy if acute lymphoblastic leukaemia or CNS disease/other clinical indication.
- CT/PET scan for lymphoma patients and other clinically indicated patient group.
- Double lumen central venous catheter.
- ECG – a 12-lead electrocardiograph.

Sufficient cell collections are required with a minimum PBSC (HPC-A) of 2×10^6/kg CD34[+] or BM (HPC-M) of 2.0×10^8/Kg MNC cells for infusion unless instructed otherwise by the transplant consultant for autologous transplantation and PBSC (HPC-A) of 4×10^6/kg CD34[+] or BM (HPC-M) of 4.0×10^8/Kg for donor harvested cell infusion. Donor cell collection results are not normally known prior to admission as the donor cells are not often cryopreserved and are coordinated a day prior to infusion (local policy may differ slightly), but clearance and agreement of the donor must be confirmed prior to patient admission.

4.8 Venous Access Devices: Principles of Placement and Care

Since the introduction of vascular access devices (VAD) in the seventeenth century and the first intravenous (IV) infusion procedures during the cholera epidemic in 1832 (Rivera et al. 2005), IV therapy is slowly developing towards a part of the treatment that all haematology patients will experience. In most countries infusion therapy is underestimated with a high incidence of complications. Although the positive effect of an infusion team is well proven (Brunelle 2003; Rutledge and Orr 2005), IV therapy still is a major burden for most patients. Health-care workers still miss the state-of-the-art knowledge and skills to make the right choice for the right patients and to use the VAD as it should. For venous access, we now have several VAD options to choose from. The most recent overview of VAD shows all options available now (Chopra et al. 2013) (Fig. 4.1).

In many centres the first option for vascular access is inserting a peripheral intravenous cannula (PIVC) for the initial IV therapy. If inserted by experienced health professionals in the right vein for the right indication, a PIVC is often the first VAD the patient is offered. Unfortunately PIVC's are still used for irritating infuses for as long as veins are accessible. Even small veins at the back of the hands, wrists and the ante cubital veins are used even if this is restricting the patient

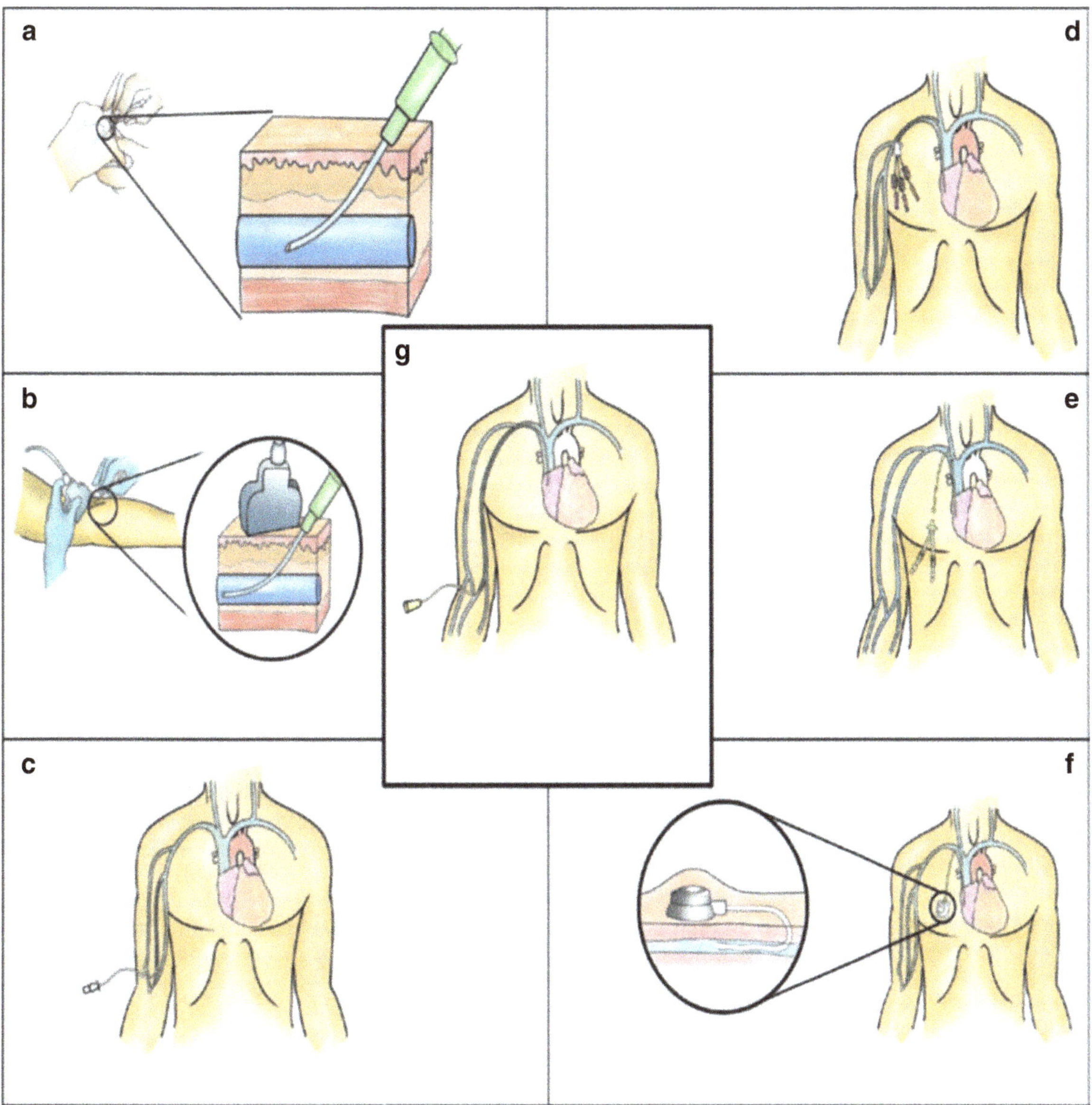

Fig. 4.1 Types of vascular access devices. (**a**) Peripheral IV catheter. (**b**) US-guided peripheral IV catheter. (**c**) Midline catheter, (**d**) Nontunneled central venous cathe-ter. (**e**) Tunneled central venous catheter. (**f**) Implanted port. (**g**) Peripherally inserted central catheter

in mobility of hands and arms and often causing chemical phlebitis. Once peripheral veins are no longer accessible with conventional techniques and several hospital 'experts' accessed the last veins, an alternative is found in a tunnelled sub-clavian or jugular central venous access device (CVAD), mainly the so-called Broviac and Hickman catheters, named after the inventors of these VADs. A venous access port (VAP) is hardly seen in haematology treatment. The more invasive procedure for subcutaneous implanta-tion of these VADs and the high risk during explanting of this type of VAD, these risks make the VAP in haematology not a real option.

During the EBMT congresses, the attention for vascular access is mainly limited to care and maintenance of CVADs in the annual nurses' group congress program. It is suggested that vas-cular access gets more attention in the EBMT program both for doctors and nurses and a multi-disciplinary approach should be chosen. Vascular access should not be limited to care and

Fig. 4.2 Algorithm intravenous access for non-acute treatment in adults, University Medical Center Utrecht, 2008

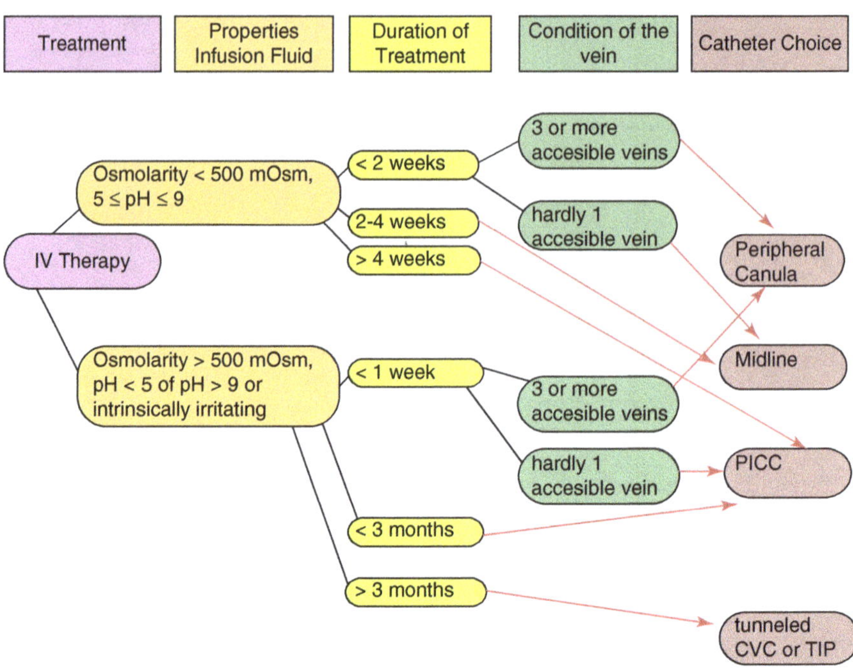

maintenance after insertion of the VAD but should be focused on wellbeing and patient safety. An algorithm for choosing the right VAD for the right patient should start with the diagnosis and treatment plan. The best VAD should be chosen based on the pH and osmolarity of the drugs used during the whole treatment period and the vein condition and should include the option for (partial) home infusion treatment. In 2008 a model was introduced for non-acute patients VAD choice in the UMC Utrecht, the Netherlands (Giesen et al. 2008) (Fig. 4.2).

Extensive expertise, best materials, equipment and skills are needed to offer state-of-the-art insertion of the preferred VAD. The *Infusion Therapy Standards of Practice* suggests establishing or maintaining an infusion team for peripheral and central venous access device (CVAD) insertion, management and removal (Gorski et al. 2016). This chapter will mainly focus on insertion and care for VADs used in haematology patients. Based on haematology patient characteristics, only the tunnelled CVAD such as centrally inserted central catheters (CICCs) and peripherally inserted central catheters (PICCs) will be addressed.

4.8.1 Vascular Access Devices

Access to the venous system is required for all haematology patients. Access can be limited to drawing blood for research and diagnostic purposes and/or for administration of fluids, drugs and blood components. For drawing blood by venipuncture, a steel needle is used that will be removed immediately after the blood samples are collected using a vacuum collecting system.

For IV therapy, there are two options that can be used. Option one is a PIVC (Fig. 4.1a): a short flexible catheter that ends in a peripheral vein with limited blood flow. As seen in Fig. 4.1, a PIVC should only be used for non-vesicant drugs with an osmolarity <600 mOsm/L for a short period of time. An alternative PIVC might be a midline catheter. This VAD is inserted in the upper arm and the tip lies in the cephalic, brachial or basilic vein.

Option two is a CVAD with the tip of the catheter ending in a central vein with high blood flow. The definition for all CVADs is that the distal tip ends in a large vein close to the heart, the superior vena cava (SVC) or inferior vena cava (IVC) for femoral catheters. In adults, both SVC and IVC have a blood flow up to 2–2.5 litre per minute and dilution of drugs happens so fast that the endothelium is not damaged.

Within the range of CVAD, a PICC (Fig. 4.1g) is seen more frequently in haematology patients, often as an alternative for a tunnelled CICC such as a Hickman catheter.

The insertion of a PICC is safe and non-invasive and can be performed even with low platelet counts. The PICC is first described in 1975 by Hoshal (1975) and has evolved to a VAD that can be the first option if central venous access in haematology patients is needed. A PICC can be used as an alternative to subclavian, internal jugular or femoral venous catheters. CICCs such as subclavian or internal jugular catheters may cause a pneumothorax, and femoral catheters are relatively more prone to infections. PICCs do not have these disadvantages.

A recent published algorithm in the MAGIC paper is based on latest evidence and supported by VA experts from many countries. This and other parts from this publication might also be helpful to use in your practice (Chopra et al. 2013) (Fig. 4.3).

Early studies show that a PICC is a safe and reliable option for central venous access (Maki et al. 2006; van Boxtel et al. 2008) (Table 4.1).

More recent results even come close to zero infections for PICCs if a bundle of preventive measures are taken (Harnage 2013). This bundle includes:

- Site selection
- Skin disinfection with 2% chlorhexidine in 70% gluconate
- Hand hygiene
- Maximum barrier precautions
- Daily control on indication
- Daily control on complications

Many clinicians still have the old-fashioned ideas that a PICC has a high incidence of infections and thrombosis, often based on their own

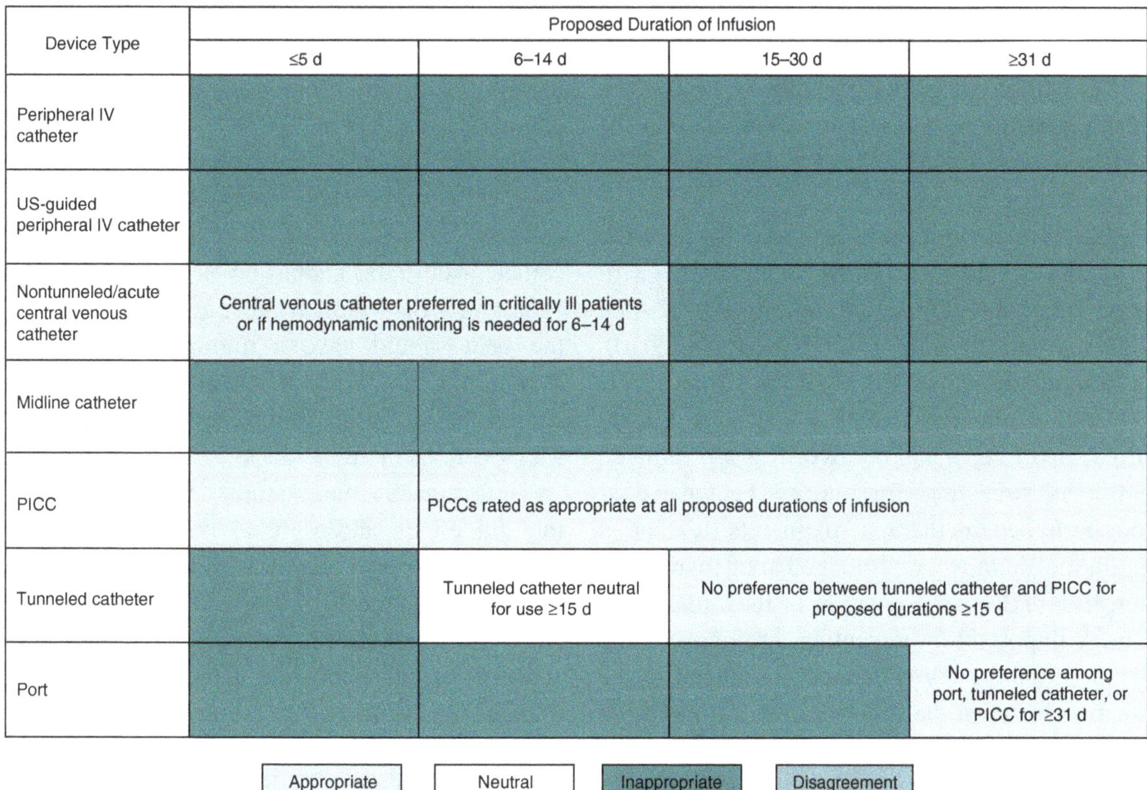

Device Type	Proposed Duration of Infusion			
	≤5 d	6–14 d	15–30 d	≥31 d
Peripheral IV catheter				
US-guided peripheral IV catheter				
Nontunneled/acute central venous catheter	Central venous catheter preferred in critically ill patients or if hemodynamic monitoring is needed for 6–14 d			
Midline catheter				
PICC		PICCs rated as appropriate at all proposed durations of infusion		
Tunneled catheter		Tunneled catheter neutral for use ≥15 d	No preference between tunneled catheter and PICC for proposed durations ≥15 d	
Port				No preference among port, tunneled catheter, or PICC for ≥31 d

Fig. 4.3 Venous access device recommendations for infusion of non-peripherally compatible infuses

Table 4.1 CRBSI in PICCs

	No. of catheters	Catheter days	No. of BSI	CRBSI per 100 devices	CRBSI per 1000 cath. days
UMC inpatient	418	13.258	11	2.63	0.82
UMC outpatient	92	4397	1	1.09	0.23
UMC in- and outpatient	510	17.655	12	2.35	0.68
Maki inpatient	625	7137	35	2.4	2.1
Maki outpatient	2813	98.702	15	3.5	1.0
Maki in- and outpatient	3566		112	3.1	1.1

Table 4.2 Blood flow reduction based on vein diameter versus catheter size

Vein	Initial flow	2 Fr		4 Fr		6 Fr		8 Fr	
Cephalic (4 mm)	10	5	48%	3	28%	1.5	14%	0.5	0.5%
Brachial (5 mm)	25	13	53%	9	36%	6	22%	9	12%
Basilic (6 mm)	52	29	56%	21	41%	15	28%	9	18%
Axillary (8 mm)	164	100	61%	79	48%	62	38%	47	28%
Subclavian (10 mm)	400	256	64%	212	53%	175	44%	143	36%

experience with drum catheters and the Intra Cath. Since the introduction of ultrasound-guided PICC insertion around 2004 and the introduction of ECG tip confirmation techniques, only well-designed studies, later than 2005, should be analysed and used for local policies on VAD selection and insertion.

The correct position of a CVAD tip is at the lower third of the SVC (Gorski et al. 2016), cavo-atrial junction (CAJ) or right atrium (RA) (Espen 2009), lower third SVC or RA (RCN 2010), cavo-atrial region or RA (SIR 2010) and SVC adjacent to the RA (ASPEN 2010). A CVAD (PICC and CICC) can be used over a prolonged period of time, e.g. for multiple, extensive or long-term chemotherapy regiments, extended antibiotic therapy or prolonged total parenteral nutrition (TPN). The position of the catheter tip is very important in preventing thromboses. The distal tip of the CVAD should be placed at the junction between the superior vena cava and the right atrium to have the lowest incidence of thrombosis (Debourdeau et al. 2009). In a study from Cadman, CVADs with the tip in a distal position (lower third of the SVC or right atrium) had a 2.6% thrombosis. CVADs with tips in a proximal position were 16 times more likely to thrombose than those with the tip in a distal position. None of the 58 CVADs with the tip located in the right atrium thrombosed or caused complications (Cadman et al. 2004).

Another important criterion to prevent thrombosis is the vein-catheter ratio when choosing the catheter size. Based on the Nifong study, the catheter-vein ratio should be at least 1 to 3. For example, for a 4 French catheter, the diameter of the vein should have a minimal diameter of 4 mm. For a 5 French catheter, the diameter should be at least 5 mm, etc. (Nifong and McDevitt 2011) (Table 4.2).

Unfortunately many studies used for preparing guidelines and/or local policies for VAD selection are based on poorly designed retrospective studies. At the 2016 World Congress Vascular Access (WoCoVA), Pittiruti presented a thorough analysis of all published papers on catheter-related thrombosis (CRT). Relevant criteria, such as vein-catheter ratio and tip position, are often not taken as outcome criteria. In the review by Pilker et al., the authors included at least five studies dealing with PICCs inserted without US in their analysis for PICC-related thrombosis.

One of the studies used the same size of PICCs regardless of the vein's diameter. Only three of the studies had declared diagnostic criteria used for thrombosis. No study was prospective and/or randomised (Pikwer et al. 2012). The 'meta-analysis' from Chopra included any type of clinical papers (retrospective, non-randomised, etc.) and even abstracts and papers published on non-peer-reviewed journals. At least 14 of the 64 studies reported are old-fashioned with PICCs inserted without micro-introducer and without ultrasound, at the ante cubital fossa (Chopra et al. 2013). Fallouh and colleagues in their paper have not conducted any systematic assessment of the studies; they just discuss some studies from the literature (Fallouh et al. 2015). The review by Zochios is carried out without any systematic methodology. It describes a few studies about PICC-related thrombosis. Moreover, most of the studies quoted in his review are affected by bias related to the insertion technique, to the type of device used (inappropriate calibre) and to the retrospective design (Zochios 2015) (Fig. 4.4).

In those recent studies on haematology patients with a PICC, the CRT rate varies between 0 and 5.8%. If studies are well analysed, it is still evident that the expected rate of CRT with PICCs is not really different from the expected rate of CRT with CICCs. If an insertion bundle like the GAVeCeLT (Gruppo Aperto di Studio 'Gli Accessi Venosi Centrali) bundle for CRT prevention is implemented, the best options to prevent CRT are given:

1. Proper choice of the vein
2. Minimal trauma during venipuncture
3. Appropriate tip location
4. Proper securement

Bellesi 2013 (hemato-BMT)	5	%
Mitrovic 2014 (hemato)	3.8	%
Martella 2015 (hemato)	0	%
Sriskanadarajah 2015 (hemato)	5.8	%
Morano 2015 (hemato)	2.6	%

Fig. 4.4 Thrombosis rates in haematology patients with a PICC

Before starting the actual insertion procedure, the selected vein should be well examined, and the diameter of the vein should be documented.

As for all VAD insertion techniques, materials and procedures and care and maintenance are very important. To offer high-quality IV treatment and improve patient safety and satisfaction, insertion and the use of VADs should be limited to well-trained and certified health-care providers. Vascular access should be a specialty based on clear criteria-certified training programs and state-of-the-art materials and procedures (Moreau et al. 2013).

Although the insertion protocol might be slightly different in each country, a state-of-the-art protocol should be available and executed only by VA experts.

4.8.2 Care and Maintenance

If a CVAD is placed in the correct vein and the tip of the catheter is right position, the VAD should function properly with the lowest rate of complications possible. The care professional using the catheter should be sure that the catheter is fully functional before any drugs are administered. One has to be sure about functionality in order to take responsibility for any infusion. A back flash of blood is a good parameter, but not always possible with a poor tip position or minor thrombus at the catheter tip, allowing infusion but no aspiration of blood. If this problem is occurring since the CVAD insertion, it is most likely that the catheter is too short. If occurring after some time and normal functioning in the beginning, it might be a 'little' thrombus at the catheter tip. An x-ray of the chest might be part of the assessment. A urokinase or alteplase instillation in the catheter will help to restore patency if a thrombus at the tip is preventing aspiration of blood. The weekly care of the catheter and insertion site is different for a well-healed tunnelled CVAD with a subcutaneous cuff. This Hickman-type CVAD does not need a dressing covering the insertion site (Gorski et al. 2016). A PICC and other non-tunnelled CVADs need weekly dressing change. If sterile gauze is used in case of skin irritation or allergy, dressing change is every 2 days.

4.8.3 Flushing and Locking

Optimal functioning of a CVAD should be possible by using a strict flushing and locking protocol. In most protocols for preventing occlusion in CVADs, a heparin solution is still used. In a recent study in Leuven, Belgium, a randomised trial concluded that normal saline is a safe and effective locking solution in implantable ports if combined with a strict protocol for device insertion and maintenance (Goossens et al. 2013). This conclusion supports the hypothesis that a catheter lumen will not occlude if materials such as a neutral or positive displacement needle-free connectors are used and the technique of flushing and locking does not allow blood or any drug to stick to the catheter wall. Preventing any adhesion to the catheter wall also reduces the biofilm and bacteremia.

4.8.4 Securement

Use of tape or sutures is not effective for securement or VAD stabilisation. Suturing should be avoided to prevent needle stick injuries and infections. There are different types of securement devices. Frequently used is an adhesive attaching the catheter to the skin covered with a semipermeable folio. These securement devices should be changed together with the weekly dressing change. If dressing change is not well performed, there is a major risk of pistoning of the catheter increasing the risk of insertion site infections. A recently introduced subcutaneous securement device, an anchoring device, holds the catheter in place and stays in situ during dwell time of the catheter. This device is easy to remove after removal of the catheter by folding the base or with a firm pull of each part after cutting the base in two. The nitinol anchor pieces will stretch and not damage the skin or cause any pain. As for all insertion and care protocols, training is required for inserting and removal.

4.8.5 Occlusion

The care professional using the catheter should be sure that the catheter is fully functional before any drugs are administered. One has to be sure about functionality in order to take responsibility for any infusion. A back flash of blood is a good parameter, but not always possible with a poor tip position or minor thrombus at the catheter tip, allowing infusion but no aspiration of blood. If this problem is occurring since the CVAD insertion, it is most likely that the catheter is too short and aspiration is blocked when the opening of the CVAD is sucked against the vein wall. An x-ray should be made to confirm the diagnoses. If partial occlusion (easy infusion, but no blood return) occurs right after taking blood samples form the catheter lumen, it is most likely that the lumen is blocked by hemolyses of blood in the catheter or it might be a 'little' thrombus at the catheter tip. An x-ray of the chest might be part of the assessment. A urokinase or alteplase instillation in the catheter will help to restore patency if a thrombus at the tip is preventing aspiration of blood. CVADs should be regularly assessed for patency and proper function as defined by the ability to flush the catheter without resistance and the ability to yield a blood return. If the VAD is occluded, restoration should be done after assessment of the origin of dysfunction. If blood return is not possible from right after insertion, it might be that the catheter is too short.

The use of a thrombolytic agent such as urokinase can be used to restore patency. A 10,000ie vial should be diluted in 2 ml saline solution. The estimated volume of the catheter lumen should be instilled and left for 30–60 min before aspirating the solution. Slow infusion of 10,000ie urokinase can also be performed. Using this protocol is only on doctor's order and dependent on the coagulation status of the patient.

For restoration of a totally blocked catheter lumen, a vacuum protocol can be used to restore patency. A three-way stopcock is placed directly at the blocked lumen. An empty 20 ml syringe is connected to one side. A 2 ml syringe with 10,000ie urokinase is connected to the other side. With the stopcock opened between the 2 ml syringe and the lumen, a firm vacuum is created. While vacuuming, the stopcock is switched to the urokinase catheter. Repeat this a second time. Leave this situation for 30–60 min and check patency. If not successful, this procedure may be repeated once. In most cases the patency will be restored when done properly. If not, it might still have an effect after a few hours. This procedure should only be performed after training and doctor's order. It prevents removal of the CVAD and is a safe, cost-effective and patient-friendly method. If the origin of the occlusion is an acidic drug precipitate (low pH, less than 6), use a 0.1 N hydrochloric acid solution for declotting. For alkaline drug precipitate (pH greater than 7), sodium bicarbonate 8.4% or sodium hydroxide 0.1 mmol/L should be used. If the occlusion is from a lipid residue, 70% ethanol in a sufficient volume should been used to fill the catheter lumen; for paediatric patients, a dose of 0.55 mL/kg has been used with no more than 3 mL maximum. Use ethanol with caution with polyurethane CVADs as ethanol may damage the catheter material; refer to vascular access device (VAD) manufacturers' directions for use regarding exposure to any form of alcohol (Gorski et al. 2016).

4.8.6 CVAD Removal

If the indication for the VAD is no longer there or if the VAD is source of unsolvable complications, removal is indicated. Depending on the type of CVAD, removal can be done in the operating suite, bedside or at the patients home.

A venous access port (VAP) removal can only be performed as a sterile surgical procedure, mainly done in the operating suite. Also being an invasive procedure is the removal of a tunnelled, cuffed CVAD. A PICC however, even if the PICC is tunnelled, can be removed at the bedside or outside the hospital. After removing the dressing and the adhesive securement device, the PICC can easily be removed by gently pulling the catheter. After removal and checking on complete removal, there will not be much blood spilling, but compression of the insertion site is needed to prevent air embolism. The insertion site is covered with a dressing of sterile gauze or folio. If there is too much resistance at removal, it might help to apply warmth and try again after 10 min. If still not possible to remove the catheter, a specialised colleague should be consulted. If sepsis is suspected, the 'sterile' tip of the CVAD should be collected and sent for culturing.

If a PICC is removed at the end of indication without problems, the same site might be used for future access through the same vein. Thorough assessment, including scanning the route of the catheter, should be performed prior to insertion of the CVAD.

4.8.7 Pre-transplant Disease Assessment

Diagnosis and prognosis are based on the morphological examination of the blood and bone marrow blasts, the immunophenotype and the cytogenetic and molecular study (Willekens 2013).

Remission can be defined as the disappearance of clinical signs (anaemia, infections, bleeding, gingival hypertrophy, hepatomegaly, cutaneous leukaemia, etc.), but correction of cytopenias and disappearance of medullary blasts with a normal/normalising maturation of the bone marrow function should be observed. Moreover, recent and sophisticated methods (flow cytometry, molecular biology) can make it possible to follow the 'minimal residual disease' (MRD).

Diagnosis and remission can be determined by one or more of the following:

- Haematological status: review of the blood and bone marrow would indicate percentage of normal/abnormal cell population.
- Cytogenetics: karyotype becomes normal – cytogenetic abnormalities disappear (sensitivity: 1/100).
- Molecular: molecular biology (minimal residual disease) – undetectable transcript (sensitivity: 1/10000 to 1/100000).
- Imaging: CT/PET scan, MRI scan.
- Blood and urine tests (myeloma).

4.9 The Advocacy Role of HSCT Nurses

Patient preparation for HSCT involves the use of chemotherapy and/or radiotherapy to eradicate the underlying disease of the patient. This initial step leads to immunosuppression in order to trigger aplasia of the bone marrow and thus prevent graft rejection (Ortega 2004).

Throughout the procedure, the patient needs special care to overcome the complications associated with treatment. Nurses must be aware of the possible complications in order to play a role in preventing or early detection of alarming signs, such as sepsis, fluid overload and organ dysfunction, taking appropriate measures to minimise adverse effects and restoring the clinical balance of the patient. This care is very complex and requires a high level of skill to be able to provide those (Ortega et al. 2009).

Specific technical care activities require nursing knowledge and specific skills in the field of haematopoietic stem cell transplantation such as instrument manipulation, knowledge of technologies and use of special protocols to effectively intervene in complex situations that deal with acute complications (Dallaire 1999, 2008).

Nurses as 'health care provider' (Loren et al 2013) should be part of the interdisciplinary team The treatment team should be knowledgeable about fertility preservation so that they can educate patients and families about available fertility preservation options. It is important to consider and discuss all available fertility options with patients at the time of diagnosis (Fernbach et al. 2014).

Health-care providers should be prepared to discuss the negative impact of cancer therapy on reproductive health with their patients in the same way as any other risks of cancer treatment are discussed (Rodriguez-Wallberg and Oktay 2014).

Nurses provide a key role in patient education, providing pre- and post-transplant advocacy and counselling, planning hospitalisations and consultations and responding to patients' telephone calls. They also act as educators and role models to nursing students where appropriate and share knowledge and skills in accordance with local policies and JACIE guidelines. The presence of dedicated nurse staff and psychologists in the counselling task force is a mandatory.

Educating or teaching helps establish a relationship in order to encourage the individual to make free and informed choices. The nature of the disease and the transplant itself require patients to learn about it in order to cope with the consequences of treatment and to be involved in decision-making processes. Counselling and providing education is mandatory at each stage of the pathway.

Nurses should be able to work within a team, communicating with both the nursing colleagues and doctors, ensuring excellent medical care of the patient giving useful and clear information to the whole team. They help to identify early symptoms and are aware of the treatments to administer and the side effects to monitor and to accurately inform the medical teams of any changes or concerns.

Whatever the department or place of practice, the nurse's missions and activities are diverse and varied. Our primary task is the realisation of care intended to maintain or restore the health of the person.

4.10 Ethical Dilemmas

Ethics involves the meaning of words such as right, wrong, good, bad, ought and duty on a basis where people either individually or collectively decide that actions are right or wrong and whether one ought to do something or has a right to do something (Rumbold 1993).

In 1994, Tschudin states ethical dilemmas have become a major part of nursing with the ever more holistic and patient-centred care. Nurses are often drawn into case discussions, and their views are considered and valued. Medical ethics must allow access to care for all, without discrimination of any kind. Medical confidentiality or patient freedom is part of the rules of medical ethics.

Constant advances in haematology have raised challenging ethical dilemmas concerning end of life, palliative care, patient information, donor concerns and impartiality and issues related to the risk we run to our patients.

In 2009, according to Langlois, ethical dilemmas often experienced by oncology and HCST nurses include:

- Therapeutic relentlessness – continuation of treatment, when the outcome is futile
- End-of-life intervention leading to death and euthanasia or cessation and withdrawal of treatment
- Transplantation in complex situation: refractory disease and older people

To cope with the therapeutic pathway of the patient, nurses must understand these complex situations. Regular staff meetings with a psychologist, palliative care unit and ethical committees and internal discussion in transplant ward will allow nurses to better understand this complex area by giving their nursing perspective to the team.

Ethical competencies in the transplant team allow us to solve new and unforeseen moral problems by knowing how to innovate in order to find the most legitimate and fairest behaviour possible in the face of a specific contextual situation.

The haematological pathway is often complex and uncertain. Treatments such as allogeneic HSCT can be associated with rapid changes in the care from curative to palliative (Howell 2010).

The resolution of an ethical dilemma for the nurse is related to the level of professional competence and understanding of the ethical concern allowing a better understanding of the context and of the complexity of the clinical situation. Ensuring that fully informed consent is provided by the patient is ethical dilemma which often occurs in medicine. Brykczynska (2000) identifies that the problem most often facing the haematology nurse regarding informed consent is not a lack of understanding as to what constitutes 'informed consent', or even how informed a patient needs to be for 'informed consent' to exist, but the vexed issue of conflict of interests.

Cancer invokes strong feelings and passions, and it is not infrequent to find a conflict of interest between members of the family, members of the health-care team and even members of the public as to whether to proceed with treatment or not. Emmanuel Kant's theory cited in Kemp Smith (1973) states that to act morally always treat other human beings as 'ends in themselves' and never merely as 'means'; by this Kant means that it is unethical to treat people as if they are objects. According to Kant it is fundamentally immoral to exploit a person without considering them an end in their own right. In transplantation where the side effects initially are extremely difficult and debilitating to the patient, it is sometimes difficult to justify such moral behaviour especially when nurses are striving not to inflict harm and to promote good.

What is often lacking, especially in nursing, is the courage and confidence to go through with a moral decision, which is basically an issue of personal moral development and personal integrity (Brykczynska 1997). It is the personal integrity of a particular nurse that will effect a change for the better or worse for an individual patient (Corner 1997).

4.11 Ethical Issues in Minors

Parents may act to preserve fertility of cancer patients who are minors if the child assents, and the intervention is likely to provide potential benefits to the child. Parents may act to preserve reproductive options of minor children undergoing gonadotoxic treatment as long as the minor assents, the intervention does not pose undue risk and the intervention offers a reasonable chance of net benefit to the child (Ethics Committee, ASRM).

When the child is immature, the decision to cryopreserve (or not) may be taken by the parents, unless it poses grave prejudice to the well-being/welfare of the child. The importance of preserving the possibility of having genetically related offspring in the future is generally recognised, and the parents will have to decide whether this benefit outweighs the current risk of intervention for their child.

Interdisciplinary consulting is mandatory; all specialties present in the caring team (oncologists, paediatricians, reproductive specialists, psychologists/counsellors) should be heard during decision-making about the best procedure. Experimental interventions in children can only be ethical if they can be considered to be therapeutic and in the best interests of the child. These considerations apply especially to development of techniques for prepubertal and peri-pubertal boys; although testicular tissue can be cryopreserved, how it should be used is not known at present (Anderson et al. 2015).

References

Agarwal SK, Chang RJ. Fertility management for women with cancer. Cancer Treat Res. 2007;138:15–27. Review. PMID:18080654

Anderson RA, Mitchell RT, Kelsey TW, Spears N, Telfer EE, Wallace HB. Cancer treatment and gonadal function: experimental and established strategies for fertility preservation in children and young adults. Lancet Diab Endocrinol. 2015;3(7):p556–67.

Anserini P, Chiodi S, Spinelli S, Costa M, Conte N, Copello F, et al. Semen analysis following allogeneic bone marrow transplantation. Additional data for evidence-based counselling. Bone Marrow Transplant. 2002;30:447–51.

Baker KS, Steffen L, Zhou X, Kelly A, Lee JM, Petryk A, Sinaiko AR, Dengel DR, Mulrooney DA, Steinberger J. Total body irradiation (TBI) increases cardio- metabolic risk and induces carotid vascular stiffness in survivors after hematopoietic cell transplant (HCT) for childhood hematologic malignancies. Blood. 2009;114(22):1291.

Bellesi S, Chiusolo P, De Pascale G, Pittiruti M, Scoppettuolo G, Metafuni E, Giammarco S, Sorà F, Laurenti L, Leone G, Sica S. Peripherally inserted central catheters (PICCs) in the management of onco-hematological patients. Support Care Cancer. 2013;21(2):531–5.

Borgmann-Staudt A, Rendtorff R, Reinmuth S, Hohmann C, Keil T, Schuster FR, et al. Fertility after allogeneic haematopoietic stem cell transplantation in childhood andadolescence. Bone Marrow Transplant. 2012;47(2):271–6.

Bourguignon LYW, Jy W, Majercik MH, Bourguignon GJ. Lymphocyte activation and capping of hormone receptors. J Cell Biochem. 1988;37:131–50. https://doi.org/10.1002/jcb.240370202.

van Boxtel AJH, Fliedner MC, Borst DM, Teunissen SCCM. Peripherally inserted central venous catheters: first results after the introduction in a Dutch university medical Center. J Vasc Access. 2008;13(3):128–33.

Brunelle D. Impact of a dedicated infusion therapy team on the reduction of catheter-related nosocomial infections. J Infus Nurs. 2003;26(6):362–6.

Brykczynska G 1997 Caring: the compassion and wisdom of nursing.

Brykczynska G. Cited in: nursing in haematological oncology, Grundy M. London: Balliere Tindall; 2000.

Cadman A, Lawrance JA, Fitzsimmons L, Spencer-Shaw A, Swindell R. To clot or not to clot? That is the question in central venous catheters. Clin Radiol. 2004;59(4):349–55.

Charlson ME, Pompel P, Ales K, MacKenzie CR. A new method of classifying prognostic co-morbidity in longitudinal studies; development and validation. J Chronic Dis. 1987;40(5):373–83.

Chemaitilly W, Sklar CA. Endocrine complications in long-term survivors of childhood cancers. Endocr Relat Cancer. 2010;17:R141–59.

Chopra V, Anand S, Hickner A, Buist M, Rogers MA, Saint S, Flanders SA. Risk of venous thromboembolism associated with peripherally inserted central catheters: a systematic review and meta-analysis. Lancet. 2013;382:311–25.

Clayman ML, Galvin KM, Arntson P. Shared decision making: fertility and pediatric cancers. Cancer Treat Res. 2007;138:149–60. Review. No abstract available. PMID: 18080663

Cooke L, Chung C, Grant M. Psychosocial care for adolescent and young adult hematopoietic cell transplant patients. J Psychosoc Oncol. 2011;29(4):394–414. PubMed PMID: 21966725; PubMed Central PMCID: PMC3268701

Corner J 1997 The passion of family-focused palliative care using the delphi technique.

Cotogni P, Barbero C, Garrino C, Degiorgis C, Mussa B, De Francesco A, Pittiruti M. Peripherally inserted central catheters in non-hospitalized cancer patients: 5-year results of a prospective study. Support Care Cancer. 2015;23:403–9.

Crawshaw M, Sloper P. A qualitative study of the experiences of teenagers and young adults when faced with possible or actual fertility impairment following cancer treatment. 2006. Available at: http://www.york.ac.uk/inst/spru/pubs/pdf/fertility.pdf. Accessed 28 Dec 2006.

Dallaire C. Les grandes fonctions de la pratique infirmière. In: Soins infirmiers et société. Québec: Gaëtan Morin Éditeur. p. 1999.

Dallaire C, Dallaire M. Le savoir infirmier dans les fonctions infirmières. In: Le savoir infirmier : au cœur de la discipline et de la profession; 2008.

Dalle JH, Lucchini G, Balduzzi A, Ifversen M, Jahnukainen K, Macklon KT, Ahler A, Jarisch A, Ansari M, Beohou E, Bresters D, Corbacioglu S, Dalissier A, Diaz de Heredia Rubio C, Diesch T, Gibson B, Klingebiel T, Lankester A, Lawitschka A, Moffat R, Peters C, Poirot C, Saenger N, Sedlacek P, Trigoso E, Vettenranta K, Wachowiak J, Willasch A, von Wolff M, Yaniv I, Yesilipek A, Bader P. State-of-the-art fertility preservation in children and adolescents undergoing haematopoietic stem cell transplantation: a report on the expert meeting of the Paediatric Diseases Working Party (PDWP) of the European Society for Blood and Marrow Transplantation (EBMT) in Baden, Austria, 29–30 September 2015. Bone Marrow Transplant. 2017;52(7):1029–35. https://doi.org/10.1038/bmt.2017.21. Epub 2017 Mar 13

Debourdeau P, Kassab Chahmi D, Le Gal G, Kriegel I, Desruennes E, Douard MC, Elalamy I, Meyer G, Mismetti P, Pavic M, Scrobohaci ML, Lévesque H, Renaudin JM, Farge D, Working group of the SOR; French National Feberation of Cancer Centers. SOR guidelines for the prevention and treatment of thrombosis associated with central venous catheters in patients with cancer: report from the working group. Ann Oncol. 2009;20(9):1459–71.

Diesch T, von der Weid NX, Szinnai G, Schaedelin S, De Geyter C, Rovó A, on behalf of the Swiss Pediatric Oncology Group SPOG. Fertility preservation in pediatric and adolescent cancer patients in switzerland: a qualitative cross-sectional survey. Cancer Epidemiol Int J Cancer Epidemiol Detect Prev. 2016;44:141–6.

Dilley KJ. Managing fertility in childhood cancer patients. Cancer Treat Res. 2007;138:50–6. PMID: 18080656

Dvorak CC, Gracia CR, Sanders JE, Cheng EY, Baker KS, Pulsipher MA, Petryk A. NCI, NHLBI/PBMTC fi rst international conference on late effects after pediatric hematopoietic cell transplantation: endocrine challenges-thyroid dysfunction, growth impairment, bone health, & reproductive risks. Biol Blood Marrow Transplant. 2011;17(12):1725–38. https://doi.org/10.1016/j.bbmt.2011.10.006. S1083–8791(11)00409–5 [pii]

Ethics Committee of American Society for Reproductive Medicine. Fertility preservation and reproduction in patients facing gonadotoxic therapies: a committee opinion. Fertil Steril. 2013;100(5):1224–31.

Ethics Committee of the American Society for Reproductive Medicine: Fertility and Sterility® Vol. 100, No. 5, November 2013 0015–0282/$36.00 Copyright © 2013 American Society for Reproductive Medicine, Published by Elsevier Inc.

European Association for Children in Hospital, 2016-last update, EACH Charter & Annotations. Available: https://www.each-for-sick-children.org/each-charter/introduction-each-charter-annotations.html [10/13, 2016].

Fallat ME, Hutter J, The Committee on Bioethics, Section on Hematology/Oncology, and Section on Surgery. Preservation of fertility in pediatric and adolescent patients with cancer: American Academy of Pediatric; 2008.

Fallouh N, McGuirk HM, Flanders SA, Chopra V. Peripherally inserted central catheter-associated deep vein thrombosis: a narrative review. Am J Med. 2015;128:722–38.

Fernbach MSN, Fernbach A, Lockart B, Armus CL, LM B, Levine J, Kroon L, Sylvain G, Rodgers C. Evidence-based recommendations for fertility preservation options for inclusion in treatment protocols for pediatric and adolescent patients diagnosed with cancer. J Pediatr Oncol Nursing. 2014;31:211–22. first published on May 5, 2014

Flink DM, Sheeder J, Kondapalli LA. A review of the oncology patient's challenges for utilizing fertility preservation services. J Adolesc Young Adult Oncol. 2017;6:31–44.

Galán S, de la Vega R, Miró J. Needs of adolescents and young adults after cancer treatment: a systematic review. Eur J Cancer Care. 2016.

Gameiro S, et al. ESHRE guideline: routine psychosocial care in infertility and medically assisted reproduction — a guide for fertility staff. Hum Reprod. 2015:1–11.

Giesen MAM, Boxtel AJH, et al. (2008) Keuze intraveneuze toegangsweg voor niet acute behandeling bij volwassenen University Medical Centrum Utrecht (unpublished).

Goossens GA, Jérôme M, Janssens C, Peetermans WE, Fieuws S, Moons P, Verschakelen J, Peerlinck K, Jacquemin M, Stas M. Comparing normal saline versus diluted heparin to lock non-valved totally implantable venous access devices in cancer patients: a randomised, non-inferiority, open trial. Ann Oncol. 2013;24(7):1892–9.

Gorski L, Hadaway L, et al. Infusion therapy standards of practice. J Infus Nurs. 2016;39:1S.

Harnage S. Seven years of zero central-line- associated bloodstream infections. Br J Nurs. 2013;21(21):S6. (IV Therapy Supplement)

Hoshal VL. Total intravenous nutrition with peripherally inserted silicone elastomer central venous catheters. Arch Surg. 1975;110(5):644–6.

Howell DA. 2010 BMC palliative care.

Jacob A, Barker H, Goodman A, Holmes J. Recovery of spermatogenesis following bone marrow transplantation. Bone Marrow Transplant. 1998;22:277–9.

Jakes AD, Marec-Berard P, Phillips RS, Stark DP. Critical review of clinical practice guidelines for fertility preservation in teenagers and young adults with cancer. J Adolesc Young Adult Oncol. 2014;3(4):144–52.

Johnston AJ, Streater CT, Noorani R, Crofts JL, Del Mundo AB, Parker RA. The effect of peripherally inserted central catheter (PICC) valve technology on catheter occlusion rates: the 'ELeCTRiC' study. J Vasc Access. 2012;13(4):421–5.

Kant I. Critique of pure reason. In: Kemp Smith N, editor. Immanuel Kant's critique of pure reason. London: Macmillian; 1973.

Kari B, Levine DR. (2016). Fertility preservation and ethical issues in pediatric oncology patients. Retrieved Sep 16, 2016, from https://www.cure4kids.org/ums/home/seminars/seminars_list/seminar_detail/?ppts_id=3399.

Karnofsky DA, Abelmann WH, Craver LF, Burchenal JH. The use of the nitrogen mustards in the palliative treatment of carcinoma - with particular reference to bronchogenic carcinoma. Cancer. 1948;1(4):634–56.

Katz SL, Webb SA, Bioethics Committee. Informed consent in decision-making in pediatric practice. Pediatrics. 2016;138(2)

Lansky SB, List MA, Lansky LL, Ritter-Sterr C, Miller DR. The measurement of performance in childhood cancer patients. Cancer. 1987;60(7):1651–6.

Leader A, Lishner M, Michaeli J, Revel A. Fertility considerations and preservation in haemato-oncology patients undergoing treatment. Br J Haematol. 2011;153(3):291–308.

Loren AW, Mangu PB, Beck LN, Brennan L, Magdalinski AJ, Partridge AH, Quinn G, Wallace WH, Oktay K. Fertility preservation for patients with cancer: American Society of Clinical Oncology clinical practice guideline update. J Clin Oncol. 2013;31(19):2500–10. https://doi.org/10.1200/JCO.2013.49.2678. Epub 2013 May 28. Review. PMID: 23715580

Majhail NS, Rizzo JD, Lee SJ, Aljurf M, Atsuta Y, Bonfim C, Burns LJ, Chaudhri N, Davies S, Okamoto S, Seber A, Socie G, Szer J, Van Lint MT, Wingard JR, Tichelli A, Center for International Blood and Marrow Transplant Research, American Society for Blood and Marrow Transplantation, European Group for Blood and Marrow Transplantation, Asia-Pacific Blood and Marrow Transplantation Group, Bone Marrow Transplant Society of Australia and New Zealand, et al. Recommended screening and preventive practices for long-term survivors after hematopoietic cell transplantation. Bone Marrow Transplant. 2012;47(3):337–41.

Maki DG, Kluger DM, Crnich CJ. The risk of bloodstream infection in adults with different intravascular devices: a systematic review of 200 published prospective studies. Mayo Clin Proc. 2006;81:1159–71.

Martella F, Salutari V, Marchetti C, Pisano C, Di Napoli M, Pietta F, Centineo D, Caringella AM, Musella A, Fioretto L. (2015) a retrospective analysis of trabectedin infusion by peripherally inserted central venous catheters: a multicentric Italian experience. Anti-Cancer Drugs. 2015;26(9):990–4.

Mitrović Z, Komljenović I, Jaksic O, Prka Z, Crnek SS, Stojsavljević RA, Pirsic M, Haris V, Kusec R, Dautovic D, Pejsa V. The use of peripherally inserted central catheter (PICC) in patients with hematological malignancies – a single center experience. Lijec Vjesn. 2014;136(5–6):136–40.

Moureau N, Lamperti M, Kelly LJ, Dawson R, Elbarbary M, van Boxtel AJH, Pittiruti M. Evidence-based consensus on the insertion of central venous access devices: definition of minimal requirements for training. Br J Anaesth. 2013:1–10.

Müller J, Sønksen J, Sommer P, Schmiegelow M, Petersen PM, Heilman C, et al. Cryopreservation of semen from pubertal boys with cancer. Med Pediatr Oncol. 2000;34(3):191–4.

Nahata L, Cohen LE, Richard NY. Barriers to fertility preservation in male adolescents with cancer: It's time for a multidisciplinary approach that includes urologists. Urology. 2012;79(6):1206–9.

Nifong TP, McDevitt TJ. The effect of catheter to vein ratio on blood flow rates in a simulated model of peripherally inserted central catheters. Chest. 2011;140(1):48–53.

Nobel Murray A, Chrisler JC, Robbins ML. Adolescents and young adults with cancer: oncology nurses report attitudes and barriers to discussing fertility preservation. Clin J Oncol Nurs. 2015;20(4): E93–9.

Ortega ETT, et al. Compêndio de enfermagem em transplante de células-tronco hematopoéticas : rotinas e procedimentos em cuidados essenciais e em complicações. Curitiba: Maio; 2004.

Ortega ETT, et al. Assistência de enfermagem em transplante de células-tronco hematopoéticas. In: Transplante de células-tronco hematopoéticas. São Paulo. p. 2009.

Patient Information Forum. Making a case for nformation. www.pifonline.org.uk. 2010.

Pikwer A, Åkeson J, Lindgren S. Complications associated with peripheral or central routes for central venous cannulation. Anaesthesia. 2012;67:65–71.

Recommendations on Fertility preservation for boys and young men with childhood cancer. Nordic network for gonadal preservation after cancer treatment in children and young adults, finalized March 2011, revised Feb 2015.

Recommendations on Fertility preservation for girls and young women with childhood cancer. Nordic network for gonadal preservation after cancer treatment in children and young adults, finalized May 2012, revised Feb 2015.

Rivera AM, Strauss KW, van Zundert A, Mortier E. The history of peripheral intravenous catheters: how little plastic tubes revolutionized medicine. Acta Anaesthesiol Belg. 2005;56(3):271–82.

Rodriguez-Wallberg KA, Oktay K. Fertility preservation during cancer treatment: clinical guidelines. Cancer Manag Res. 2014;6:105–17.

Rumbold G. Ethics in nursing practice. 2nd ed. London: Balliere Tindall; 1993.

Rutledge D, Orr M. Effectiveness of intravenous therapy teams. J Clin Innovat. 2005;8(2):1–24.

Sanders JE, Woolfrey AE, Carpenter PA, Storer BE, Hoffmeister PA, Deeg HJ, Flowers ME, Storb RF. Late effects among pediatric patients followed for nearly 4 decades after transplantation for severe aplastic anemia. Blood. 2011;118(5):1421–8.

Schmidt KT, Larsen EC, Andersen CY, Andersena AN. Risk of ovarian failure and fertility preserving methods in girls and adolescents with a malignant disease. BJOG. 2010;117:163–74.

Sklar C, Boulad F, Small T, Kernan N. Endocrine complications of pediatric stem cell transplantation. FrontBiosci. 2001;6:G17–22.

Smith FO, Reaman GH, Racadio JM, et al. Hematopoietic cell transplantation in children with cancer, pediatric oncology. Berlin Heidelberg: Springer-Verlag; 2014. https://doi.org/10.1007/978-3-642-39920-6_7.

Sorror M, Maris M, Storb R, Baron F, Sandmaier B, Maloney D, Storer B. Hematopoitic cell transplantation (HCT) – specific cormobidity index: a new tool for risk assessment before allogeneic HCT. Blood. 2005;106(8):2912–9.

Sriskandarajah P, Webb K, Chisholm D, Raobaikady R, Davis K, Pepper N, Ethell ME, Potter MN, Shaw BE, Thromb J. Retrospective cohort analysis comparing the incidence of deep vein thromboses between peripherally-inserted and long-term skin tunneled venous catheters in hemato-oncology patients. Thromb J. 2015;13:21.

Suhag V, Sunita BS, Sarin A, Singh AK, Dashottar S. Fertility preservation in young patients with cancer. South Asian J Cancer. 2015;4(3):134–9.

Tal R, Botchan A, Hauser R, Yogev L, Paz G, Yavetz H. Follow-up of sperm concentration and motility in patients with lymphoma. Hum Reprod. 2000;15:1985–8.

The ESHRE Task Force on Ethics and Law. Taskforce 7: ethical considerations for the cryopreservation of gametes and reproductive tissues for self-use. Hum Reprod. 2004;19(2):460–2.

Tomlinson D, Kline NE. In: Tomlinson D, Kline NE, editors. Pediatric oncology nursing advanced clinical handbook. Berlin/Heidelberg: Springer; 2005.

Tschudin V. Deciding ethically: a practical approach to nursing challenges. London: Balliere Tindall; 1994.

Viviani S, Bonfante V, Santoro A, Zanini M, Devizzi L, Di Russo AD, et al. Long-term results of an intensive regimen: VEBEP plus involved-field radiotherapy in advanced Hodgkin's disease. Cancer J Sci Am. 1999;5:275–82.

Wallace WHB, Anderson RA, Irvine DS. Fertility preservation for young patients with cancer: who is at risk and what can be offered? Lancet Oncol. 2005;6(4):209–18.

Wallace WH, Smith AG, Kelsey TW, Edgar AE, Anderson RA. Fertility preservation for girls and young women with cancer: population-based validation of criteria for ovarian tissue cryopreservation. Lancet Oncol. 2014;15(10):1129–36.

Wooddruf TK, Sneider KA. In: Wooddruf TK, Sneider KA, editors. Oncofertility fertility preservation for cancer survivors. New York: Springer; 2007.

Zebrack B, Bleyer A, Albritton K, Medearis S, Tang J. Assessing the health care needs of adolescent and young adult cancer patients and survivors. Cancer. 2006;107:2915–23. https://doi.org/10.1002/cncr.22338.

Cell Source and Apheresis

5

Aleksandra Babic and Eugenia Trigoso

Abstract

Peripheral blood stem cells have largely replaced harvested bone marrow stem cells both in the autologous and allogeneic settings. Advantages of peripherally harvested cells include higher stem cell dose, more rapid engraftment, reduced donor/patient discomfort, and better graft-versus-leukemia effect in the allogeneic setting. Within the apheresis machine, whole blood is separated into its components by centrifugation, and the red cell-depleted, stem cell-rich buffy coat is extracted for use as a stem cell product, simultaneously returning the other blood components back to the donor. Prediction of procedure length is based on the required cell dose target but still remains challenging. Moreover, the number of apheresis procedures needed should be as few as possible in order to reduce costs and patient/donor discomfort and to increase safety. The volume of blood which needs to be processed in order to collect an adequate number of stem cells depends on several factors such as method of stem cell mobilization, vascular access, and collection efficiency.

Another issue to take into consideration is cell storage: according to GITMO's study (Perseghin et al. 2014) in most Italian centers, even up to 83.4% correspond to useless storage and only the remaining 16.6% to useful storage. Therefore, SIdEM and GITMO proposed a policy for autologous HPC disposal that fulfills clinical, ethical, and economic criteria.

A. Babic (✉)
Istituto Oncologico della Svizzera Italiana,
Bellinzona, Switzerland
e-mail: aleksandra.babic@eoc.ch

E. Trigoso
Paediatric Transplant Unit, Hospital Universitario y
Politécnico LA FE, Valencia, Spain

© EBMT and the Author(s) 2018
M. Kenyon, A. Babic (eds.), *The European Blood and Marrow Transplantation Textbook for Nurses*,
https://doi.org/10.1007/978-3-319-50026-3_5

JACIE standards on peripheral blood stem cell (PBSC) collection by apheresis require that collection, manipulation, and clinical use of peripheral blood stem cells must be validated and monitored rigorously. The validation procedure consists of systematic review of all apheresis procedures performed at the collection facility of a transplant program.

Keywords

Stem cell source • Peripheral stem cell mobilization • SC mobilization and apheresis • Vascular access • Quality and apheresis

5.1 Cell Source: Where Do We Get the Cells From?

Hematopoiesis refers to the production of all types of blood cells including formation, development, and differentiation of blood cells. In adults, hematopoiesis primarily occurs in bone marrow contained in the pelvis, sternum, vertebral column, and skull. All blood cells are derived from progenitor stem cells – pluripotent stem cells. These cells have the capacity for unlimited self-renewal and the ability to differentiate into all types of mature blood cells starting from the common myeloid or the common lymphoid progenitor (Fig. 5.1). This process occurs continually in order to maintain adequate concentrations of circulating components necessary for normal immune system function and hemostasis.

Cells in the myeloid lineage, such as red blood cells, platelets, and white blood cells, are responsible for hemopoiesis (tissue nourishment, oxygenation, coagulation) and immune function such as innate and adaptive immunity. The lymphoid lineage components, namely, T cells and B cells, provide the foundation for the adaptive immune system.

Hematopoietic stem cell (HSC) products for autologous or allogeneic transplantation are available from bone marrow, peripheral blood, and umbilical cord blood (UCB) sources. Bone marrow was the original source of cells for transplantation because of the easier process of collection. UCB has been found and established to have an important role in treatment due to relative immunologic naiveté of the donor with the feasibility of multiple antigen-mismatched transplantations where there is a lack of related or unrelated volunteer donor. UCB had limited use in adult transplantation because of the small cell dose collected which may result in greater risk of post-transplant opportunistic infection due to a longer time to hematologic recovery and a higher risk of primary engraftment failure. However, the use of "double cords" has to a certain extent ameliorated some of the difficulties by improving engraftment times. Nevertheless, late infections remain a concern, and lack of available donor lymphocytes means that other products are often favored over UCB in some settings.

Peripheral blood stem cells (PBSC) have largely replaced the bone marrow in both autologous and allogeneic transplantation setting. The rapid engraftment kinetics of PBSC compared to the bone marrow is widely recognized. Median times to achieve an absolute neutrophil count greater than 500/ul after autologous PBSC transplantation are approximately 11–14 days in autologous setting (Klaus 2007).

In allogeneic settings the choice of HSC product source for transplantation may depend on donor availability. The appropriate donor selection, quality control, and risk assessment are paramount not only for patient and donor safety but also impact on transplant outcome. In the absence of a sibling HLA-identical donor, the search and identification of an unrelated donor may take up to 5 months. Depending on recipients underlying disease and "urgency" for HSCT, haploidentical donors or cord blood unit(s) might be selected (Ruggeri et al. 2015).

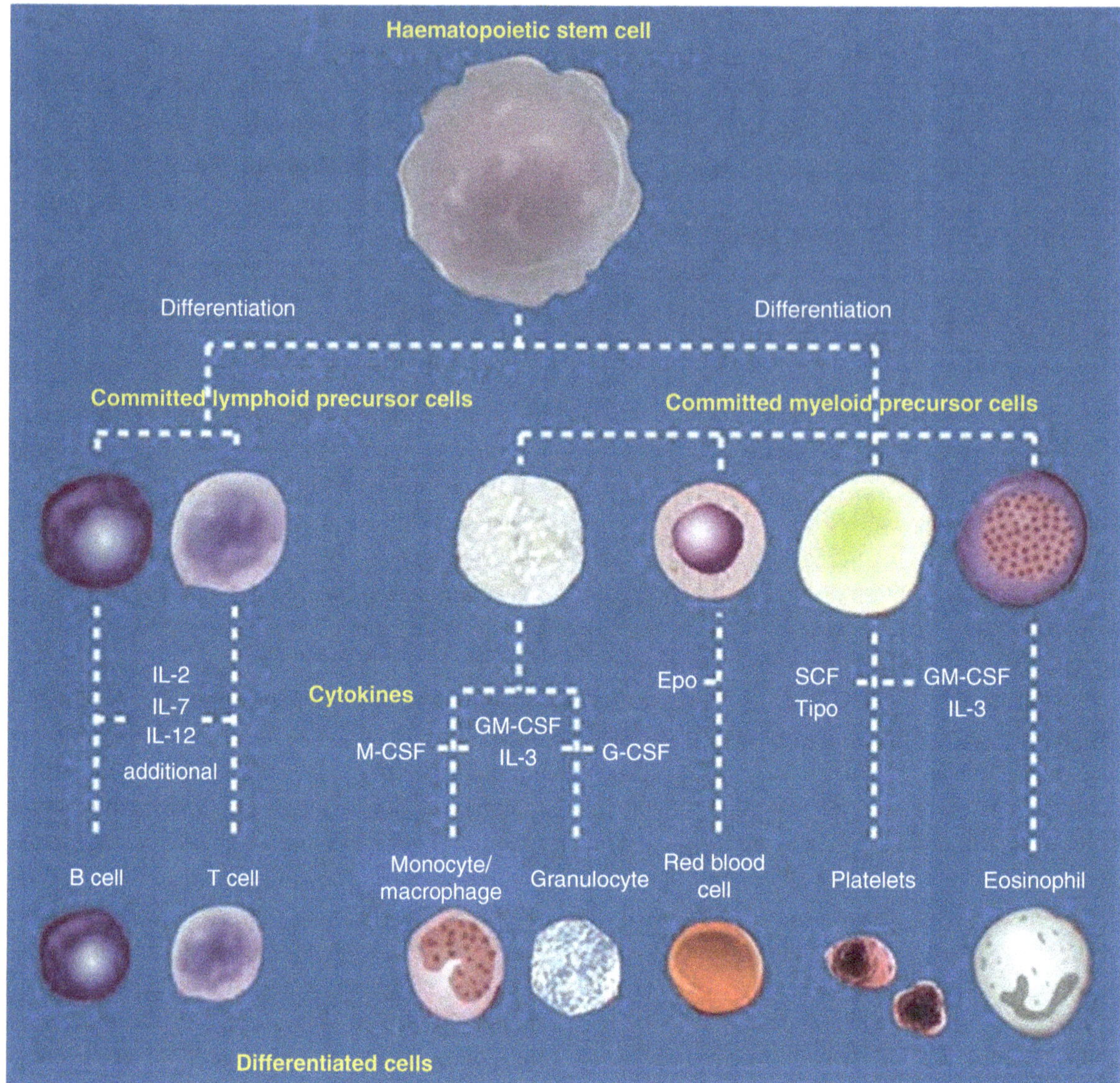

Fig. 5.1 Stem cell maturation cascade (Adapted from EBMT NG (2009)) (*Epo* erythroprotein, *G-CSF* granulocyte colony-stimulating factor, *GM-CSF* granulocyte-macrophage colony-stimulating factor, *IL* interleukin, *M-CSF* macrophage colony-stimulating factor, *SCF* Stem cell factor, *Tpo* thrombopoietin)

Nurses who assist patients during the donation procedure should be particularly aware of factors that influence risk for donation which include:

- Age
- Gender
- Low weight
- Duration of procedure
- Type of anesthesia (BM donation)
- CD34+ cell dose requested
- Vascular access (PBSC)

5.1.1 Cell Collection

- *Bone Marrow Collection*
  The bone marrow is harvested from the posterior iliac crest region under general or regional anesthesia in a hospital operating room. For the healthy donor, the risk of serious complication from either general or local anesthesia is similar (Hoffman et al. 2008). With adequate fluid and sometimes blood replacement, overnight hospitalization is often not required.

Multiple aspirations are performed with collection of approximately 5 ml of liquid marrow blood from each puncture site. The usual volume harvested from healthy donors is approximately 10–15 ml of marrow per kilogram of recipient body weight in order to achieve the desired CD34+ cell doses. This results in an average blood loss of 800–1000 ml for an adult donor. Some patients and donors receive pre-donated blood transfusions to alleviate symptoms of volume depletion usually with preharvested autologous blood, but salt or colloid solutions are acceptable replacements too. Anesthesia and blood loss present the greatest risk of serious complications associated with bone marrow harvesting, and therefore patients and marrow donors must undergo a detailed medical examination including questionnaire of health history. After confirming they wish to proceed to be a donor, they are asked to sign the written consent to undergo donation.

- *Peripheral Blood Stem Cells (PBSC)*
  The concentrations of hematopoietic stem cells (HSC) in the peripheral blood are normally very low compared to 10–100 times greater concentration in the bone marrow (EBMT NG 2009). Therefore it is necessary to increase the circulating concentrations of HSC for adequate PBSC collections. HSC mobilization into the peripheral blood can be stimulated by different disease-related and relatively predictable mobilization regimens. Rapid and widespread adoption of PBSC as a source of HSC for transplantation is due to rapidly available results of CD34+ count by the laboratory. Before commencing a leukapheresis, we count the number of CD34+ cells in peripheral blood, and if the number is adequate, the collection procedure may be performed.

- *Cord Blood Collection*
  UCB is collected from the placental vein after infant delivery and transection of the cord. UCB can be collected either by the obstetrician before delivery of the placenta or by laboratory personnel after delivery of the placenta. The timing of cord clamping after delivery of the infant is associated with the

volume of cord blood collected with earlier clamping relating to greater collection volumes. Cell dose is an important predictor of outcome after UCB transplantation, and many cord blood units are discarded because of small cell doses. Greater cell quantities are found for infants with greater birth weight, independent of gender and gestational age. Many cord blood banks reduce the volume of the product by depleting red cells and plasma in order to minimize storage space and reduce possible infusion-related toxicities from mature blood cells contained in unfractioned cord blood units. UCB will maintain viability for period of at least 15 years if appropriately cryopreserved (Hoffman et al. 2008; Schoemans et al. 2006). Allogeneic transplant access can be severely limited for patients of racial and ethnic minorities without suitable sibling donors. Whether umbilical cord blood (UCB) transplantation can extend transplant access because of the reduced stringency of required HLA match is not proven.

Patients had highly diverse ancestries including 35% non-Europeans. In Barker's article from 2010 (Barker n.d.), of 525 patients undergoing combined searches, 10/10 HLA-matched URDs were identified in 53% of those with European ancestry but only 21% of patients with non-European origins. However, the majority of both groups had 5–6/6 UCB units. Availability of UCB significantly extends allotransplant access, especially in non-European patients, and has the greatest potential to provide a suitable stem cell source regardless of race or ethnicity. Minority patients in need of allografts, but without suitable matched sibling donors, should be referred for combined URD and CB searches to optimize transplant access.

5.2 Mobilization of Stem Cells and Apheresis

Administration of hematopoietic cytokines, such as granulocyte colony-stimulating factor (G-CSF), causes a transient increase (mobilization) of HSC in the peripheral bloodstream and enables the collection of adequate numbers of PBSC for transplantation.

Pluripotent stem cells express the cell surface marker antigen CD34 (CD34+ cells). Cytokine-mobilized PBSC components contain much greater numbers of cells expressing the CD34 antigen which then acts as a surrogate marker for the engraftment capacity of the stem cell component.

5.2.1 Cytokines

Several cytokines have been identified to play an important role in hematopoiesis. When progenitor cells are exposed to these cytokines, the maturation cascade producing committed mature blood cell components can occur. Examples of important cytokines are listed in Fig. 5.1. These cytokines are externally administered to patients in an effort to enhance the yield of stem cells within a short time period. An example of such a cytokine is glycosylated granulocyte colony-stimulating factor (G-CSF).

Chemokines are a subset of cytokines and can induce activation and migration of specific types of white cell and assist the process of stem cells homing to the marrow compartment. Stem cell CXCR4 is responsible for anchoring stem cells to the marrow matrix through interactions with adhesion molecules such as stem cell-derived factor-1 alpha (SDF-1α). Blockade of this receptor with a receptor antagonist such as plerixafor has produced elevations of circulating hematopoietic progenitor cells, which has aided stem cell collections in patients with multiple myeloma and lymphoma "poor mobilizers," those not able to reach the sufficient number of CD34+ cells for commencing a leukapheresis.

Because of its efficacy compared to other cytokines and its low toxicity profile, G-CSF is the cytokine most commonly used to increase the level of myeloid progenitor cells in the blood.

Recombinant methionyl human G-CSF (filgrastim) and recombinant human G-CSF (leno-grastim) are the two forms of this cytokine available for clinical use.

In clinical practice, for autologous PBSC, the most frequent mobilization procedure is the administration of filgrastim in combination with chemotherapy. Nowadays we are observing increased use of mobilization regimens without chemotherapy (chemo-free mobilization regimens) in patients affected by multiple myeloma (Afifi et al. 2016).

5.2.2 The Role of CD34+

CD34+ is the indicator most frequently used in clinical practice to determine the extent and efficiency of peripheral blood stem cell collections (Brando et al. 2000). Once specific cell dose targets are achieved, cell collections are completed and stored for future use. Standard target levels can vary among treating centers, and a patient's specific goal is based on the underlying disease, the source of stem cells, and the type of transplant to be performed. In general, a target level of 2×10^6 CD34+ cells/kg recipient body weight is considered the minimum for transplant with optimal levels being $> 5 \times 10^6$ CD34+ cells/kg for a single transplant and $> 6 \times 10^6$ CD34+ cells/kg for a tandem transplant (Pierelli et al. 2012).

Peripheral blood stem cell is considered the preferred cell source due to patient convenience, decreased morbidity, and faster engraftment of white blood cells and platelets (Table 5.1).

Poor stem cell yields after mobilization might occur. The most important risk factor for inadequate mobilization is the amount of myelosuppressive chemotherapy a patient has received prior to their autologous collection. Agents which are toxic to stem cells such as cyclophosphamide (doses > 7.5 g), melphalan, carmustine, procarbazine, fludarabine, nitrogen mustard, and chlorambucil are particularly detrimental to stem cell collection yields. Other risk factors associated with low CD34+ cell collections include advanced age (> 60 years), previous radiation therapy, short time interval between chemotherapy and mobilization, extensive disease burden, and tumor infiltration of the bone marrow (Olivieri et al. 2012).

Table 5.1 A comparison between mobilization methods

Mobilization regimen	Characteristics
Filgrastim	Low toxicity
	Outpatient administration
	High efficacy in most patients
	Bone pain
	Lower stem cell yield compared to filgrastim + chemotherapy
	Shorter time from administration to collection compared to filgrastim + chemotherapy
Filgrastim + chemotherapy	Higher stem cell yield compared to filgrastim alone
	Fewer stem cell collections
	Potential for anticancer activity
	May impair future mobilization for stem cells
	Highly toxic in many patients
	Inconsistent results
	Longer time from administration to collection compared to filgrastim
Filgrastim + plerixafor	Low toxicity
	High efficacy in most patients
	Predictable mobilization permitting easy apheresis scheduling
	Gastrointestinal side effects

Adapted from EBMT NG (2009)

5.2.3 Chemo-mobilization

Chemo-mobilization is a combination of myelo-suppressive chemotherapy with filgrastim which appears to work synergistically to mobilize HSC, although the exact mechanism for this observation has not been fully elucidated. Filgrastim is thought to stimulate HSC mobilization by decreasing SDF-1 gene expression and protein levels while increasing proteases that can cleave interactions between HSC and the bone marrow environment. These growth factors are typically given as subcutaneous injections at a total daily dose of 3–24 mcg/kg/day.

5.2.4 Alternative Mobilization Strategies

Despite different mobilization regimen attempts, some patients are not able to achieve enough CD34+ cells to start apheresis. Those groups of patients are defined "poor mobilizers." In this case the use of plerixafor, CXCR4 antagonist that reversibly inhibits the interaction between CXCR4 and SDF-1, is needed. The use of plerixafor in combination with G-CSF has been shown to improve CD34+ cell collections in lymphoma and multiple myeloma patients (Olivieri et al. 2012).

Because no single chemotherapy mobilization regimen has demonstrated superiority, some clinicians may elect to mobilize patients during a cycle of a disease-directed chemotherapy regimen. With this approach, examples of regimens utilized have included cyclophosphamide, doxorubicin, vincristine, and prednisone (CHOP) and ifosfamide, carboplatin, and etoposide (ICE).

A comparison between mobilization methods is listed on Tables 5.2, 5.3, and 5.4.

5.2.5 PBSC Collection by Apheresis

The quantity of CD34+ cells in a PBSC component varies greatly, and its achievement by apheresis procedure depends on:

- Mobilization protocol
- Patient condition
- Timing of the PBSC collection
- Equipment
- Operator-dependent technique
- Volume of blood processed

The timing of PBSC collection has a critical role, and based on the mobilization regimen, we are able to appropriately schedule the apheresis procedures. For growth factor mobilization alone, the first collection procedure is calculated on days 4–5 when the peak of CD34+ cell count is expected to be achieved. After mobilization with chemotherapy regimens and growth factor, the expected day can vary between days 12 and 15 (Pierelli et al. 2012).

The first day collection procedure is determined by WBC count and CD34+ cell count.

Table 5.2 Advantages and disadvantages of hematopoietic stem cell collection methods

Collection method	Advantages	Disadvantages
Bone marrow	Single collection No need for special catheter placement No need for growth factors	Performed in an acute care setting as it requires general anesthesia Slower neutrophil and platelet engraftment Associated with higher rates of morbidity
Peripheral blood	Does not require general anesthesia and can be performed in an outpatient setting Faster recipient neutrophil and platelet engraftment Associated with lower rates of donor morbidity Tumor cell contamination of product may be less	Collection may take several days Sometimes requires placement of large double lumen catheter for collection Citrate toxicity

Adapted from EBMT NG (2009)

Table 5.3 Complications from chemotherapeutic agents commonly used for mobilization

Chemotherapeutic agent or regimen	Common side effects
Cyclophosphamide Note: must be combined with mesna administration	Appetite loss Color change in the skin Diarrhea Leukopenia Mouth sores Nausea, vomiting Skin rash Stomach discomfort or pain Texture change in nails Thrombocytopenia Weakness Hemorrhagic cystitis
Etoposide	Myelosuppression Infusion-related side effects (such as hypotension, flushing, chest pain, fever, diaphoresis, cyanosis, urticaria, angioedema, and bronchospasm) Nausea and vomiting Alopecia

Adapted from EBMT NG (2009)

Established thresholds for apheresis initiation may vary across centers but typically range from 10 to 20 CD34+ cells/mL. Once mobilization has reached an optimal level according to WBC and CD34+ levels, a patient can attend their scheduled sessions in the apheresis area. Optimized scheduling will avoid unnecessary collection procedures and unnecessary PBSC processing and will save freezing space.

The apheresis objective is to collect a product with requested PBSC counts with low cross cellular contamination in the smallest possible collect volume (ideally 80–90 ml/bag) and in as few procedures as possible. This will ensure cost optimization and enhance patient comfort and safety.

Clinical nurses working in the apheresis unit are responsible for educating the patient about the stem cell collection process and monitoring patients for any adverse reactions. The apheresis nurse challenges are:

- To understand how and when to administer agents used in the mobilization process
- To schedule mobilization regimen which occurs with or without chemotherapy
- To explain what medications the patient should and should not take during mobilization
- To expect adverse events and to be aware of their management for all agents used in mobilization
- To manage venous access catheter used for apheresis
- To be aware of the importance of laboratory monitoring and how to manage electrolyte imbalances
- To be aware of stem cell collection target level and options for patients who mobilize poorly or fail to mobilize

Patients are connected to the apheresis machine by their centrally or peripherally inserted venous catheters. One lumen is used to withdraw blood out of the patient and into the machine. Here the blood is centrifuged in a bowl housed within the cell separator machine. The desired stem cells are then siphoned off before

Table 5.4 Common apheresis complications

Side effect	Cause	Signs and symptoms	Corrective action
Citrate toxicity	Anticoagulant (citrate) given during apheresis	*Hypocalcemia* Common: dizziness, tingling in hands and feet Uncommon: chills, tremors, muscle cramps, tetany, seizure, cardiac arrhythmia	Slowing rate of apheresis, increasing the blood/citrate ratio, calcium replacement therapy
		Hypomagnesemia Common: muscle spasm or weakness Uncommon: decrease in vascular tone and cardiac arrhythmia	Slowing rate of apheresis, increasing the blood/citrate ratio, magnesium replacement therapy
		Hypokalemia Common: weakness Uncommon: hypotonia and cardiac arrhythmia	Slowing rate of apheresis, increasing the blood/citrate ratio, potassium replacement therapy
		Metabolic alkalosis Common: worsening of hypocalcemia Uncommon: decrease in respiration rate	Slowing rate of apheresis, increasing the blood/citrate ratio
Thrombocytopenia	Platelets adhere to internal surface of the apheresis machine	Low platelet count, bruising, bleeding	Priming apheresis machine with blood products in place of normal saline, platelet transfusion
Hypovolemia	Patient intolerant of large shift in extracorporeal volumes	Dizziness, light-headedness, tachycardia, hypotension, diaphoresis, cardiac arrhythmia	Slowing rate of apheresis session or temporarily stopping, intravenous fluid boluses
Catheter malfunction	Blood clot forms or catheter is not well positioned to allow for adequate blood flow	Inability to flush catheter, fluid collection under the skin around catheter site, pain and erythema at catheter site, arm swelling, decrease in blood flow	Repositioning of catheter, gentle flushing of catheter, treatment of blood clot

Adapted from EBMT NG (2009)

the remaining blood components are returned to the patient through the second lumen of their catheter. This second lumen can be used to administer intravenous fluids, electrolyte supplements, and medications to the patient if necessary. Each apheresis session lasts approximately 2–4 h during which an average of 7–10 l of blood, or twice the average total human blood volume, is exchanged or processed. Collections can occur on a daily basis until target CD34+ levels are achieved, which can last for up to 3–4 days depending on patient charac-

teristics and mobilization regimen used (Figs. 5.2 and 5.3).

5.3 Vascular Access

Appropriate catheter selection and placement is scheduled prior to the first stem cell collection (Toro et al. 2007). Catheters used for apheresis procedures must be able to tolerate large fluctuations in circulating blood volume on more than one occasion. Peripheral catheters are preferred

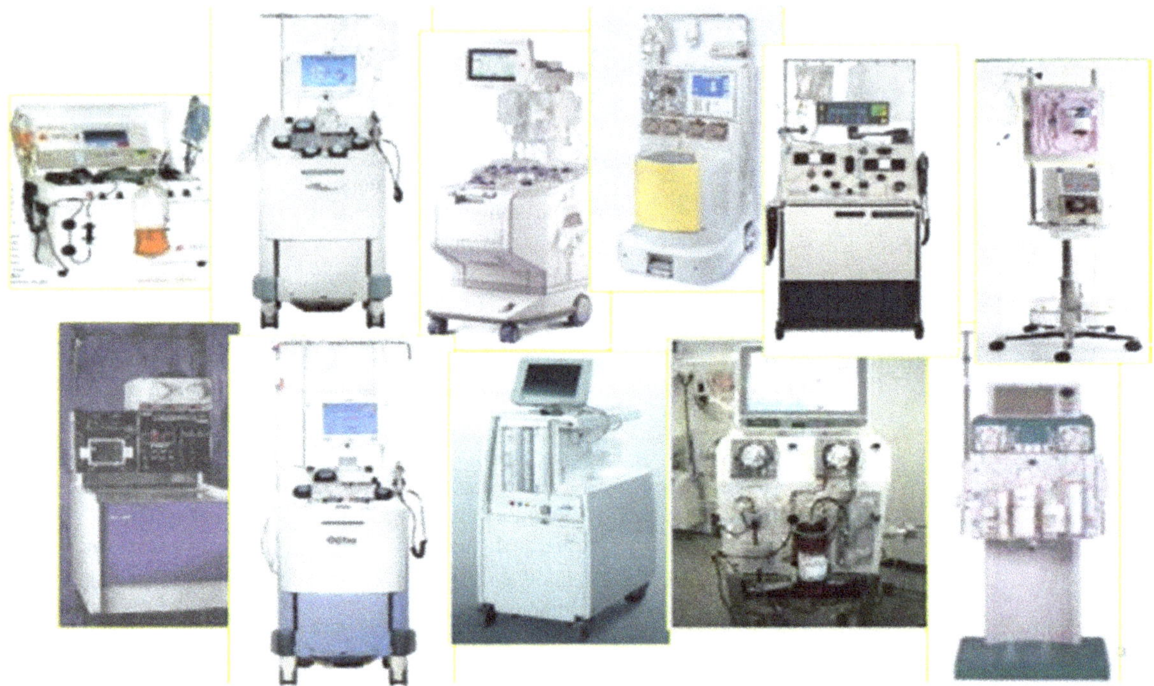

Fig. 5.2 Frequently used apheresis machines (https://www.google.it/search?q=apheresis+machines&biw=1920&bih=1018&tbm=isch&tbo=u&source=univ&sa=X&sqi=2&ved=0ahUKEwj2lui0gKvPAhUmLMAKHRDNAf8QsAQILQ)

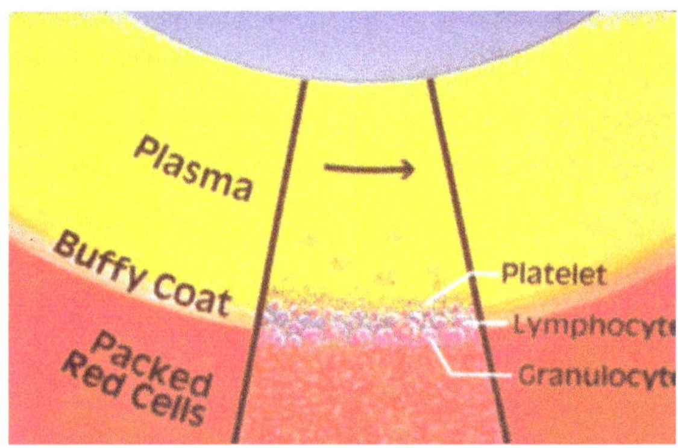

Fig. 5.3 Separation of components by G-force (https://www.google.it/search?q=separation+of+components+by+G-force&client=safari&rls=en&source=lnms&tbm=isch&sa=X&ved=0ahUKEwiHmv36gKvPAhVbF8AKHUf8BVEQ_AUICSgC&biw=1920&bih=1018#tbm=isch&q=apheresis+separation+of+components+by+G-force&imgrc=dKciXWNMkHikzM%3A)

where possible and placed in the cubital vein for drawing. If available, a port-a-cath or other previously inserted central catheters can be used for blood return.

In the absence of adequate peripheral veins, a large-bore, double lumen device can be inserted. These can be used temporarily during cell collections only, or they can be placed permanently and used throughout the transplant process. As with most centrally placed catheters, when placed in the area of the upper extremities, patients should be monitored for signs and symptoms of hypotension, shortness of breath, and decreased breath sounds as these can be indicative of venous wall perforation and require urgent attention. Hemothorax and pneumothorax, which are rare but serious complications, can occur and also require immediate attention. In some cases, catheters for apheresis may be placed in a femoral vein. In case of catheter positioning in the jugular vein, radiographic evaluation is used to verify catheter placement prior to clearance for its use. Instructions on caring for the catheter to prevent infection and maintain patency should be extensively reviewed with the patient and/or caregivers. Internal SOPs need to be observed.

5.4 Adverse Reactions

Apheresis procedures are relatively safe for the patient. While the procedure-related mortality rates are low at an estimated 3 deaths per 10,000 procedures, apheresis-associated morbidity is more frequently reported (Halter et al. 2009).

5.4.1 Citrate Toxicity

One of the most common adverse effects seen during the cell collection process is citrate toxicity, frequently manifested by hypocalcemia. Sodium citrate is used during apheresis to prevent blood from clotting while it is being processed by the machine. Citrate is known to bind to ionized serum calcium leading to hypocalcemia. Signs and symptoms of this complication can include:

- Burning
- Numbness and tingling in the extremities and/or the area around the mouth
- Muscle twitching
- Abdominal cramps
- Shivering

5.4.2 Treatment

Citrate toxicity complication can be managed by slowing the apheresis flow rate and providing patients with oral calcium supplements. In severe cases, intravenous supplementation of calcium may be given to the patient in order to prevent severe reactions such as tetany, seizure, and cardiac arrhythmia. Serum monitoring of calcium levels prior to each apheresis session is often helpful in decreasing the likelihood of hypocalcemia.

Other effects stemming from citrate toxicity include hypomagnesemia, hypokalemia, and metabolic alkalosis. Magnesium, like calcium, is a bivalent ion that is bound by citrate. Declines in serum magnesium levels often are more pronounced and take longer to normalize compared to aberrations in calcium levels. Signs and symptoms of hypomagnesemia are muscle weakness or spasm, decreased vascular tone, and abnormal cardiac contractility. Oral and intravenous supplementation with magnesium and potassium is often effective.

5.4.3 Hypovolemia

Because large fluctuations in blood volume can be experienced throughout each collection, patients are at risk of hypovolemia. Prior to starting the collection, baseline pulse and blood pressure should be measured and continually rechecked at designated intervals of approximately 1 h. It is also recommended that hemoglobin and hematocrit be monitored after the procedure as well.

5.4.4 Risk Factors

Patients at risk for developing hypovolemia include those with anemia, a previous history of cardiovascular compromise, and children or adults with a small frame.

5.4.5 Preventative Measures

Preventative measures are aimed at minimizing the extracorporeal volume shift by priming the apheresis machine with red blood cells and fresh frozen plasma in place of normal saline.

5.4.6 Clinical Manifestations

Clinical manifestations of hypovolemia can include dizziness, light-headedness, tachycardia, hypotension, and diaphoresis. Most concerning is the development of a cardiac dysrhythmia which can be life-threatening.

5.4.7 Treatment

Sessions should be interrupted and symptoms should subside before proceeding with collections. Hypovolemia may also be managed with providing intravenous fluid boluses and slowing the rate of flow on the apheresis machine.

5.4.8 Thrombocytopenia

Thrombocytopenia is another complication encountered during stem cell collections. When the patient's blood is in the cell separator machine, platelets can stick to the bowl used during the centrifuge process. Decreases in platelet concentrations can be precipitous, and obtaining platelet counts prior to each collection is essential.

5.4.9 Treatment

If platelet levels are low, patients may receive a platelet transfusion prior to the procedure. Also helpful, but not necessarily therapeutic, in managing thrombocytopenia is returning the collected platelet-rich plasma to the patient at the conclusion of the collection session.

5.5 Patient Assessment and Preparation

Prior to initiation of the stem cell collection process, patient candidates for autologous transplantation procedure must be thoroughly evaluated and determined fit to be able to tolerate all involved procedures.

5.5.1 Medical Assessment

The medical evaluation is the first step that a patient must complete when undergoing treatment. This involves the patient's primary medical oncologist making a referral to a transplant center or service. The physician provides the transplant team with information which often includes specifics relating to the care of the patient up to

this time point including past medical history, cancer status, summary of cancer treatments and response, and complications experienced during therapy. Accompanying this information are any available radiographic information and laboratory testing results. After review of the patient's medical information, the transplant team will initiate their own procedure-specific tests and evaluations to assess a patient's eligibility to proceed with stem cell collection and transplant. This involves restaging the patient to verify or establish their current disease status, ascertaining the function of various organ systems (e.g., renal, hepatic, pulmonary, etc.), documenting the absence of certain comorbid conditions and diseases (e.g., the presence of human immunodeficiency virus), and evaluating the overall performance status and psychosocial condition of the patient.

5.5.2 Patient Education

Education of the patient and their respective family and/or caregivers is integral to preparatory phase. Often a member of the nursing profession (clinic nurse, nurse educator, or nurse coordinator) will coordinate the education process for the patient and carers.

5.5.3 Donor Assessment and Preparation

Allogeneic related or non-related donors are submitted initially to interview and medical history questionnaire evaluation, including vaccination and travel history, blood transfusion, and risk for transmission of communicable disease together with physical and psychological exams that involves multidisciplinary teamwork and coordination as well.

The risks of donation shall be evaluated, discussed, and documented as a possible need for central venous access, the risk of hemoglobinopathy prior to administration of the mobilization therapy for collection of HPC, apheresis, and vascular access or anesthesia for collection of HPC by bone marrow harvesting.

Allogeneic donor eligibility, as defined by applicable laws and regulations, shall be determined by a physician after history, exam, medical record review, and testing. The donor eligibility determination shall be documented clearly in the recipient's medical record before the recipient's preparative regimen is initiated and before the allogeneic donor begins the mobilization regimen (EBMT NG 2009; Pierelli et al. 2012; JACIE n.d.).

The collection procedure shall be explained in terms the donor can understand the risks and benefits of the procedure, tests and procedures performed, and the rights according to applicable laws and regulations. Alternative collection methods need to be explained, and confidentiality must be guaranteed (EBMT NG 2009; JACIE n.d.). The donor shall have the right to refuse to donate but shall be informed of the potential consequences to the recipient of such refusal. Informed consent from the allogeneic donor shall be obtained by a licensed health-care professional who is not the primary health-care professional overseeing care of the recipient.

5.6 Quality in Apheresis

FACT-JACIE International Standards Accreditation (sixth edition) (JACIE n.d.) requires that the clinical program has access to personnel who are formally trained, experienced, and competent in the management of patients receiving cellular therapy. The Apheresis Collection Facility shall be licensed, registered, or accredited as required by the appropriate governmental authorities for the activities performed. The quality management plan should include, or summarize and reference, policies and standard operating procedures addressing personnel requirements for each key position in the Apheresis Collection Facility.

5.6.1 Training and Competencies

Core competencies are specified within the JACIE standards, and evidence of training in these competencies must be documented. This may be achieved by evidence of in-service training, attendance at conferences, etc. While initial supervised training is easily documented, annual competency maintenance can be difficult to demonstrate. Ongoing training for clinical personnel should reflect their experience, individual competencies and proficiencies, orientation for new staff, and necessary training. Training also needs to be undertaken in a timely manner to demonstrate annual updating (Babic et al. 2015).

5.7 Cell Source and Apheresis in the Pediatric Population

Abstract   Hematopoietic stem cell transplantation has become a well-established treatment for many malignant and nonmalignant disorders in children. Small body weight, venous access, and ethical dilemmas in minors represent a challenge in the pediatric population.

Keywords   Apheresis • Cell source • Children • Pediatric population

5.7.1 Introduction

During the past three decades, bone marrow transplantation and transplantation of peripheral blood stem cells have become a well-established treatment for many malignant and nonmalignant disorders in children and in adult patients (Bader et al. 2005).

Research has shown a continued and constant increase in the annual numbers of hematopoietic stem cell transplant (HSCT) and transplant rates (number of HSCT/10 million inhabitants) for both allogeneic and autologous HSCT (Passweg et al. 2013).

Indications for pediatric HSCT have changed considerably during the last 7 years. These changes provide tools for decision-making in health-care planning and counseling (Miano et al. 2007).

There is accumulating evidence of the role of hematopoietic SCT in non-hematological disorders such as autoimmune diseases (Sureda et al. 2015).

Some common nonmalignant diseases treated with hematopoietic stem cell transplant are (Nuss et al. 2011):

- *Hematologic* (severe aplastic anemia, Fanconi anemia, thalassemia, sickle-cell disease, Diamond-Blackfan anemia, Chédiak-Higashi syndrome, chronic granulomatous disease, congenital neutropenia)
- *Solid tumors* (Ewing's sarcoma, soft tissue sarcoma, neuroblastoma, and Wilms' tumor, where there is high risk or 4CR1, osteogenic sarcoma, and brain tumors)
- *Immunodeficiency* (severe combined immuno-deficiency disease, Wiskott-Aldrich syndrome, functional T-cell deficiency)
- *Genetic* (adrenoleukodystrophy, metachromatic leukodystrophy, Hurler syndrome, Hunter disease, Gaucher syndrome)
  – Cell Source in Pediatric Population

There are three commonly used sources of hematopoietic stem cells:

- BM
- Cytokine-mobilized PB progenitor cells (PBSC)
- UCB cells

The proportion of autologous to allogeneic HSCT is different in pediatric population (29% autologous) compared with adults (62% autologous) and is mainly used for treating solid tumors (Passweg et al. 2013).

Stem cells may be collected from the bone marrow (BM), peripheral blood, or umbilical cord blood (UCB). Each of these sources has several advantages and disadvantages.

Despite the increased use of peripheral blood and umbilical cord blood, BM is the primary graft source in *pediatric patients.*

For children and adolescents aged 8–20, allogeneic transplantation of HLA antigen-identical sibling peripheral blood stem cells is associated with higher mortality than the bone marrow (Eapen, et al JCO 2004). In contrast, previous work showed that peripheral blood was superior to the bone marrow as a stem cell source for adult and adolescent (aged 12–55) recipients of matched related donor grafts (Bensinger et al. N Engl J Med. 2001). More pediatric patients receive BM than PBSC, irrespective of donor type. This is explained by the higher incidence of nonmalignant conditions and the higher risk for chronic GvHD with peripheral blood as a stem cell source (Passweg et al. 2013).

The bone marrow remains the most common graft source for unrelated donors accounting for 49% in 2013. The use of umbilical cord blood is declining steadily, after peak in 2009, from 46% to 32% of all unrelated donor transplants performed in this age group (Sureda et al. 2015).

However, the recently completed NMDP/CIBMTR randomized study of unrelated marrow versus PBSC, which included pediatric patients, found that there were no significant differences in mortality between recipients of PBSC compared to the bone marrow.

The donor's preferences must also be taken into account as there are differences in the side effects experienced by the donors from a BM or PBSC harvest (Sureda et al. 2015; Pasquini and Zhu 2016).

From 2012 onward, there was an increase in the numbers of transplants from other relatives, which is likely due to rapid adoption of the strategy of posttransplant cyclophosphamide in the haploidentical setting. In 2014, the numbers of transplants using other relatives surpassed the total numbers of umbilical cord transplant performed in the USA, accounting for 11% of all allogeneic transplants performed in the USA (Pasquini and Zhu 2016).

Box: Bone marrow stem cell source in nonmalignant diseases in pediatric population

- *The BM remained the preferred source of stem cells for allogeneic transplants for nonmalignant disorders (62%). For diseases that do not require graft-versus-tumor effect, such as aplastic anemia, sickle-cell disease, or metabolic disorders, many consider it advantageous to use the bone marrow.*

Disadvantages include the need for general or epidural anesthesia and the risk of infection, bleeding, and bone damage. Also this population, although a minority, is still a significant minority that includes a number of unique diagnoses such as the hemoglobinopathies, immune deficiencies, immune dysregulation, and metabolic diseases, all of which are not common or present at all in the adult HSCT population (Passweg et al. 2013).

Annual numbers for allogeneic transplants in pediatric population demonstrate increase in the overall utilization of alternative donors.

From 2003 to 2011, there was a steady increase in the numbers of transplants using umbilical cord blood as a result of several published studies demonstrating its benefit in both children and adults.

Umbilical cord blood (UCB) characteristically differs from the marrow in a number of ways. The median doses of total nucleated cells (TNC), CD34+ cells, and CD3+ cells in UCB unit are approximately ten times lower than that of a bone marrow graft (Moscardo et al. 2004; Barker and Wagner 2003).

The indications for the use of UCB as a source for stem cells in children are identical to the indications for matched unrelated donor transplants (Sureda et al. 2015).

5.7.2 Apheresis in Pediatric Population

Experience with pediatric stem cell apheresis collections is limited. Challenges of apheresis in small children (<20 kg) include:

- Small total blood volume
- Vascular access issues
- Concerns about tolerable anticoagulant doses
- Limitations in product volumes that can be safely collected

Therefore, in many countries worldwide, children under the age of 18 years are not allowed to donate hematopoietic stem cells (HSCs) for unrelated recipients (Sörensen et al. 2013).

Adequate peripheral vascular access is difficult to find in young children, so we often need to consider a central apheresis catheter placement with its attendant risks.

Placement of central venous catheter (5–7 Fr with double offset lumens) is widely used for apheresis procedure; therefore, some PBSC donors receive a general anesthesia, and others have conscious sedation.

The apheresis team must consider the size and type of catheter that will yield the highest flow rate during apheresis, as well as patient or donor comfort. Often the catheter used for apheresis may be used for venous access during the high-dose therapy, reinfusion of stem cells, and recovery phases. We should try to avoid adverse events such as pain, hemorrhage, and inadequate sedation. A trained team in pediatric apheresis is mandatory as well as central line placement by ultrasound technique.

5.7.3 Key Differences: Pediatric vs Adult

Apheresis procedure in children differs from adult in *device (machine set) priming.*

Priming of the apheresis circuit with heterologous packed red blood cells is widely undertaken where donors weigh less than 20 kg. We should consider the risk of heterologous blood product administration in healthy donors – such as transfusion reaction and the risk of system overload if primed blood for some reason is reinfused. Usually we prime with RBC crossmatched, irradiated and leukocyte-depleted in patient and prime with 4% albumin solution in donors.

In the pediatric setting, the most common *adverse event* is pain, observed after central venous catheter (CVC) placement for PBSC collection. Pain at the site of puncture occurs more frequently in donors with a central (58%) than peripheral vein access (38%) (Hequet, 2015).

Often reported side effects after pediatric apheresis are:

- Hematoma formation
- Hypotension and cyanosis
- Allergic reaction to red blood cells
- Thrombocytopenia

Rare side effects reported are:

- Low-grade fever during the mobilization
- Hypovolemic signs: tachycardia >120 (most cases), hypotension, systolic blood pressure < 80 mmHg, pallor, and diaphoresis
- Nausea related to citrate effects during the apheresis procedure

In the absence of consensus and in order to prevent signs and symptoms of hypocalcemia, some centers administrate orally calcium gluconate (adult patients), and some centers routinely replace calcium i.v. during the entire apheresis procedure (mostly in pediatric apheresis). Nurses who perform pediatric procedures need to achieve competence in machine settings to allow the proper anticoagulation of the patient during the procedure (ACD-A or heparin or combination anticoagulation). The nurse must be competent in blood priming and in use of diluted or undiluted packed red blood cells, in prevention of hypocalcaemia and fluid balance, etc.

5.7.4 Ethical Dilemmas

The approach to minor donors is different in many countries.

> A donor is a person, no matter how small (Styczynski et al. 2012; Pulsipher et al. 2005).

Styczynski and colleagues compared donor and recipient children's age, both being small where donors were with smaller body weight than recipient and at higher risk for requiring a blood transfusion, additional apheresis procedures, pain, and cardiovascular complications after anesthesia. Most pediatric physicians who perform transplants believe it is acceptable to expose minors to the risks of a stem cell donation when donation offers a substantial prospect of benefit to a close family member and when proper consent is obtained (often from parents of both, donor and recipient).

The key issue that must be addressed with childhood HSC donors is their initial inability to understand and to voluntarily consent the procedure. Understanding increases as they age into an ability to assent and then finally to legally consent. Because HSC donation can benefit their sibling more than any other tissue sources and because the procedure can be performed with limited risk, sibling donation under parental consent has been considered appropriate to date (Bitan et al. 2016).

Summarizing:

- Advocacy and medical review of donors by individual(s) without dual responsibility to the recipient are recommended.
- Regarding the relationship between a pediatric donor and a family recipient, it is recommended to focus on avoiding psychological harm rather than predicting whether donation will result in a psychological benefit to the donor.
- Pediatric donors may be considered for research that carries minimal risk above the standard procedure or studies aimed at improving the safety and efficacy of the donation process.
- Donors with medical conditions that may increase the risk of complications associated with donation are not ever to be considered fit for donation.
- Centers should always avoid performing human leukocyte antigen typing on potential donors with medical/psychological reasons not to donate (Bitan et al. 2016).

5.7.5 Psychosocial Risks and Benefits

The primary benefit to the donor is the psychosocial value of helping a sibling or other close family members. This benefit may accrue even if the transplant is unsuccessful, because the donor and family can at least be reassured that the stem cell transplant was tried. There is a small but growing literature on the psychosocial risks and harms caused by hematopoietic stem cell donation by children. Data show that many children experience distress related to their role as a donor. Many pediatric donors believe that they did not have a choice about whether to serve as a marrow donor, report being poorly prepared for the procedures, and describe feeling responsible for the recipient's course after transplantation (Weisz 1996).

References

Afifi S, Adel NG, Devlin S, et al. Upfront plerixafor plus G-CSF versus cyclophosphamide plus G-CSF for stem cell mobilization in multiple myeloma: efficacy and cost analysis study. Bone Marrow Transplant. 2016;51:546–52.

Babic A, Wannesson L, Trobia M. Transplant unit personnel competency maintenance: online testing by sharepoint application. Lazzaro – EBMT 2015, oral presentation N003.

Bader P, Niethammer D, Willasch A, Kreyenberg H, Klingebiel T. How and when should we monitor chimerism after allogeneic stem cell transplantation? Bone Marrow Transplant. 2005;35(2):107–19. Review. PubMed PMID: 15502849.

Barker JN. Availability of cord blood extends allogeneic hematopoietic stem cell transplant access to racial and ethnic minorities. n.d.. http://www.sciencedirect.com/science/article/pii/S1083879110003502.

Barker JN, Wagner WJ. Umbilical-cord blood transplantation for the treatment of cancer (review). Nat Rev Cancer. 2003;3(7):526–32.

Bitan M, van Walraven SM, Worel N, Ball LM, Styczynski J, Torrabadella M, Witt V, Shaw BE, Seber A, Yabe H, Greinix HT, Peters C, Gluckman E, Rocha V, Halter J, Pulsipher MA. Determination of eligibility in related pediatric hematopoietic cell donors: ethical and clinical considerations. Recommendations from a Working Group of the Worldwide Network for Blood and Marrow Transplantation Association. Biol Blood Marrow Transplant. 2016;22(1):96–103.

Brando B, Barnett D, Janossy G, et al. Cytofluorimetric methods for assessing absolute numbers of cell subsets in blood. European Working Group on Clinical Cell Analysis. Cytometry. 2000;42(6):327–46.

Klaus J. Effect of CD34. cell dose on hematopoietic reconstitution and outcome in 508 patients with multiple myeloma undergoing autologous peripheral blood stem cell transplantation. Eur J Haematol. 2007;78(1):21–8.

Haematopoietic stem cell mobilisation and apheresis: a practical guide for nurses and other allied health care professionals (EBMT NG), 2009.

Halter J, Kodera Y, Ispizua AU, et al. Severe events in donors after allogeneic hematopoietic stem cell donation. Haematologica. 2009;94(1):94–101.

Hequet OJ. Hematopoietic stem and progenitor cell harvesting: technical advances and clinical utility. J Blood Med. 2015;6:55–67.

Hoffman R, et al. Hematology, Basic principles and practice. In: Practical aspects of stem cell collection, vol. 2: Churchill Livingstone-Elsevier; 2008. p. 1695–7. ISBN: 978-0-443-06715-0.

International standards for hematopoietic cellular therapy product collection, processing, and administration – Foundation for the Accreditation of Cellular Therapy (FACT) and Joint Accreditation Committee -ISCT and EBMT (JACIE). n.d..

Miano M, Labopin M, Hartmann O, Angelucci E, Cornish J, Gluckman E, Locatelli F, Fischer A, Egeler RM, Or R, Peters C, Ortega J, Veys P, Bordigoni P, Ior AP, Niethammer D, Rocha V, Dini G. Haematopoietic stem cell transplantation trends in children over the last three decades: a survey by the paediatric diseases working party of the European Group for Blood and Marrow Transplantation for the Paediatric Diseases Working Party of the European Group for Blood and Marrow Transplantation. Bone Marrow Transplant. 2007;39:89–99. https://doi.org/10.1038/sj.bmt.1705550.

Moscardo F, Sanz GF, Sanz MA. Unrelated-donor cord blood transplantation for adult haematological malignancies (review). Leuk Lymphoma. 2004;45(1):11.

Nuss S, Barnes Y, Fisher V, Olson E, Skeens M. In: Hematopoietic cell transplantation. In: Baggott C, Fochtman D, Foley GV, Kelly KP, editors. Nursing care of children and adolescent with cancer and blood disorders. 4th ed: APHON Association of Pediatric Hematology/Oncology Nurses; 4th edition 2011. p. 405–66.

Olivieri A, Marchetti M, Lemoli R, et al. Proposed definition of "poor mobilizer" in lymphoma and multiple myeloma: an analytic hierarchy process by ad hoc working group Gruppo Italiano trapianto di Midollo Osseo. Bone Marrow Transplant. 2012;47(3):342–51.

Pasquini MC, Zhu X. CIBMTR.Summary slides – HCT trends and survival data current uses and outcomes of hematopoietic stem cell transplantation: CIBMTR summary slides. Available at: http://www.cibmtr.org. Accessed 05 Sept 2016.

Passweg JR, Baldomero H, Bregni M, Cesaro S, Dreger P, Duarte RF, Falkenburg JH, Kröger N, Farge-Bancel D, Gaspar HB, Marsh J, Mohty M, Peters C, Sureda

A, Velardi A, Ruiz de Elvira C, Madrigal A. European Group for Blood and Marrow Transplantation. Hematopoietic SCT in Europe: data and trends in 2011. Bone Marrow Transplant. 2013;48(9):1161–7. https://doi.org/10.1038/bmt.2013.51. PubMed PMID: 23584439; PubMed Central PMCID: PMC3763517.

Perseghin P, et al. A policy for the disposal of autologous hematopoietic progenitor cells: report from an Italian consensus panel. Transfusion. 2014;54(9):2353–60. https://doi.org/10.1111/trf.12619. Epub 2014 Mar 24

Pierelli L, Perseghin P, Marchetti M, et al. Best practice for peripheral blood progenitor cell mobilization and collection in adults and children: results of a Società Italiana Di Emaferesi e Manipolazione Cellulare (SIDEM) and Gruppo Italiano Trapianto Midollo Osseo (GITMO) consensus process. Transfusion. 2012;52(4):893–905.

Pulsipher MA, Levine JE, Hayashi RJ, Chan KW, Anderson P, Duerst R, Osunkwo I, Fisher V, Horn B. Safety and efficacy of allogeneic PBSC collection in normal pediatric donors: the pediatric blood and marrow transplant consortium experience (PBMTC) 1996–2003. Bone Marrow Transplant. 2005;35(4):361–7. PubMed PMID: 15608659

Ruggeri A, Labopin M, Sanz G, et al. Comparison of outcomes after unrelated cord blood and unmanipulated haploidentical stem cell transplantation in adults with acute leukemia. Leukemia. 2015;29(9):1891–900. Epub 2015 Apr 17

Schoemans H, Theunissen K, Maertens J, et al. Adult umbilical cord blood transplantation: a comprehensive review. Bone Marrow Transplant. 2006;38:83–93.

Sörensen J, Jarisch A, Smorta C, Köhl U, Bader P, Seifried E, Bönig H. Pediatric apheresis with a novel apheresis device with electronic interface control. Transfusion. 2013;53(4):761–5.

Styczynski J, Balduzzi A, Gil L, Labopin M, Hamladji R, Marktel S, Akif Yesilipek M, Fagioli F, Ehlert K, Matulova M, Dalle J-H, Wachowiak J, Miano M, Messina C, Diaz MA, Vermylen C, Eyrich M, Badell I, Dreger P, Gozdzik J, Hutt D, Rascon J, Dini G, Peters C. Risk of complications during hematopoietic stem cell collection in pediatric sibling donors: a prospective European Group for Blood and Marrow Transplantation Pediatric Diseases Working Party study. Blood. 2012;119(12):2935–42.

Sureda A, Bader P, Cesaro S, Dreger P, Duarte RF, Dufour C, Falkenburg JH, Farge-Bancel D, Gennery A, Kröger N, Lanza F, Marsh JC, Nagler A, Peters C, Velardi A, Mohty M, Madrigal A. Indications for allo- and auto-SCT for haematological diseases, solid tumours and immune disorders: current practice in Europe, 2015. Bone Marrow Transplant. 2015;50(8):1037–56. Epub 2015 Mar 23

Toro JJ, Morales M, Loberiza F, Ochoa-Bayona JL, Freytes CO. Patterns of use of vascular access devices in patients undergoing hematopoietic stem cell transplantation: results of an international survey. Support Care Cancer. 2007;15:1375–83.

Weisz VR. Risks and benefits of pediatric bone marrow donation: a critical need for research. Behav Sci Law. 1996;14(4):375–91. https://www.ncbi.nlm.nih.gov/pubmed/9156419

Principles of Conditioning Therapy and Cell Infusion

6

Sara Zulu and Michelle Kenyon

Abstract

Prior to haematopoietic stem cell transplant (HSCT), conditioning therapy is used for disease eradication, creation of space for engraftment and immunosuppression. Conditioning therapy includes combinations of chemotherapy, radiotherapy and/or immunotherapy. Chemotherapy is delivered in different phases: induction, consolidation and maintenance. Total body irradiation (TBI) is widely used as part of conditioning regimens preceding allogeneic HSCT and is able to target sanctuary sites where some drugs cannot reach. Cancer immunotherapy treatment harnesses the body's natural defences to fight the cancer, by involving components of the immune system. Conditioning therapy can have acute and chronic side effects due to the toxicity of the treatment. Nursing implications involve patient education and information, toxicity assessments, close monitoring and action plans. Stem cell infusion is usually a safe procedure but can cause adverse reactions ranging from flushing and nausea to life-threatening reactions. There should be written policies for the administration of cellular therapy products, and nurses must have training and competency in order to safely administer haematopoietic stem cells.

Keywords

Haematopoietic stem cell transplant • HSCT • Conditioning therapy
Chemotherapy • Total body irradiation • TBI • Immunotherapy • Stem cell
infusion

S. Zulu (✉)
Cancer Services, Royal Free Hospital, London, UK
e-mail: sara.zulu@nhs.net

M. Kenyon
Department of Haematological Medicine,
King's College Hospital NHS Foundation Trust,
London, UK

6.1 Conditioning

Conditioning therapy in haematopoietic stem cell transplant (HSCT) is central to the preparation or 'conditioning' of the patient for the transplant. The three main goals of conditioning therapy are:

M. Kenyon, A. Babic (eds.), *The European Blood and Marrow Transplantation Textbook for Nurses*,
https://doi.org/10.1007/978-3-319-50026-3_6

Table 6.1 Examples of myeloablative, non-myeloablative and reduced intensity regimens

Myeloablative	Non-myeloablative	Reduced intensity
Bu/Cy/Mel (busulfan, cyclophosphamide, melphalan)	Flu/Cy/ATG (fludarabine, cyclophosphamide, ATG)	Flu/Bu (fludarabine, busulfan)
TBI/TT/Cy (TBI, thiotepa, cyclophosphamide)	Flu/TBI (fludarabine, TBI)	Flu/Mel (fludarabine, melphalan)
Cy/VP/TBI (cytarabine, etoposide, TBI)	TLI/ATG (total lymphoid irradiation, ATG)	Flu/Cy (fludarabine, cytarabine)

Adapted from EBMT-ESH Handbook

1. Eradication of disease
2. Creation of 'space' in the bone marrow for donor stem cells to engraft
3. Immunosuppression to decrease the risk of rejection of the donor cells by the host cells

Conditioning therapies include combinations of chemotherapy, radiotherapy and/or immunotherapy, using different regimens. The aim of conditioning regimens is to reduce relapse and rejection and can be fine-tuned to reduce treatment-related mortality. This can be done with 'reduced intensity' or non-myeloablative regimens which are less toxic or with myeloablative regimens which are a higher dose to wipe out or 'ablate' the marrow (see Table 6.1).

6.2 Chemotherapy

Dividing cells such as bone marrow stem cells proliferate and replicate in order to retain their function. Cytotoxic chemotherapy works by destroying rapidly dividing cells, including malignant cells. This is done by preventing the cells from dividing or by causing cell death (apoptosis) during different phases of the cell cycle.

The cell cycle comprises of five phases:

1. G0 phase—This is the resting phase which can last for months.
2. G1 phase—This is the growth phase, where RNA and protein synthesis occurs.
3. S phase—DNA is replicated so that when the cell divides, the new cell will have a copy of the genetic information. This phase lasts from 18 to 20 h.
4. G2 phase—Further protein synthesis occurs preparing the cell for mitosis; this phase lasts from 2 to 10 h.
5. M phase—The cell splits into two new cells. This phase lasts about 30–60 min.

There are three different means of classifying chemotherapy drugs: according to their cell cycle activity, their chemical groups or their mode of action. This chapter will focus on the mode of action classification, which is summarised in the table below.

6.2.1 Combination Chemotherapy

As previously mentioned all cells go through five phases during the reproduction cycle. Certain cytotoxic chemotherapy drugs work only at a specific phase of the cycle, whilst other drugs are not phase specific. In cytotoxic drug combination with synergy like pre-BMT conditioning (Table 6.2), it is logical to attack multiple phases of the cell replication cycle to prevent mutation and resistance from occurring. Combination chemotherapy allows for maximum cell kill, as each drug targets cells independently at different stages of the cell cycle. If the toxicities of the combination chemotherapy drugs do not replicate, the optimal dose could be administered without the high-grade toxicities.

6.2.2 Cycles and Scheduling

Chemotherapy is administered in cycles according to a schedule, in order to allow for recovery of the bone marrow and immune system after

Table 6.2 Chemotherapy classifications according to their mode of action

Cytotoxic classification	Mode of action	Examples
Alkylating agents	They prevent replication by substituting alkyl groups for hydrogen atoms in cells. This causes the DNA strands to break leading to mutation or cell death	Melphalan Iphosphomide Busulfan
Antimetabolites	These agents disrupt cellular metabolism resulting in disrupted DNA and apoptosis. Act in the S phase of the cell cycle	Methotrexate Cytarabine Fludarabine
Antitumor antibiotics	They inhibit synthesis and replication by binding to DNA and RNA ·	Daunorubicin Doxorubicin
Plant alkaloids	These are extracts from the pink periwinkle plant. They bind to microtubular proteins causing apoptosis acting mainly in the M phase	Vincristine Vinblastine
	These agents are derived from the root of the mandrake plant and act in the G2 and S phase interfering with topoisomerase II enzyme reaction	Etoposide
Miscellaneous	They cause lysis of lymphoid tumours. Act in the G0 phase of the cell cycle	Corticosteroids Enzymes (L-asparaginase)
	Rituximab causes lysis of T- lymphocytes that have the CD20 antigen on their cell surface.	Monoclonal antibodies (rituximab)

Adapted from EBMT-ESH Handbook (2012)

administration (Brown and Cutler 2012; Grundy 2006). Malignant cells are expected to have a lengthier time to recover than normal cells. In this way, by scheduling the treatment, 'normal' cells can recover from toxicity, whilst the malignant cells will be reduced with continued cycles of treatment. Administration of chemotherapy in cycles allows for the possibility of a larger dose of drugs to be given over a short period of time.

In leukaemia and lymphoma treatment, chemotherapy is usually divided into different phases:

- Induction: The first aim of the treatment is to achieve remission. Chemotherapy is administered in order to eradicate the malignant cells.
- Consolidation (intensification): After remission is achieved, further treatment is given in order to prevent a recurrence of malignant cells. Consolidation chemotherapy can include radiotherapy or a stem cell transplant.
- Maintenance: Treatment is given in order to 'maintain' remission and prevent relapse. Maintenance treatment may include chemotherapy, hormone therapy or targeted therapy.

6.2.3 Modes of Administration

Cytotoxic therapy can be delivered via different routes. The four most used in HSCT are:

1. *Intravenous* (*IV*): This is the most common route of administration in HSCT. The drug is delivered directly into the blood stream via a cannula or a central venous access device. Risks to IV administration include extravasation and chemical phlebitis (chemical reaction to the vein causing hardening of the view or cording).
2. *Subcutaneous*: This is administered as an injection under the skin. Risks include irritation to the surrounding tissue, trauma (which could be due to low platelet count) or infection.
3. *Oral:* This route is usually self-administered. It is important that the patient is able to swallow, has sufficient manual dexterity and is compliant. Risks including vomiting after a given dose can reduce bioavailability.
4. *Intrathecal* (*IT*): This is administration by lumbar puncture into the cerebrospinal fluid to treat or prevent disease in the central nervous system (CNS). Intrathecal administration can be fatal if the incorrect type of cytotoxic agent

is used, i.e. vinca alkaloids. National guidance has been publicised for the safe administration of IT chemotherapy.

6.2.4 Side Effects and Nursing Implications

- Chemotherapy side effects can be acute or chronic.
- Chemotherapy not only destroys malignant cells but also rapidly dividing 'normal' cells. The 'normal' cells that are most frequently affected include bone marrow cells, hair follicles, mucosal lining of the GI tract and skin, fertility and germinal cells.
- Nursing implications involve patient education and information, toxicity assessments, close monitoring and action plans.
- Chapters 9 and 10 discuss acute complications and supportive care in more detail.

6.3 Radiotherapy

Radiotherapy in HSCT is used as part of lymphoma treatment, as prophylaxis and treatment of disease and as palliative treatment for myeloma and lymphoma. Radiotherapy uses ionising radiation to control or kill malignant cells.

6.3.1 Total Body Irradiation

Total body irradiation (TBI) alongside high-dose chemotherapy helps to kill off leukaemia, lymphoma or myeloma cells in the bone marrow. This allows the patient to be in a preparation phase to receive the donor stem cells as part of the recovery stage of the treatment.

TBI is widely used as part of myeloablative, reduced intensity and non-myeloablative conditioning regimens preceding HSCT. As well as eradicating disease, immunosuppressive effect and creating space for donor cells to engraft; TBI is able to target sanctuary sites such as the CNS or gonads where some drugs cannot reach.

Most centres use a linear accelerator machine as a source of radiation. Patients are positioned either on their side or in a lateral position at a calculated distance from the machine. TBI is delivered in various doses and scheduling. The dose can be single (1–8 Gy total dose), fractionated (10–14 Gy total dose over 3 days) or hyperfractionated (14–15 Gy total dose over 4 days). As with chemotherapy scheduling, fractionated doses of TBI minimise toxicity (Apperly et al. 2012).

Some centres use lead shielding blocks to protect parts of the body such as the lungs and eyes; however, shielding organs could potentially shield leukaemic cells, so many centres opt not to do this.

6.3.2 Side Effects and Nursing Implications

Side effects of TBI can be acute or chronic. As TBI is usually given in combination with chemotherapy, it can be difficult to differentiate between the causes of the toxicities. Immediate side effects of TBI include bone marrow suppression, alopecia, nausea, vomiting, parotid swelling and erythema.

Chronic side effects of TBI include cataracts, infertility and interstitial pneumonitis. Nursing implications involve patient education and information, toxicity assessments, close monitoring and action plans (Apperly et al. 2012).

Chapters 9 and 10 discuss acute complications and supportive care in more detail.

6.4 Immunotherapy

The immune system has a natural ability to detect and destroy abnormal cells and in doing so prevents the development of many cancers.

However, cancer cells are sometimes able to avoid detection and destruction by the immune system by using a variety of strategies.

Cancer cells may:

- Reduce the expression of tumour antigens on their surface, making it harder for the immune system to see them
- Express proteins on their surface that inactivate or neutralise immune cells

- Encourage cells in the surrounding environment to release substances that suppress immune responses and help to promote tumour cell growth and survival

6.4.1 Cancer Immunotherapy

This is a type of cancer treatment that is designed to harness the body's natural defences to fight the cancer by involving or using components of the immune system.

Some cancer immunotherapies consist of antibodies that bind to, and inhibit the function of, proteins expressed by cancer cells. Other cancer immunotherapies include vaccines and T-cell infusions.

A number of approaches are described briefly below.

6.4.1.1 Immune Checkpoint Blockade

Immune checkpoints are pathways embedded into the immune system that keep immune responses in check. They help to limit the strength and duration of immune responses and prevent strong responses that might damage normal as well as abnormal cells. Tumours appear to hijack certain immune checkpoint pathways and their proteins and use them to suppress normal immune responses.

This therapy targets the immune checkpoint pathways so that when the immune checkpoint proteins are blocked, the 'brakes' on the immune system are released and it behaves normally once again and destroys the cancer cells.

Immune checkpoint blockade with antibodies that target cytotoxic T-lymphocyte-associated antigen 4 (CTLA-4) and the programmed cell death protein 1 pathway (PD-1/PD-L1) has shown promising results in a variety of malignancies.

6.4.1.2 Immune Cell Therapy

Adoptive cell therapy (ACT) is a treatment that uses a cancer patient's own T cells. These cells are collected from the blood of the patient and then grown in the laboratory or expanded in vitro. These cells are activated by treatment with cytokines and then infused back to the patient.

An emerging form of ACT is chimaeric antigen receptor (CAR) T-cell therapy. A patient's T cells are collected from the blood and modified to express CAR protein. These cells are grown in the laboratory to produce large numbers of CAR T cells, which are then infused back into the patient.

In the blood, the CAR T cells bind to the cancer cells, become activated and attack and destroy them.

6.4.1.3 Therapeutic Antibodies

Therapeutic antibodies are 'drug'-based antibodies produced to destroy cancer cells.

One group of therapeutic antibodies is called antibody–drug conjugate (ADC). An antibody is connected to a toxic ingredient such as a drug, toxin or radioactive substance. When the antibody–drug conjugate (ADC) binds to the cancer cell, it is absorbed, and the toxic substance is released killing the cell.

Not all therapeutic antibodies are connected to toxic substances. Some antibodies cause cancer cells to commit suicide (apoptosis), and others can make the cancer cells more recognisable to certain immune cells (complement) and help to facilitate cell death.

6.4.1.4 Therapeutic Cancer Vaccines

Another approach to immunotherapy is the use of cancer vaccines. These vaccines are usually made from a patient's own cancer cells or from substances produced by cancer cells. It is intended that when a vaccine containing cancer-specific antigens is injected into a patient, these antigens will stimulate the immune system to attack cancer cells without causing harm to normal cells.

Further Reading

http://www.nature.com/
Search on:
Cancer Reviews.
Immunology Reviews.

6.5 Paediatric Considerations

Conditioning

There are differences between adult and paediatric patient's conditioning. Children can generally tolerate side effects better than adults, and higher doses may be used. On the other hand, conditioning regimens affect growth and endocrine development of the child.

Studies so far indicate that reduced intensity conditioning (RIC) in haematopoietic cell transplantation may have an important role in treating children with primary immune deficiencies: such regimens can be used without severe toxicity in patients with pre-transplant infections or severe pulmonary or hepatic disease. RIC has extended the role of allogeneic transplantation to many patients who until recently were considered ineligible for this procedure (Chiesa and Veys 2014).

Disease-specific treatment protocols can be found, for example, in the EBMT Handbook 2012, Chap. 20. Chemotherapy and radiation therapy side effects will be discussed in more detail in Chap. 8.

6.5.1 Chemotherapy

Children in general tolerate side effect better than adults, so higher total doses may be used (Satwani et al. 2008).

When treating paediatric patients' prescriptions should be made by body surface area (BSA) mg/m^2 or mg/kg using *recent weight and height*.

6.5.2 Total Body Irradiation

TBI has severe side effects when administered to children and adolescents, and it should be avoided, whenever possible. The risk for secondary malignancies is significantly higher compared to pharmacological conditioning (ALL). Most teams use conditioning regimens (AML) that do not involve TBI (EBMT Handbook 2012).

When TBI is used, it is commonly given in fractions (two doses per day) to minimise the side effects.

Paediatric patients need age-appropriate preparation for radiotherapy. This can be done by the play therapist, but if there is no such professional, it should be done by a nurse. Preparations should be started well in advance to allow the patient and parents ask questions. It is possible to listen to music or fairy tales whilst having TBI. Immobilisation is a prerequisite for accurate radiotherapy, so anaesthesia is required for younger children.

6.6 Stem Cell Infusion

Haematopoietic stem cells (HSCs) can be procured from the patient (autologous) or from a donor (allogeneic or cord blood).

HSCs procured from the patient are almost always sourced from peripheral blood during apheresis (see Chap. 5).

HSCs procured from a donor can be sourced from the peripheral blood (apheresis), bone marrow or umbilical cord.

After harvesting, HSCs can be stored using cryopreservation. Dimethyl sulfoxide (DMSO) is a common cryopreservative used in the storage of HSCs.

6.6.1 Adverse Reactions

An adverse reaction is a noxious and unintended response suspected or demonstrated to be caused by the collection or infusion of a cellular therapy product or by the product itself.

The stem cell infusion is a generally safe procedure, but it can cause a variety of adverse reactions ranging from flushing and nausea to life-threatening reactions. It is imperative that the healthcare team is trained for early identification and managing of possible adverse reactions. Nurses must obtain baseline vital signs including temperature, breath sounds, pulse oximetry, weight and fluid status prior to the cell infusion.

Possible adverse reactions are:

Fresh *stem cells*
   Allergic reaction
   Haematolytic transfusion reaction
   Fluid overload
   Micropulmonary emboli
   Infection

Preserved stem cells

    Bad taste in the mouth, nausea and vomiting (DMSO)

    Arrhythmia hypertension

    Haemoglobinuria

    Allergic reaction

    Haemolytic transfusion reaction

    Fluid overload

    Micropulmonary emboli

    Infection (Costa et al. 2014; Tomlinson and Kline 2010; Truong et al. 2016; Vidula et al. 2015)

6.6.2   Nursing Care: Pre-, During and Post Stem Cell Infusion

6.6.2.1 Pre-infusion Assessment

Maintain a safe environment Ensure that your patient is prepared and the room is organised out in a way that you have access to the patient and you have access to everything you need including oxygen and suction. The patient should be nursed on a bed during the stem cell infusion, in case of severe allergic reaction.

Baseline observations Record baseline observations in order to assess the patient's physiological status during and post infusion.

Preparing patient for transfusion If patients are receiving cells previously cryopreserved with DMSO, they should receive a premedication with antihistamine, corticosteroids, antipyretics and anti-emetics. The nurse should discuss the procedure including length of time, how they may feel and what to tell the nurse if they experience any of the common side effects. Encourage your patient to tell you how they feel during the entire procedure, to ensure adverse incidents are spotted, to offer reassurance or to ensure side effects are managed.

IV line care Check the IV line for patency. On the whole, patients undertaking a stem cell infusion will have a permanent, central line in situ. Common lines used for this treatment are PICC lines and Hickman lines. Ensure aseptic non-touch technique is used to prevent the risk of infection.

Toileting Discuss with the patient and encourage toileting prior to starting the procedure in order to minimise interruption to the stem cell infusion and also ensure safety for the patient.

Psychological support Day zero can be a momentous occasion for someone who requires a stem cell transplantation. Patients may experience a range of emotions, from elation through to distress, anxiety, vulnerability and helplessness. Using simple techniques such as discussing the procedure, and listening and offering reassurance may help to reduce patients anxiety.

6.6.2.2 During Stem Cell Infusion

IV line care Ensure aseptic non-touch technique is used to prevent the risk of infection.

Physiological monitoring Should be carried out at least every 10–15 min and increased if there are any concerns with the patients' condition during the infusion. O_2 saturations are monitored constantly during infusion. Treat problems as they arise (i.e. drop in saturations, give O_2 as prescribed).

Assess for potential side effects Patients can have mild to severe reactions to a stem cell infusion. Autologous stem cells tend to be cryopreserved. Patients can experience allergic reactions including nausea, flushing, rash, chest tightness, shortness of breath and chills. For anaphylaxis, follow your centre guidelines for managing an anaphylaxis event. For other side effects, the infusion can be slowed down according to how the patient tolerates the infusion. Reassure the patient and treat the side effects as they occur.

6.6.2.3 Post Stem Cell Infusion

Physiological monitoring Assess for later effects of the cell infusion. Observations should be performed half hourly for the next 2 h, then hourly for another 2 h, and four hourly thereafter.

Documentation Document the care event in patients' medical records, and complete the cell infusion record.

6.6.3   JACIE Standards

The JACIE process has been explained in detail in Chap. 1. JACIE Standards give instruction on how to safely administer the product. Nurses must have training and competency for administration of cellular therapy products. There shall be also written policies for administration of cellular therapy products (JACIE Standards B3.7).

There shall be a policy addressing safe administration of cellular therapy products. These policies should determine the appropriate volume and dose of red cells, cryoprotectants and other additives and volume of ABO-incompatible red cells in allogeneic cellular therapy products. Two qualified persons shall verify the identity of the recipient, the product and the order for administration (JACIE standards B7.6).

For more detailed information, please visit the www.jacie.org

References

Apperly J, Carreras E, Gluckman E, Masszi T, The EBMT handbook. 6th ed. Paris: European School of Haematology; 2012.

Brown M, Cutler T. Haematology nursing. Hoboken, NJ: Wiley-Blackwell. 2012.

Chiesa R, Veys P. Reduced-intensity conditioning for allogeneic stem cell transplant in primary immune deficiencies. Expert Rev Clin Immunol. 8:255–67. Published online: 10 Jan 2014. Download citation https://doi.org/10.1586/eci.12.9

Costa Bezerra Freire N, et al. Adverse reactions related to hematopoietic stem cell infusion. J Nursing UFPE Online. 9:391–8.

FACT-JACIE international standards for hematopoietic cellular therapy, 6th ed. 2015.; www.jacie.org

Grundy M. Nursing in haematological oncology. 2nd ed. Edinburgh: Ballière Tindall; 2006.

Mulay SB, et al. Infusion technique of hematopoietic progenitor cells and related adverse events. Transfusion. 2014;54:1997–2003.

Satwani P, Cooper N, Rao K, et al. Reduced intensity conditioning and allogeneic stem cell transplantation in childhood malignant and non-malignant diseases. Bone Marrow Transplant. 2008;46:173–82.

Tomlinson D, Kline NE, editors. Pediatric oncology nursing: advanced clinical handbook. 2nd ed. New York/Dordrecht/Heildelberg: Springer; 2010.

Truong TH, Moorjani R, Dewey D, Guilcher GMT, Prokopishyn NL, Lewis VA. Adverse reactions during stem cell infusion in children treated with autologous and allogeneic stem cell transplantation. Bone Marrow Transplant. 2016;51:680–6.

Vidula N, et al. Adverse events during hematopoietic stem cell infusion: analysis of the infusion product. Clinical Lymphoma, Myeloma And Leukaemia. 2015;15:e157–62.

Further Reading

Pan London Guidelines for the Safe Prescribing, Handling and Administration of Systemic Anti Cancer Treatment Drugs. www.londoncanceralliance.nhs.uk.

Good practice guide for pediatric radiotherapy, Children's cancer and leukaemia group, Society and college of radiographers, The Royal College of Radiologists, 2012.

BMT Settings, Infection and Infection Control

John Murray, Iris Agreiter, Laura Orlando, and Daphna Hutt

Abstract

Despite improvements over the past several decades, infection remains a significant risk to all haematological patients receiving therapy. Those requiring allogeneic transplant and especially those that have HLA disparity or T-cell-depleted grafts have an even higher risk of infective complications due to delayed recovery of T- and B-cell function. Early identification with prompt effective treatment is paramount to improve all patients' survival. Patient safety through robust adherence to hand hygiene and maintenance of the environment with cleaning and disinfection are the backbone of an effective preventative program. Basic nursing care and a sound knowledge base of the risks, presentation, diagnosis and treatment will improve patient care.

Keywords

Viral infection · Bacterial infection · Fungal infection · Handwashing · Isolation

J. Murray (✉)
Haematology and Transplant Unit, The Christie NHS Foundation Trust, Manchester, UK
e-mail: John.Murray@christie.nhs.uk

I. Agreiter
Department of Haematology and BMT Unit, Hospital San Maurizio, Bolzano, Italy
e-mail: IRIS.AGREITER@sabes.it

L. Orlando
Division of Haemato-oncology, European Institute of Oncology, Milan, Italy
e-mail: lauraorlando25@libero.it

D. Hutt
Department of Pediatric Hematology-Oncology and BMT, Edmond and lily Safra Children Hospital, Sheba Medical Center, Tel-Hashomer, Israel
e-mail: dhutt@sheba.health.gov.il

7.1 Introduction

Infection is a major cause of mortality and morbidity in the haematopoietic stem cell transplant (HSCT) population due to regimen-related toxicity. Improvements over the past couple of decades especially in supportive care have helped to reduce this risk. The development of neutropenic fever is a frequent occurrence, and centres have algorithms for identifying and treating infection promptly. In this chapter we will discuss the common viral, bacterial and fungal infections that our transplant patients develop.

© EBMT and the Author(s) 2018
M. Kenyon, A. Babic (eds.), *The European Blood and Marrow Transplantation Textbook for Nurses*,
https://doi.org/10.1007/978-3-319-50026-3_7

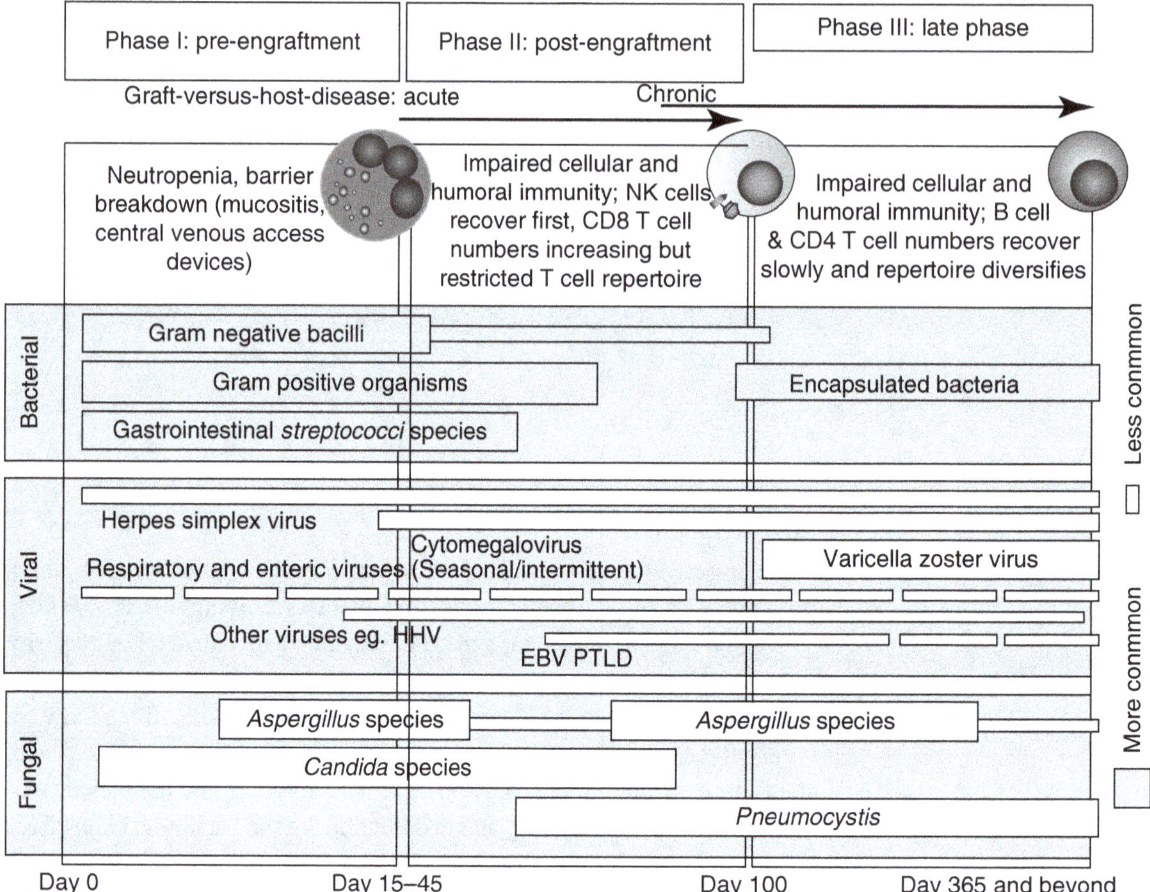

Fig. 7.1 Phases of opportunistic infections among allogeneic HCT recipients. HHV6 human herpesvirus 6, NK natural killer, PTLD post-transplant lymphoproliferative disease (Mackall et al. 2009)

Mackall et al. (2009) displays the variety of infections in Fig. 7.1 that may occur and the approximate timeframe for their development which aids the clinical team to refine and direct investigations and potential treatments appropriately.

7.2 Viral Infections

Viral infection is spread by close contact with infectious secretions, either by large particle aerosols, formites or subsequent self-inoculation. Coughing and sneezing will produce aerosol particles, and a virus can also be picked up after contact with contaminated surfaces.

7.2.1 Cytomegalovirus

7.2.1.1 Introduction

Cytomegalovirus (CMV) disease is a serious potential complication of allogeneic stem cell transplantation leading to life-threatening complications. CMV is usually acquired in childhood. It is a virus that is present worldwide, and whilst in developed countries approximately 50% of the population is seropositive, this rises to almost 100% in developing countries. CMV is shed intermittently from the oropharynx and from the genitourinary tract of both immunocompetent and immunosuppressed people. Prior to allograft the serostatus (IgG) of the patient and potential donors are assessed to gauge risk (Zaia et al. 2009).

CMV belongs to the human herpesvirus family HHV5 and comes from the subfamily Betaherpesvirinae. Betaherpesvirinae infects the mononuclear cells, establishes latency in the leukocytes and once reactivated replicates slowly. CMV is able to lie dormant for protracted lengths of time, and immunity to the CMV complex involves both the humoral and cell-mediated pathways. Patients treated with stem cell transplantation in the context of haematological malignancies can reactivate the latent virus, either from native host leucocytes, from those derived from the donor, or from both. The risk of reactivation varies dependent upon the patient and/or donor's previous exposure to CMV. CMV status can be shown as follows:

Risk factors for reactivation

	Recipient	Donor
High risk	Positive	Negative
Medium risk	Negative	Positive
Medium risk	Positive	Positive
No risk	Negative	Negative

The patient's CMV status is indicated on the left and donor CMV status on the right.

Careful measures are taken to minimize the risk of primary infection with CMV when prescribing blood products in allograft patients. All blood products should be obtained from CMV-seronegative donors and leukocyte depletion.

Risk Factors for *CMV Reactivation*

- CMV serostatus of recipient/donor (+/− or +/− > > −/+)
- Previous CMV reactivation
- Time post-transplant – increased in early post-transplant period (to day 100)
- T-cell-depleted transplant conditioning protocols (e.g. Campath 1-H)
- Systemic immunosuppression (particularly corticosteroids, antibodies directed against T-cells, e.g. ATG/Campath 1-H)
- Recipient age – increased in older patients
- Graft versus host disease (GvHD)

Risk Factors for *Primary CMV Infection*

- Person-to-person transmission
- Low risk in use of blood not screened negative for CMV (Meijer et al. 2003)

7.2.1.2 Presentation

CMV can occur as a primary infection or as a reactivation of the previously latent virus. When a CMV IgG-negative patient develops CMV, this is termed a primary infection. When a patient, or donor, is known to be CMV antibody positive and then develops CMV, this is termed reactivation. The diagnosis of CMV disease requires the presence of symptoms and signs compatible with end-organ damage, together with the detection of CMV. If left untreated, asymptomatic CMV infection can progress to CMV disease.

7.2.1.3 Diagnosis

It is important to diagnose reactivation early and institute timely treatment; therefore regular monitoring of CMV levels is of paramount importance. Polymerase chain reaction (PCR) is the most sensitive and quantitative method of monitoring at-risk patients especially in the early post-transplant period (until at least day 100 post-transplant) and longer in those on systemic immunosuppression.

CMV infection most commonly affects the lung, gastrointestinal tract, eye, liver or central nervous system, with CMV pneumonia being the most serious complication with >50% mortality (Tomblyn et al. 2009).

All bone marrow transplant patients and donors will have their CMV status tested in clinic pre-transplant along with the CMV status of the donor.

7.2.1.4 Monitoring and Surveillance

For disease monitoring post-transplant, all patients who are seropositive themselves or whose graft is seropositive must receive twice weekly (if an in-patient) monitoring of CMV levels by whole blood (EDTA sample) for PCR (or once weekly in the outpatient setting). This monitoring must continue whilst the patient is considered high risk of reactivation; the first 100 days post-transplant or until systemic immunosuppression has been discontinued, and there is no evidence of graft versus host disease.

7.2.1.5 Treatment

Treatment of CMV reactivation will be undertaken following two consecutive positive CMV PCR levels at, or greater than, the limit of sensitivity, 500 copies/ml or one result of greater than 1000 copies/ml (or depending on local policy). Treatment will also be initiated regardless of PCR if signs of organ-specific disease are identified. Some centres may adopt a policy of preemptive treatment; please refer to your own institution guidelines for advice.

The treatment regimen is often undertaken as an in-patient. In which case, first-line therapy is with intravenous ganciclovir 5 mg/kg twice daily for a minimum of a week. Second-line treatment may be given if there is significant ganciclovir-related bone marrow suppression (neutrophil count less than 1) or treatment failure with rising viral levels or evidence of viral resistance after at least 1 week of treatment.

Second- and third-line treatment is with foscarnet 90 mg/kg twice daily and cidofovir 5 mg/kg weekly for 2 weeks followed by fortnightly until negative. Foscarnet may be adopted as a first-line treatment if the patient reactivates within the first month of transplant when blood counts have not fully recovered as it is less myelotoxic than ganciclovir. It does, however, have more renal complications, and regular electrolyte replacement is often required.

Similarly, cidofovir leads to renal impairment, and a urine sample should be tested prior to infusion for the presence of protein. If proteinuria is greater than 2 on dipstick, or renal function has deteriorated (please refer to hospital/unit guidelines), then cidofovir should not be given.

In asymptomatic patients, or in those with viral levels responsive to the above treatments that are fit for discharge, oral therapy with valganciclovir may be used. Outpatient use of valganciclovir in asymptomatic reactivation is usually confined to those with low-level reactivation around log 3.

Treatment with Ganciclovir and Valganciclovir, Dosing and Administration for Nursing Staff

For detailed instructions consult the summary of product information at website address

http://emc.medicines.org.uk/emc/assets/c/html/displaydoc.asp?documentid=3497

http://emc.medicines.org.uk/emc/assets/c/html/displaydoc.asp?documentid=9315

(accessed 28/7/17)

The normal dose for ganciclovir is 5 mg/kg given every 12 h by intravenous infusion in 100 ml normal saline over an hour, rounded dose to the nearest 25 mg. The drug is an irritant; it is alkaline and may cause chemical phlebitis, so care should be taken to observe the cannula and ensure that it is functioning well prior to each use.

The normal dose for valganciclovir is 900 mg taken every 12 h orally. Valganciclovir is the oral prodrug of ganciclovir, so the same considerations should be made as when using ganciclovir.

Both ganciclovir and valganciclovir should be used with caution in patients with impaired renal function; there is additive toxicity in patients taking other nephrotoxic drugs (e.g. ciclosporin, amphotericin B). In such patients, the dose should be adjusted and must not be given or used together with imipenem-cilastatin due to the increased risk of convulsions.

Ganciclovir and valganciclovir treatment commonly results in cytopenias, and extreme caution should be applied when using it in patients with impaired bone marrow function (neutrophils $<1 \times 10^9$/l or platelets $<50 \times 10^9$/l), and the drug is contraindicated with severely impaired bone marrow function (neutrophils $<0.5 \times 10^9$/l or platelets $<25 \times 10^9$/l). Dose adjustment must be made if there is any degree of renal impairment. Creatinine clearance must be calculated, using the Cockcroft-Gault equation for dosing decisions or another formula at your own institution.

Toxicity

Teratogenicity has been shown in animal models and therefore care should be used in handling the drug. It should not be administered by pregnant staff. Bone marrow suppression is very common, and blood counts should be monitored daily during therapy and visualized prior to infusion. Patients with significant cytopenias should be treated with haemopoietic growth factors and/or discontinuation of therapy if growth factor support is not available or clinically safe. A patient developing a cytopenia must be discussed with the treating consultant for a clinical decision to be made with regard to continuation of therapy.

Gastrointestinal toxicity is common with nausea, vomiting and diarrhoea and should be recorded. Other drugs, e.g. ciclosporin, amphotericin B or MMF, may also potentiate the toxicity of ganciclovir; for further details consult the SmPC email link or discuss with your pharmacist or lead clinician.

Treatment with Foscarnet Dosing and Administration

For detailed instructions consult the summary of product characteristics

http://www.medicines.org.uk/emc/medicine/174 (accessed 28/7/17)

The normal dose is 90 mg/kg   given every 12 h by intravenous infusion. The drug is an irritant; it is alkaline and causes chemical phlebitis; therefore it must be diluted if administered via a peripheral vein; the undiluted solution (24 mg/ml) may be used if administered via a central venous catheter.

Foscarnet should be used with caution in patients with impaired renal function; there is additive toxicity in patients taking other nephrotoxic drugs, e.g. ciclosporin and amphotericin B. To minimize the risk of renal impairment, an additional 500 ml of fluid (saline or dextrose) should be co-administered with each dose of foscarnet.

Toxicity

Nephrotoxicity is a major side effect, with 12–30% of patients showing a significant decline in renal function. Electrolyte disturbance occurs frequently with low magnesium, calcium, phosphate and potassium most commonly requiring regular monitoring at least once daily whilst on treatment and following therapy. Hypocalcaemia complicating the use of foscarnet has been implicated in patients developing seizures on therapy. Local irritation to veins may occur, and it is advised that central venous access should be used if possible together with maintenance of good hydration and diuresis during treatment. Local ulceration in the genital area may also occur in both men and women, and patients should be informed of this at the start of treatment and asked to be vigilant and inform staff if and when this occurs. Strict hygiene should be advised to reduce risk of skin ulceration.

Gastrointestinal toxicity is common with nausea, vomiting and diarrhoea. CNS toxicity is not infrequent, and patients may suffer with headache, dizziness, anorexia and altered mental state. Haematological toxicity is also common and mainly results in anaemia; leucopenia is less common, whilst thrombocytopenia occurs infrequently.

Treatment with Cidofovir Dosing and Administration

For detailed instructions consult the summary of product characteristics

http://www.mhra.gov.uk/spc-pil/?prodName=CIDOFOVIRTILLOMED 75 MG/ML CONCENTRATE FOR SOLUTION FOR INFUSION&subsName=CIDOFOVIR DIHYDRATE&pageID=SecondLevel (accessed 28/7/17)

The normal dose is 5 mg/kg given once weekly by intravenous infusion for two doses, as an induction, and then given twice weekly as a maintenance. Maintenance treatment starts 2 weeks after completion of induction therapy and will continue until clearance of virus. Often the first dose is given as an in-patient, and further doses are given in outpatients if well staffed with appropriate training.

Cidofovir is markedly nephrotoxic and if damage occurs this is often irreversible. As such cidofovir is contraindicated in patients with pre-existing renal dysfunction. Renal toxicity occurs frequently during treatment, and renal function must be monitored closely; deterioration is likely to necessitate discontinuation of therapy. There is additive toxicity in patients taking other nephrotoxic drugs, e.g. ciclosporin and amphotericin B.

To minimize renal toxicity, hydration and probenecid must be administered with each dose of cidofovir. In patients with hypersensitivity to probenecid or sulpha-containing drugs, cidofovir is likely to be contraindicated; such cases must be discussed with the treating consultant before initiating therapy.

Cidofovir also frequently causes non-dose-dependent neutropenia, although this may resolve spontaneously whilst continuing on treatment. Dose interruption is not mandatory in patients developing neutropenia although the risk benefit of continued treatment in such patients must be discussed with the treating consultant or transplant physician.

Toxicity

Renal dysfunction is the major dose-limiting toxicity and may be irreversible. Eighty percent of patients develop proteinuria due to tubular dysfunction whilst on therapy. Gastrointestinal toxicity is common with nausea and vomiting. Haematological toxicity is common and is mainly neutropenia. Alopecia, uveitis and fever are also frequently observed during treatment with cidofovir but resolve on discontinuation.

There are currently several new emerging drugs for the treatment of CMV although these have so far not shown superiority to the above four drugs following phase 1 and 2 clinical trials. These newer therapies include maribavir, brincidofovir and letermovir. Another option for those patients who are difficult to treat could be the use of CMV-specific CTLs. Unfortunately, they are expensive and difficult to obtain.

7.2.2 EBV

7.2.2.1 Introduction

Epstein-Barr virus (EBV) is a latent herpesvirus that is thought to infect as much as 95% of the adult population by the age of 40 years. It is an enveloped and double-stranded DNA virus and human herpesvirus 4 (HHV4). Primary infection with EBV usually results in mild, self-limiting illness of the oropharynx in childhood and the clinical syndrome of infectious mononucleosis in adults and is often asymptomatic.

During the primary infection, an immunocompetent individual will mount a vigorous response. Once the initial infection has cleared, the linear EBV genome becomes circular forming an episome in infected B cells and becomes established as a latent infection awaiting reactivation. This has relevant implications for clinical approaches as antiviral agents such as ganciclovir inhibit the replication of the linear EBV-DNA but are ineffective against episomal DNA. These drugs therefore fail to prevent B-cell proliferation and are of no clinical use in treatment plans (Rasch et al. 2014).

Epstein-Barr virus post-transplant lymphoproliferative disease (EBV-PTLD) results from outgrowth of EBV-infected B cells that are normally controlled by an effective EBV-specific cytotoxic T-cell response that occurs in the immunocompromised host (Deeg and Socie 1998; Heslop 2009). PTLDs are classified as either early-onset lesions which develop within 1 year or late onset occurring greater than a year post-transplant (Ibrahim and Naresh 2012).

7.2.2.2 Presentation and Manifestations

The clinical manifestations of PTLD vary widely and may include nonspecific symptoms such as fever, malaise, sweats, weight loss and in some cases obvious enlargement of lymphoid tissue (Ibrahim and Naresh 2012).

Post-transplant lymphoproliferative disease (PTLD) is a rare but potentially life-threatening disease with an incidence of 1–11% and a mortality of >80% in the pre-rituximab era (Landgren et al. 2009). It is defined as a lymphoid proliferation or lymphoma that develops as a consequence of immunosuppression in a recipient of a solid organ or bone marrow transplant. The immunosuppression required to preserve graft function post-transplant leads to an impairment of T-cell immunity. This allows an uncontrolled proliferation of EBV-infected B cells. This results in monoclonal or polyclonal plasmacytic hyperplasia, B-cell hyperplasia, B-cell lymphoma or immunoblastic lymphoma. Immune surveillance is impaired; the balance between latently infected B-cell proliferation and the EBV-specific T-cell response is disrupted and leads to the infected B cells developing into PTLD (Heslop 2009).

The early detection of EBV viral load by polymerase chain reaction (PCR) in whole blood is widely accepted as the preferred method of monitoring patients and should commence on the day of cell infusion. Viral levels should be monitored weekly for 3–6 months and longer in those with GvHD or on immunosuppression. Those at greater risk are recipients of T-cell-depleted HSCT, HLA mismatches or patients conditioned with antithymocyte globulins (Landgren et al. 2009). Other risk factors that have been identified as predictive for the development of PTLD include recipient pre-transplant EBV seronegativity and donor EBV seropositivity (Styczynski et al. 2009).

It is presumed that EBV is transmitted from donor to recipient via the graft at a time of considerable immunosuppression for the recipient, or the patient develops primary EBV infection unrelated to donor EBV status. It is therefore advisable if possible to choose a seronegative donor if one is available. Reactivation is common but does not always lead to end-organ disease requiring treatment (Styczynski et al. 2009).

Cohen (1991) reviewed cases of PTLD in the literature involving renal, cardiac, heart-lung, liver and bone marrow transplantation. Allogeneic bone marrow transplantation-related PTLD had an incidence of 1.6%. This was much higher if the patient had received mismatched T-cell-depleted bone marrow (24%) or if the patient had received anti-T-cell monoclonal antibodies for graft versus host disease (17%). The mean time interval from transplantation to a diagnosis of PTLD was 5 months, with the majority by 3 months.

The pathological diagnosis of PTLD is based on the WHO classification and includes four main categories and is the basis for the UK BCSH guidelines:

1. Early lesions
   Are those that show features when biopsied of infectious mononucleosis and plasmacytic hyperplasia. These are the first signs in the spectrum of PTLD diagnosis.
2. Polymorphic PTLD
   Comprises small- and medium-sized lymphocytes and Reed-Sternberg-like cells. Underlying cell structure is destroyed and may show malignant features.
3. Monomorphic PTLD
   Comprises large lymphocytes and plasma cells that are uniform in appearance with most being B cells with a clonal abnormality.
4. Classic Hodgkin lymphoma
   This is a rare form of PTLD usually found in renal transplant patients
   (Swerdlow et al. 2008).

In practice, a clear separation between the different subtypes is not always possible; early lesions, polymorphic PTLD and monomorphic PTLD probably represent a spectrum of diseases (Parker et al. 2010). More recently Styczynski et al. (2009) published definitions of EBV that are in common use across Europe.

EBV-DNA-emia:	Detection of EBV-DNA in the blood
Primary EBV infection:	EBV detected in a previously EBV-seronegative patient
Probable EBV disease:	Significant lymphadenopathy (or other end-organ disease) with high EBV blood load, in the absence of other aetiologic factors or established diseases
Proven EBV disease:	(PTLD or other end-organ disease): EBV detected from an organ by biopsy or other invasive procedures with a test with appropriate sensitivity and specificity together with symptoms and/or signs from the affected organ

7.2.2.3 Diagnosis

Early diagnosis is important so that treatment can be initiated promptly. The exact copy or log number to commence therapy has not yet been fully established. Action from a blood test alone is not indicated and should be in parallel with clinical symptoms such as fever and lymphadenopathy and imaging studies (Heslop 2009).

Whether PTLD presents as localized or disseminated disease, the tumours are aggressive and rapidly progressive and often are fatal. Clinical presentation is very variable and includes fever (57%), lymphadenopathy (38%), gastrointestinal symptoms (27%), infectious mononucleosis-like syndrome that can be fulminant (19%), pulmonary symptoms (15%), CNS symptoms (13%) and weight loss (9%). Patients may report fever, weight loss, anorexia, lethargy, sore throat, swollen glands, diarrhoea and abdominal pain, shortness of breath, neurological symptoms or symptoms that initially would not suggest a diagnosis of PTLD. CNS involvement is of particular concern as it offers a dismal prognosis (Deeg and Socie 1998).

The most common sites for involvement are the lymph nodes (59%), liver (31%), lung (29%), kidney (25%), bone marrow (25%), small intestine (22%), spleen (21%), CNS (19%), large bowel (14%), tonsils (10%) and salivary glands (4%). T-cell lymphoproliferative disorders not associated with EBV infection tend to occur at extranodal sites.

7.2.2.4 Monitoring

Reactivation usually occurs in the first 6 months and up to 1 year post-transplant and is predominantly derived from donor B cells before reconstitution of the EBV-specific cytotoxic T-lymphocyte response but can occur later if patients are still heavily immunosuppressed, e.g. when taking ciclosporin (Kuriyama et al. 2014).

7.2.2.5 Treatment

Withdrawal of immunosuppression in the first instance and if patients are still positive then treatment with rituximab monoclonal antibody (anti-CD20) once a CT scan and if possible biopsy has been taken is the standard therapy for transplant PTLD.

The removal of immunosuppression to restore immune response is usually not effective for treating those who develop PTLD very close to their transplant date due to their profound immunosuppressed state. The regenerating immune system is not able to recover fast enough to eradicate the malignant cells. It also carries a risk of

graft rejection. Those who are significantly further away from transplant may reduce the EBV load by removal of immunosuppression alone.

Rituximab has been shown to improve outcome when initiated early as it targets B-cell-specific surface antigens present on the EBV-transformed malignant cells. Rituximab is a chimeric murine/human monoclonal anti-CD20 antibody. As CD20 cells are not only expressed on malignant cells, normal B cells are destroyed in a patient who will already be immunocompromised and may lead to other viral infections. The effect of rituximab on the B-cell compartment can be up to 6 months following treatment and should therefore be used with caution and under strict surveillance in specialist centres. Failure to respond to single-agent rituximab leads to the option of chemotherapy in the form of CHOP (cyclophosphamide, doxorubicin, vincristine and prednisolone).

Additional options such as adoptive T-cell therapies are still unavailable in many centres, but some series of studies suggest that this may offer response to those in whom standard rituximab has failed. EBV-specific cytotoxic T cells (CTL) aim to selectively restore the impaired immune function by the adoptive transfer of EBV-specific cytotoxic T cells. CTLs can be generated by using EBV-infected lymphoblastic cell lines to sufficiently stimulate donor-derived T cells, expand them over a 3–4-week period and then give to the patient. This is a time-consuming process and one that the patient can often not wait for. A quicker process for rapidly generating CTLs by overnight stimulation of donor mononuclear blood cells with EBV-specific peptides, selection of Ag-specific T cells by IFN-gamma surface capture assays and subsequent immunomagnetic selection has been developed although not widely available. There is an associated high risk of developing acute or chronic GvHD post infusion, and so risk benefit should be discussed with the patient (Rasch et al. 2014).

Rituximab is given by IV infusion and is not a vesicant. It is initially given slowly to reduce the risk of a reaction with each subsequent cycle given quicker as tolerated. A reaction to rituximab is thought to be mediated by a cytokine release from both normal and malignant B cells.

The most common adverse events (AEs) with rituximab include infusion reactions, the majority of which are mild to moderate (grades 1 and 2) in nature. Seventy-seven percent of any grade infusion reactions occur during the first infusion, and the incidence decreases with each subsequent infusion. These infusion reactions generally resolve with the slowing or interruption of the infusion and with supportive care. The incidence of grade 3 or 4 infusion-related events in patients is reported to be 9% for the first infusion of rituximab. The majority of severe reactions occur approximately 30–120 min after starting the first infusion.

7.2.3 HHV6

7.2.3.1 Introduction
Human herpesvirus 6 (HHV6) is a ubiquitous virus, and more than 90% of the population over the age of 2 years are seropositive as it is easily passed person to person via saliva. It is usually latent and is commonly reactivated in approx. 30–70% of post-allogeneic stem cell transplant patients.

7.2.3.2 Risk
Those at increased risk are HLA mismatches, and those on corticosteroid therapy for GvHD and highest of all are umbilical cord (UCBT) allografts with an incidence of 9% compared to 1% in BM or PBSC recipients. It is postulated that the higher incidence is due to the lack of memory T cells in the UCBT against HHV6 that are present in adult donors.

7.2.3.3 Presentation
HHV6 may be associated with the development of encephalitis in 1–11% of patients and also in some reports of pneumonia (Zerr et al. 2005). HHV6 can be divided into two groups HHV6 variants A and B. Primary infection with HHV6B causes exanthema subitum (roseola infantum) in infants, whilst the role of HHV6A in disease is not yet fully explored (Ljungman et al. 2000). HHV6 typically reactivates earlier than cytomegalovirus post allograft.

The evidence for the relationship between HHV6 positivity and encephalitis is not conclusive especially as HHV6 is often asymptomatic. Clinically patients present 2–6 weeks post allograft with delirium, amnesia, confusion, ataxia and seizure. During the transplant process, HHV6 has been cited by Zerr et al. (2005) to cause a delay in engraftment with up to 60% more platelet requirements in those who become positive.

7.2.3.4 Diagnosis
Memory loss is cited as the most common feature; this can develop to confusion and then finally to unconsciousness. HHV6 may accompany the syndrome of inappropriate antidiuretic hormone (SIADH). On magnetic resonance imaging (MRI) of the head, there are hyperintense lesions noted, and these are referred to as post-transplant acute limbic encephalitis (PALE). Upon examination of the cerebrospinal fluid (CSF), HHV6 DNA is observed. For a confirmed diagnosis to be made, the gold standard would be tissue biopsy. This is impossible in the acutely unwell post-transplant patient, and therefore the accepted approach is PCR testing of CSF and the exclusion of other causes for the patient's symptoms.

7.2.3.5 Treatment
Foscarnet and ganciclovir are the recommended treatments and should be started as soon as possible following symptoms suggestive of HHV6 (Ogata et al. 2015).

7.2.4 *Pneumocystis jirovecii*

7.2.4.1 Introduction
Pneumocystis jirovecii (PCP) is an atypical fungus that causes severe pneumonia in immunocompromised patients. Recognized as a protozoan initially and reclassified in 1988 as a fungus, pneumocystis cannot be propagated in culture, and few treatment options exist for those with PCP pneumonia. It is ubiquitous with almost universal seropositivity by 2 years of age (Thomas and Limper 2004). The accepted belief for

contracting PCP was as a reactivation of a latent virus. However, evidence suggests that PCP may occur following recent infection and may also be transmitted person to person. Many hospital policies do not mandate isolation, but a pragmatic approach is often taken, and HSCT recipients should avoid exposure to those with proven PCP (Gea-Bancloch et al. 2009).

7.2.4.2 Risk Factors

It is recommended that all allograft patients are adequately covered with prophylaxis for PCP for at least 6 months and up to 1 year or more if on immunosuppression with combination trimethoprim-sulfamethoxazole (TMP-SMX) as this has reduced incidence of infection to approximately 5% (Castro et al. 2005). Prophylaxis usually starts at the point of engraftment or upon discharge as TMP-SMX can cause engraftment delay.

The most effective first-line prophylaxis is a combination of trimethoprim-sulfamethoxazole given in a variety of doses dependent upon your local policy. If the patient develops any sensitivity to these drugs, then alternatives are pentamidine nebulizer, atovaquone and oral dapsone. If dapsone is to be used, then glucose 6-phosphate dehydrogenase (G6PD) deficiency should be ruled out. G6PD is highly prevalent in African, Asian, Oceanian and Southern European populations, and those with G6PD deficiency may develop acute haemolytic anaemia. Nebulized pentamidine can cause bronchospasm, and patients need to be informed of this prior to inhalation. Atovaquone is generally well tolerated but poorly absorbed unless taken with a high fat diet. Patients in the immediate post-transplant setting may struggle with this especially those with GI GvHD issues (Gea-Bancloch et al. 2009).

7.2.4.3 Presentation

Those with PCP present with symptoms of subtle onset dyspnoea, a low-grade temperature and a non-productive cough, and when examined, the chest is clear on auscultation. However, this may rapidly change with the onset of hypoxia requiring admission to a critical care unit. Imaging of the chest with X-ray reveals bilateral perihilar interstitial infiltrates that become increasingly homogenous and diffuse as the disease progresses. Computed tomography (CT) scans show extensive ground-glass attenuation or cystic lesions (Thomas and Limper 2004).

7.2.4.4 Diagnosis

Patients have a 50% mortality associated with the development of PCP; prompt diagnosis and treatment are warranted with adherence to prophylactic cover. Due to the difficulties of culturing samples, the diagnosis of PCP is made through microscopic examination of sputum or bronchoalveolar fluid or by polymerase chain reaction (PCR).

7.2.4.5 Treatment

If PCP pneumonia is suspected, treatment is with trimethoprim-sulfamethoxazole and the addition of systemic steroids to reduce the inflammatory lung processes. For those that are intolerant to trimethoprim-sulfamethoxazole, then atovaquone or a combination of clindamycin with primaquine is licenced for use (Chen et al. 2003).

7.2.5 Varicella Zoster Virus

7.2.5.1 Introduction

Varicella zoster virus (VZV) infection or chickenpox is usually a childhood disease, and transmission is either by inhalation of respiratory secretions or direct physical contact. Following exposure the virus remains latent in the dorsal root ganglion, and when it reactivates, it is referred to as "shingles" or herpes zoster. Herpes zoster is grouped painful vesicular lesions that can affect several dermatomes in immunocompetent people. In the setting of allogeneic stem cell transplantation, VZV carried a major risk of morbidity and mortality with 18–52% patients having clinically apparent infection related to reactivation of latent virus; however, with the use of aciclovir, this number has decreased (Thomson et al. 2005). Complications such as post-herpetic neuralgia, skin scarring and bacterial superadded infection are factors in morbidity (Steer et al. 2000; Boeckh et al. 2006).

7.2.5.2 Risk Factors

All stem cell transplant patients should receive prophylaxis for (VZV) with oral aciclovir or valaciclovir for 6 months to 1 year (according to local policy) or until immunosuppression is discontinued (Kanda et al. 2001). Transmission of VZV is difficult to prevent as the period prior to symptoms where an individual is contagious can be up to 48 h before the appearance of a rash. The incubation period varies from 10 to 21 days, and an individual remains contagious until all of the vesicles have crusted over. If the immunocompromised patient is in contact with an individual with VZV infection (varicella or HZ), they are at significant risk of developing varicella themselves and will require prompt action from the transplant team (Styczynski et al. 2009).

HSCT will probably destroy any previous immunity to VZV. Immunization of family contacts especially children is advised to reduce risk.

7.2.5.3 Presentation

VZV infection occurs in 40–50% if prophylaxis stopped at 6–12 months, with a peak incidence around 5 months and a spread of 2–10 months, usually occurring within 5 weeks of cessation of oral prophylaxis (Steer et al. 2000). Risk factors include unrelated donors, myeloablative conditioning, graft versus host disease (GvHD) and the use of systemic corticosteroids. Pain in the back or abdomen with distension and a rise in ALT are seen in approx. Ten % of patients prior to the development of a rash. The rash may spread to more than 1–3 dermatomes in patients with visceral dissemination and is more difficult to treat.

7.2.5.4 Diagnosis

The best method for diagnosing VZV is by polymerase chain reaction (PCR) testing of blood or a glass slide touched to a vesicle as the DNA is highly specific and sensitive.

7.2.5.5 Treatment

Treatment for those who have been exposed to a healthy individual with VZV infection is advised depending upon the serostatus of the recipient and availability of drug. Patients who are seronegative and are less than 2 years post allograft or

who have active chronic GvHD or are taking immunosuppressive medications should have intravenous varicella zoster immunoglobulins (VZIG). If this passive immunization medication is unavailable, then high-dose aciclovir, valaciclovir or famciclovir (nucleoside analogues that interfere with viral thymidine kinase activity) can be employed.

Post treatment for VZV, it is advisable to restart prophylactic aciclovir if this was previously discontinued. The length of time prophylaxis should be continued will be guided by local policy and may range from 1 year to lifelong.

7.2.6 Adenovirus

7.2.6.1 Introduction

Adenovirus (ADV) is a ubiquitous non-enveloped double-stranded DNA virus. It currently has more than 50 serotypes and is divided into six subgroups A–F (La Rosa et al. 2001). Adenovirus is more prevalent in children but is becoming more prevalent in adults in the transplant population.

7.2.6.2 Risk Factors

Adenovirus is spread by aerosolization or the faecal-oral route with approx. 80% of children aged 1–5 years old seropositive. Risk factors include mismatched or unrelated donor, acute graft versus host disease (aGvHD) and isolation of ADV from multiple sites (Ljungman et al. 2003).

7.2.6.3 Presentation

In healthy individuals, infection is self-limiting causing conjunctivitis and upper respiratory tract, urinary tract or gastrointestinal infections and remains latent in lymphocytes post exposure. Chakrabarti et al. (2002) report a 5–29% incidence of ADV after allogeneic stem cell transplantation.

7.2.6.4 Diagnosis

Those with viral-like symptoms usually have a full screen of virology requested that will include ADV. Samples taken from nasopharyngeal, rectal and corneal secretions, urine and unfixed biopsy tissue can be examined with PCR to assess viral load. Similar to those with viral reactivation of CMV and EBV, low level of ADV infection does not carry a high mortality. However, those patients that develop invasive disease, such as ADV colitis, have a significant mortality of 20–80% (Robin et al. 2007).

7.2.6.5 Treatment

Cidofovir is first-line treatment and is a monophosphate nucleotide analogue of cytosine. Cidofovir inhibits viral DNA polymerase and has a low bioavailability with 90% of the drug excreted in the urine. Patients require hyperhydration and oral probenecid pre, during and post cidofovir to protect nephrons.

7.2.7 Hepatitis B

7.2.7.1 Background

The hepatitis B virus (HBV) is a DNA virus classified in the hepadna virus family. Patients infected by HBV prior to transplantation have a higher risk (70–86%) of HBV reactivation 5 years after HSCT transplantation. An active immunization of donors and early post-transplant vaccination of recipients have been suggested to avoid HBV reactivation. Donors should optimally receive more than one immunization, a rather high Ag dose and a highly immunogenic vaccine (Lindemann et al. 2016).

The use of chemotherapy and immunosuppression can reactivate latent hepatitis B. Further, HBV infection or reactivation contributes to liver-related morbidity and mortality; it occurs in 21–53% of patients, especially after conditioning regimens containing alemtuzumab. Transplantation of HBV-negative patients with stem cells from an infected donor (HBsAg positive) is associated with a high risk of transmission; some patients develop chronic hepatitis B. Donors with active HBV (DNA detection) should receive, if possible, antiviral treatment (Ullmann et al. 2016).

7.2.7.2 Clinical Features

Post-transplant HBV infection can arise in different ways. Patients may have active HBV (HBsAg positive) prior to transplant or reactive latent HBV infection (HBsAg negative). Infection may also occur during the transplantation process, from an infected HSC donor or rarely from infected blood products. HBV DNA titer may rise to very high levels, particularly in patients receiving corticosteroids. At the time of immune reconstitution or during reduction of immunosuppressive drugs, a flare is given by a rise in serum aspartate aminotransferase (AST) and alanine aminotransferase (ALT) levels. Another clinical symptom is jaundice and fulminant liver failure as a result of HBV (liver-related mortality) (Lau et al. 2003).

7.2.7.3 Treatment

Lamivudine (100 mg/day) is the first choice for antiviral therapy for treatment, which should be continued for at least 6 months following discontinuation of immunosuppressive drugs in allogeneic haematopoietic cell transplantation patients (Tomblyn et al. 2009).

7.2.7.4 Prevention

Several studies in the literature describe prevention of HBV reactivation in the setting of immunosuppression. HBV reactivation has been variably reported as ALT elevation above upper limit of normal or by increases from baseline. Patients who undergo HSCT for haematological malignancy are an "at-risk" population because of the prolonged immunosuppression following the conditioning chemotherapy.

The nucleoside analogue antiviral drugs lamivudine, adefovir, telbivudine, entecavir and tenofovir may all be of potential use in the prevention of HBV reactivation in such patients. The majority of reports describe the use of lamivudine or entecavir, and both drugs appear to reduce the incidence of HBV reactivation. However, entecavir (and potentially tenofovir) may be superior to lamivudine because of more potent viral suppression and lower risk of antiviral resistance.

Prophylaxis for HBV reactivation with antiviral nucleoside analogues should be commenced in susceptible individuals before the initiation of chemotherapy, in order to lessen the risk of HBV reactivation and the associated adverse clinical outcomes (Pattullo 2016).

7.2.8   Hepatitis C

7.2.8.1   Background

The hepatitis C virus (HCV) is a double-stranded RNA virus classified within the Flaviviridae. Six major genotypes have been identified, from HCV1 to HCV6. It can be responsible for several systemic complications. The extrahepatic manifestations include vasculitis, fatigue, cryoglobulinemia and autoimmune disorders. HCV replication is significantly increased by immunosuppression and may cause a direct cytopathic effect in infected cells. The identification of pre-transplant HCV infection appears clinically relevant. Being infected with HCV has been indicated as an independent risk factor for post-transplant veno-occlusive disease (VOD) of the liver. Reactivation of chronic HCV infection after tapering immunosuppressive therapy can sometimes lead to fulminant hepatic failure (Locasciulli et al. 2009).

7.2.8.2   Clinical Features

HCV infection is responsible for hepatic and extrahepatic manifestations. After 1 year post HSCT, HCV infection course has an increased risk of fatal sinusoidal obstruction syndrome and later hepatic inflammation occurring 3–6 months after HCT, coincident with immune reconstitution and interruption of immunosuppressive medications. The symptom of liver decompensation among patients who had cirrhosis at the time of transplant has been described in the literature, and rarely, fatal fibrosing cholestatic HCV can occur before day 100 in recipients receiving mycophenolate mofetil (Torres et al. 2015).

HCV infection is associated with high risk for several complications, which include accelerated liver disease progression, acute HCV exacerbation and viral reactivation. The last two are common, but not associated with increased liver-related mortality rates or changes in HSCT care (Kyvernitakis et al. 2016).

A reported case of severe HCV reactivation occurred early (<30 days after HCT) with elevated ALT and bilirubin levels. Liver biopsy revealed chronic portal inflammation, bile duct injury and moderate cholestasis (Oliver et al. 2017).

HCV adversely impacts on platelet recovery, non-relapse mortality and overall survival. Sinusoidal obstruction syndrome (SOS), liver graft versus host disease (GvHD) and hepatic problems are more likely to be severe and fatal in recipients with HCV. Pre-transplant HCV infection is associated with a lower rate of platelet recovery. An excess of bacterial infections in HCT recipients with HCV infection has been reported, and these findings suggest that the defence mechanisms against bacterial infections are impaired in recipients with HCV (Nakasone et al. 2013).

7.2.8.3   Treatment

All HSCT recipients with HCV infection should be evaluated for HCV therapy before the start of conditioning therapy. Whenever possible, HCV-infected HSCT candidates should commence and complete HCV therapy before transplant. If there is an oncologic imperative for moving quickly to transplant, a therapy with direct-acting antiviral agents (DAAs) should be able to clear extrahepatic HCV from donors more quickly than interferon and ribavirin.

Treatment of post-transplant HCV infection must be an urgent consideration for patients with fibrosing cholestatic HCV, patients with cirrhosis whose condition is deteriorating and patients who underwent HSCT for HCV-related lymphoproliferative disorders. Once HCV therapy is initiated, treatment interruption is not recommended because it is associated with increased risk of treatment failure. The alternative to pre-HSCT therapy for HCV is to treat after HCT using DAAs following immune reconstitution.

All long-term HCV-infected HSCT survivors should be offered DAAs therapy.

HCV therapy should be undertaken by providers experienced in management of HCV in HSCT. There are many combinations of DAAs, depending on HCV genotype. Commonly used DAAs include daclatasvir, sofosbuvir, ledipasvir, ombitasvir, paritaprevir, ritonavir, dasabuvir, simeprivir and ribavirin. The choice of regimen should be individualized on the basis of patient-specific data, and take into consideration potential drug interactions with tacrolimus, sirolimus and ciclosporin (Torres et al. 2015).

7.2.8.4 Prevention

A vaccination against HCV does not exist. However, to prevent the complication of co-infection, people with hepatitis C should be vaccinated against hepatitis A and B. Standard precautions are recommended for the care and treatment of all patients, regardless of their perceived or confirmed infectious status and in handling of blood, all other body fluids, secretions and excretions, non-intact skin and mucous membranes (ASHM 2012).

HCV-infected donors should be evaluated for HCV therapy and treated before cell harvest, in order to prevent transmission of HCV to uninfected recipients (Torres et al. 2015).

7.2.9 Emerging Infections (Hepatitis E)

7.2.9.1 Background

Hepatitis E virus (HEV) is a single-stranded, non-enveloped RNA virus. It was discovered in 1983 by investigators of an outbreak of unexplained hepatitis in Russian soldiers in Afghanistan. In areas with poor sanitation, HEV 1 and 2 are spread orofaecally between humans, usually via contaminated water. In developed countries, HEV 3 and HEV 4 are transmitted from animal reservoirs. HEV antibodies were found in pig farmers, slaughterhouse workers, veterinarians, and farm labourers. In Western Europe the food chain is the main source of infection, where HEV is transmitted through the consumption of contaminated animal meat (undercooked pig liver). Person-to-person transmission is uncommon, although nosocomial and parenteral transmission in haemophiliac and in haemodialysis patients has been reported (Marano et al. 2015).

7.2.9.2 Clinical Features

The most common symptom of HEV is jaundice, followed by:

- Malaise/lethargy
- Nausea and vomiting
- Abdominal pain
- Loss of appetite
- Myalgia
- Fever
- Loss of weight
- Neurological features

Extrahepatic manifestations of acute and chronic hepatitis E involve the following systems and organs (Dalton et al. 2015) (Table 7.1).

7.2.9.3 HEV in Developing Countries

After an incubation period of 2–6 weeks, genotypes 1 and 2 develop to HEV infection. The source of infection is human, mostly by faecal-oral route via infected water. Outbreaks can occur at times of flooding/monsoon and can involve thousands of cases. Symptoms of HEV progress with fever, nausea, abdominal pain, vomiting,

Table 7.1 Extrahepatic manifestations of acute and chronic hepatitis E

Neurological system	Haematological system	Other organs
Guillain-Barré syndrome	Thrombocytopenia	Acute pancreatitis
Brachial neuritis	Lymphopenia	Arthritis
Transverse myelitis	Monoclonal immunoglobulin	Autoimmune thyroiditis
Bell's palsy		
Vestibular neuritis		

anorexia, malaise and hepatomegaly. Jaundice is present in about 40% of patients. Pregnant females and individuals with underlying chronic liver disease present a high mortality.

7.2.9.4 HEV in Developed Countries

Numerous studies report that autochthonous HEV is a problem across Europe and that infection has a predilection for middle-aged elderly males (mean age ≈ 60 years). Large outbreaks do not occur, most cases are sporadic and the source of infection remains uncertain in most cases. In the developed countries, we can distinguish between acute and chronic hepatitis E.

Acute

Acute HEV is mostly caused by genotypes 3 and 4. Jaundice occurs in about 75% of patients, and the clinical manifestations are the same as those of hepatitis E in developing countries. HEV infection may be misdiagnosed as drug-induced liver injury (DILI) and is responsible for extrahepatic disorders: neurological disorders, kidney injury, acute pancreatitis associated with HEV 1 and haematological disorders as thrombocytopenia and aplastic anaemia.

Chronic

No studies have assessed the prevalence or incidence of HEV infection among haematological patients receiving chemotherapy. A small number have been found to have a chronic HEV infection and include a patient with untreated hairy cell leukaemia, a patient with idiopathic CD4 T lymphopenia and patients treated for lymphoma, chronic myelomonocytic leukaemia and B-cell chronic lymphocytic leukaemia. HEV RNA was found in 8 of 328 stem cell transplant patients and 5 developed chronic hepatitis (Kamar et al. 2014).

One case of chronic HEV infection following allogeneic haematopoietic stem cell transplantation was reported in 2015 as differential diagnosis for graft versus host disease (Bettinger et al. 2015).

7.2.9.5 Treatment

In haematological patients, pegylated interferon alone and ribavirin alone for 3 months have been used (Kamar et al. 2014).

7.2.9.6 Prevention

Immunocompromised patients should be screened for HEV antibodies and RNA not only prior transplantation but also post-transplantation and during episodes of liver enzyme abnormalities.

In immunocompetent patients adequate cooking procedures for porcine and boar/deer meat are useful to prevent HEV disease (De Keukeleire and Reynders 2015).

This is a list of the more common virus that patients develop during transplantation.

Rhinovirus	Role of treatment is limited by lack of agents and RCT
Influenza	Oseltamivir +/− zanamivir (research and some limited European areas use IV peramivir, favipiravir)
Respiratory syncytial virus	Ribavirin (research and Europe again use palivizumab)
Parainfluenza	Ribavirin +/− IVIg in some centres
Metapneumovirus	Ribavirin +/− IVIg in some centres
Coronavirus	Role of treatment is limited by lack of agents and RCT
Bocavirus	Role of treatment is limited by lack of agents and RCT

7.2.10 Multiply-Resistant Bacteria: Reducing the Spread

7.2.10.1 Background

Multidrug-resistant organisms (MDRO) have emerged as significant pathogens in haematology and haematopoietic stem cell transplant recipients. Neutropenia and malignancy are independent risk factors for MDRO-invasive infections. Resistant *Escherichia coli* and *Klebsiella pneumoniae* bacteraemia and carbapenemase-producing *K. pneumoniae* (KPC) are emerging in haematology populations with associated mortality, as well as increasing rates of vancomycin-resistant *Enterococci* that are responsible for up to 41% of all gram-positive bacteraemias.

Infection prevention, antimicrobial stewardship and antimicrobial prophylaxis are essential for control and management of MDRO. Hand hygiene, environmental cleaning/disinfection, isolation and surveillance are indeed the backbone of effective prevention programs (Trubiano et al. 2013).

In 2014 the World Health Organization declared antimicrobial resistance a worldwide threat that requires urgent action.

7.2.10.2 Contact Precautions

The application of contact precautions (CP) requires that gowns and gloves should be worn when entering the patient's room and removed before leaving it. Dedicated equipment such as stethoscopes or blood pressure cuffs should remain in the patient's room and not be used for other patients. CP may include single-room isolation, an entire isolation ward or cohorting of a group of patients (with or without designated staff). The aim of CP is preventing transmission of epidemiologically important pathogens from a colonized or infected patient through direct (patient or healthcare personnel) or indirect (surfaces or roommates in the patient's environment) contact. In addition to hand hygiene, appropriate CP measures should decrease the risk of MDRO transmission.

Current controversies remain whether patients only colonized, rather than infected, with MDROs should be subjected to isolation. Another issue is the impact of CP on patient's well-being. Healthcare workers who care for patients in contact isolation enter their rooms less frequently and have significantly less direct contact with them. Patients express greater dissatisfaction with their treatment and have less documented care (Landelle et al. 2013).

A review by Cohen et al. (2015) reports that CP do not represent a statistically significant improvement in MDRO infection control. Five of the six reviewed studies did not find significant association between CP and reduction in MDRO transmission (Cohen et al. 2015).

7.2.11 Gram-Positive Bacteria

Gram-positive (gram+) pathogens cause significant morbidity and mortality in bone marrow transplant recipients.

- *Enterococci*
- Vancomycin-resistant *Enterococci* (VRE)
- *Coagulase-negative Staphylococcus* (CNS)
- *Staphylococcus aureus*
- Methicillin-resistant *Staphylococcus aureus* (MRSA)
- *Streptococcus viridans*
- *Streptococcus pneumoniae*

7.2.11.1 *Enterococci*

Enterococci are gram-positive aerobes and facultative anaerobes which are seen microscopically as single, pairs and short chains and are part or the normal flora of the gastrointestinal tract. In transplant recipients, enterococcal infections are usually nosocomial and occur generally as invasive infections in the immediate post-transplant period, mostly as a consequence of endogenous gram-positive translocation.

7.2.11.2 Vancomycin-Resistant *Enterococci* (VRE)

VRE, also known as glycopeptide-resistant *Enterococci*, are increasingly causing outbreaks in haematology units.

At many transplant centres, VRE are the predominant organism causing pre-engraftment bacteraemia among HSCT recipients.

The evidence for an association between acting contact precautions and surveillance testing or not and the incidence of VRE bacteraemia starts to stagger.

VRE are strongly associated with colonization pressure, and strategies to reduce VRE burden in colonized patients may reduce VRE transmission. Infection control efforts should include contact precautions, and the need for active surveillance testing should be guided by local epidemiology (Kamboj and Sepkowitz 2014).

However, Almyroudis et al. (2016) reported on the discontinuation of systemic surveillance and contact precautions for VRE and its impact on the incidence of VRE faecium bacteraemia in patients with haematological malignancies. In this study, the incidence of VRE bacteraemia remained stable after discontinuation of surveillance and contact precautions. Furthermore, contact isolation can be associated with medication errors, reduced visits of physicians and nurses, safety concerns such as increased falls and bedsores, anxiety and depression among patients and a significant increase in the cost of care (Almyroudis et al. 2016).

7.2.11.3   *Coagulase-Negative Staphylococcus* (CNS)

CNS are members of the Micrococcaceae family, produce catalase and divide in irregular clusters to produce packets of cells. Transplant recipients with a central venous catheter (CVC) are particularly vulnerable to CNS infections. CNS cause surgical wound infections and infections associated with lines, including CVC bacteraemia, CVC local infections and drain-associated peritonitis.

7.2.11.4   *Staphylococcus aureus*

Staphylococcus aureus occurs microscopically as single, pairs and short chains and has a strong tendency to form clusters. *Staphylococcus aureus* is mainly found in the nasopharynx and on the skin.

Methicillin-susceptible *Staphylococcus aureus* (MSSA) and methicillin-resistant *S. aureus* (MRSA) are major causes of infections after transplantations. The prevalence of vancomycin-intermediate *S. aureus* (VISA) and heterogeneous or heteroresistant VISA (hVISA) is reported to be increasing worldwide. *S. aureus* truly resistant to vancomycin (VRSA) is very rare, and no data are available for the transplant population (Garzoni 2009).

7.2.11.5   MRSA

According to the Center for Disease Control and Prevention guidelines (ref website? access date?), HSCT centres should follow stringent infection control practices handwashing, contact precautions, including wearing gloves whenever entering the MRSA-infected or colonized patient's room. MRSA is indeed transmitted via an infected or colonized patient or by a colonized healthcare worker.

Patients with MRSA should be placed under CP until all antibiotics are discontinued and until three consecutive cultures, taken >1 week apart, are negative. Screening cultures for MRSA include the anterior nares, any body site previously positive for MRSA and any wounds or surgical site (Dykewicz and Kaplan 2000).

7.2.11.6   *Streptococcus viridans*

Streptococcus viridans are facultative anaerobic, gram-positive cocci and are part of the normal microflora, found mainly in the oral cavity but also in the upper respiratory, gastrointestinal and female genital tract. Septicaemia is the most common manifestation in bone marrow transplant (BMT) recipients (Ihendyane et al. 2004).

To lessen the risk of oral sources of infection following HSCT, dental treatment and oral hygiene instructions given 3–4 weeks before the HSCT are required (Tomblyn et al. 2009).

7.2.11.7   *Streptococcus pneumoniae*

Streptococcus pneumoniae is a gram-positive diplococcus causing significant morbidity and mortality in all age groups, wherein children, the elderly and immunocompromised patients are especially vulnerable. Pneumococcal infection may occur during hospitalization for the transplant procedure but more commonly occurs as a community-acquired infection, months or years following the transplantation as meningitis or fulminant sepsis.

7.2.12 Gram-Negative Bacteria

Over the last decade, multidrug-resistant (MDR) gram-negative (gram-) pathogens have been implicated in severe healthcare-associated infections, and their occurrence has increased steadily. The emerging problem of carbapenemase-producing *Enterobacteriaceae* has become a major healthcare threat with associated mortality also in haematology populations.

The recommended strategies to prevent healthcare-associated transmission of gram-negative bacteria are prompt laboratory-based identification, adherence to contact precautions and strict hand hygiene. Further, more expensive approaches include dedicated equipment and staff, especially for patients with MDR in the respiratory tract. Cohorting patients in a specific hospital area can be effective but also very disruptive. Finally, integration of antimicrobial stewardship efforts based on dominant MDR organisms may help prevent future problems (Kamboj and Sepkowitz 2014).

The ESCMID guidelines for the management of the infection control measures to reduce transmission of multidrug-resistant gram-negative bacteria in hospitalized patients by Tacconelli et al. (2014) summarize the importance of adherence to hand hygiene, wearing contact precautions and using disposable single-use or patient-dedicated care equipment and performing active screening cultures, as well as the role of environmental cleaning and antimicrobial stewardship and the role of infrastructure and education to reduce the spread.

7.2.12.1 *Enterobacteriaceae*

Enterobacteriaceae are facultative anaerobes and are intestinal colonizers. *Enterobacteriaceae* encompass a large heterogeneous family of gram-negative bacteria, which are divided into lactose fermenters as *Escherichia coli*, *Citrobacter*, *Klebsiella spp.* and *Enterobacter spp.* and non-lactose fermenters *Salmonella*, *Shigella*, *Proteus* and *Yersinia*.

7.2.12.2 *Klebsiella pneumoniae*

K. pneumoniae is encountered as a saprophyte in humans and other mammals, colonizing the gastrointestinal tract, skin and nasopharynx. In the past it has been seen as an important causative agent of community-acquired infections, including a severe form of pneumonia. In the early 1970s, infections caused by *K. pneumoniae* became a leading cause of nosocomial infections. High carriage rates have been recorded in patient's nasopharynx and hands, as well as the gastrointestinal tract. *K. pneumoniae* has a considerable efficiency of colonization, enhanced by acquired resistance to antibiotics, which enables it to persist and spread rapidly in healthcare settings.

K. pneumoniae is a notorious "collector" of multidrug resistance mechanisms, such as the "carbapenemases" encoded by transmissible plasmids. The clinically most important carbapenemases in *Enterobacteriaceae* are the class A enzymes of the KPC type, then the zinc-dependent class B metallo-ß-lactamases (MßLs), represented mainly by the VIM, IMP and NDM types and the plasmid-expressed class D carbapenemase of the OXA-48 type. Carbapenemase-producing *Enterobacteriaceae* (CPE) cause serious infections in immunocompromised patients, in association with prolonged hospital stay and increased mortality rates, because of panresistance to antimicrobials (Tzouvelekis et al. 2012).

7.2.12.3 Carbapenemase-Producing *Klebsiella pneumoniae*

Carbapenemase-producing *Klebsiella pneumoniae* (CP-Kp) are emerging in immunosuppressed patients, and their expansion represents a challenging problem in terms of outcome and management. A retrospective study by Girmenia et al. reports that CP-Kp were documented in 87 allogeneic HSCT in 52 Italian centres, and a colonization documented before or after transplant was followed by an infection in 39% of allogeneic HSCT (Girmenia et al. 2015). An analysis of 50 cases of KPC bloodstream infections (BSI) in neutropenic patients with haematological malignancies or aplastic anaemia, conducted by Tofas et al. reports that all episodes of KPC BSI were hospital-acquired, the median duration of hospitalization before the onset of bacteraemia was

22 days and 48 of 50 CP-Kp produced KPC enzyme and 2 produced VIM enzyme (Tofas et al. 2016).

7.2.12.4 *Pseudomonas aeruginosa*

Pseudomonas aeruginosa is a glucose non-fermenting gram-negative rod. It is a strict aerobe pathogen, cosmopolitan in distribution, with a particular predilection for moist environments. *Pseudomonas aeruginosa* has shown the ability to acquire resistance to all traditionally effective agents, such as anti-pseudomonal penicillins, third- and fourth-generation cephalosporins, aminoglycosides, fluoroquinolones and carbapenems.

Patient gastrointestinal colonization serves as an important reservoir for endogenous infection, as well as the source of horizontal transmission to other patients.

In patients with haematological malignancies, enteric colonization by *Pseudomonas aeruginosa* occurs typically after chemotherapy.

7.2.12.5 *Acinetobacter baumannii*

Acinetobacter baumannii is a nonfermentative gram-negative pathogen. Its ability to survive on dry, inanimate surfaces for long periods of time suggests that the hospital environment serves as a reservoir for MDR strains. *Acinetobacter baumannii* can be resistant to many or all available antibiotics. Multidrug resistance is common in the US hospital-acquired infections, estimated up to 60%.

Colonized patients' skin may serve as effective reservoirs, and healthcare workers' hands can serve as vehicles for transmission. Commonly employed strategies to avoid the spread of *Acinetobacter baumannii* include identifying and eliminating common sources of contamination, optimizing contact isolation and hand hygiene to minimize cross-transmission, enhancing environmental cleaning to reduce contamination and reducing broad-spectrum antibiotic use (Lin et al. 2014).

7.2.13 *Clostridium difficile*

7.2.13.1 Background

Clostridium difficile is an anaerobic, gram-positive spore-forming bacterium and increas-ingly identified as the cause of nosocomial diarrhoea in growing numbers of patients. Patients who are admitted for treatment of haematological malignancies or undergoing HSCT are at high risk for *Clostridium difficile* infection (CDI). Risk factors for CDI include exposure to broad-spectrum antibiotics, which can cause changes to the microbiota of the gut, total body irradiation, long hospitalization, immunocompromised state, older age and irritation of the intestinal mucosa by chemotherapy drugs (Gu et al. 2015).

7.2.13.2 Infection Control Management

(Adapted from Debby Weston, Fundamentals of Infection Prevention and Control, 2013).

Isolation

- In the event of confirmation of a *Clostridium difficile* (CD) toxin-positive result in a patient with diarrhoea, who is not already isolated, the patient must be moved to a single room with en suite bathroom or dedicated night commode.
- An isolation notice must be displayed on the door.
- The nurse looking after the patient should inform the infection prevention control team.
- Isolation can be discontinued once the patient has been asymptomatic for 48 h and is passing "normal" stools.

Equipment and Cleaning

- Dedicated patient equipment must be used, including disposable blood pressure cuffs and tourniquet.
- Floors, night commodes, toilets and bed-frames are subject to the heaviest faecal contamination; it is important that the ward environment should not be cluttered in order to facilitate thorough and effective ward cleaning.
- On discharge or transfer of the patient, it is important that an accurate clean of the room is undertaken using 1000 ppm available chlorine and/or a sporicidal agent.

Hand Hygiene

- The patient should be assisted with hand hygiene after using the toilet or night commode and before eating if unable to wash his or her hands independently.
- Healthcare workers must wash their hands with soap and water after contact with the patient or his/her environment. Alcohol hand rubs or gels are not effective against *Clostridium difficile* spores.

Personal Protective Equipment (PPE)

- Wear gloves and apron before entering the patient's room.
- Remove apron and gloves before leaving the patient's room.
- Hands must be decontaminated before putting on and after removing gloves.
- Ensure that all healthcare workers and visitors wear and dispose of PPE appropriately.

Waste and Linen

- Any clinical waste and linen, including bedding and, if present, curtains, should be considered contaminated and managed properly.

Movement of Patients

- Patients with CD should not be transferred to other wards in the hospital, except for isolation purposes or if they require specialist care on another ward.
- When patients need to attend departments for essential investigations, the nurse looking after the patient is responsible for informing the receiving area in advance of the patient's CD-positive status; if possible, symptomatic patients should be seen at the end of the working session and should be sent for only when the department is ready to see them; it should be avoided to leave them in a waiting area with other patients.

CD spores are known to contaminate the environment, are resistant to standard disinfectants and are capable of surviving for long periods on dry surfaces. 10% bleach solutions are sporicidal and should be used for environmental decontamination during outbreaks.

The combination of strict hand hygiene and contact precautions (gloves and apron) significantly reduces the incidence of CD (Dubberke and Riddle 2009).

7.2.13.3 Treatment

First-line treatment is given by oral metronidazole (500 mg three times daily for 10–14 days) and/or vancomycin (125 mg every 6 h for 10–14 days) (Kamboj et al. 2014).

Gu et al. (2015) report a treatment with berberine when CDI first symptoms appeared and they did not have severe cases of CDI in the study. Berberine is a traditional Chinese medicine that has been used to treat bacterial or secretory diarrhoea for 12,000 years in China. Additional studies are needed to demonstrate whether berberine could be a new useful therapeutic agent to alleviate clinical symptoms of CDI (Gu et al. 2015).

Further treatments of recurrent CDI are fidaxomicin, probiotics, intravenous immunoglobulin and faecal transplants.

7.2.13.4 Faecal Microbiota Transplant

The treatment with faecal microbiota therapy consists in a technique that involves transfer of fresh stool from a healthy donor to the gastrointestinal tract of the patient suffering from severe or recalcitrant *Clostridium difficile* infection (CDI). In the case report by Neemann et al. (2012), the donated stool sample was screened for transmissible pathogens, ova and parasites, *Clostridium difficile*, *Salmonella*, *Shigella*, *Campylobacter* and *Escherichia coli*. After a brief liquefaction procedure, 30 ml of fresh stool suspended in non-bacteriostatic saline was slowly injected via nasojejunal tube into upper jejunum, followed by non-bacteriostatic saline flush. Within 2 days of faecal transplant, the patient had no further diarrhoea or haematochezia. For fulminant CDI unresponsive to metronidazole and/or vancomycin, the definitive treatment has been colectomy, but faecal microbiota therapy should be considered a potentially bowel- and life-saving intervention, if other medical modalities fail (Neemann et al. 2012).

Another case reported by Castro et al. (2015) describes a persisting CDI infection and diarrhoea 10 months after bone marrow transplantation. The patient had an allergic response to oral vancomycin and was subsequently treated with oral metronidazole and i.v. meropenem. After performing faecal microbiota transplantation with material from two different donors, the patient's bowel showed significant improvements, and any antibiotic were not needed anymore (Castro et al. 2015).

7.3 BMT Setting, Infection and Infection Control

7.3.1 Introduction

Haematopoietic stem cell transplantation (HSCT) can be defined as the transfer of haematopoietic stem cells (HSCs) from one individual to another (allogeneic HSCT) or the return of previously harvested cells to the same individual (autologous HSCT) after manipulation of the cells and/or the recipient (Tomblyn et al. 2010).

Haematopoietic stem cell transplantation (HSCT) is a major procedure, which needs the use of chemotherapy. Some patients who are undergoing allogeneic transplantation for haemato-oncological malignancies will require radiotherapy. The use of these treatments, coupled with the patient's disease, compromises the immune system. The administration of immunosuppressant to prevent graft rejection contributes also to the high risk of infections in this patient group (Brown 2010).

In recent years, improvement in HSCT supportive care measures, better understanding of the mechanism of immunosuppression, the introduction of reduced intensity conditioning (RIC) regimens and new anti-infectious agents and prophylactic strategies have decreased infectious morbidity and mortality. However, there is still scope for improvement since infection remains a leading cause of morbidity and mortality in patients undergoing HSCT (Gratwohl et al. 2005).

Principal risk factors for infections after HSCT are:
- Status of the haematological disease at HSCT
- Comorbidities of the patient
- Degree and duration of neutropenia
- Disruption of anatomical barriers (mucositis and indwelling catheters)
- Depressed T- and B-cell function and immunosuppressive therapy

Reconstitution of immune status after HSCT depends on:
- Type of transplantation (autologous or allogeneic)
- Source of progenitor cells (bone marrow, peripheral blood or cord blood)
- Conditioning regimen (myeloablative, RIC or non-myeloablative)
- Degree of histocompatibility between the donor and the recipient (sibling, unrelated or mismatch)
- Type of GvHD prophylaxis (calcineurin or mTOR inhibitors, mono or polyclonal antibodies or T-cell depletion)
- Presence and grade of GvHD and its treatment

Depending on these factors, the patient can be rendered immunodeficient for months or even years after HSCT (Rovira et al. 2012).

There is a clear relationship between the type of immunodeficiency after HSCT and the incidence of certain infections. According to this, three different periods can be distinguished, with a predominance of specific pathogens in each phase (Fig. 7.2) (Tomblyn et al. 2010; Rovira et al. 2012).

The chronology of the previously mentioned infections was described in patients receiving a myeloablative HSCT, and some differences can be observed in recipients of autologous HSCT or RIC-HSCT. Thus, in the autologous setting, bacterial infections are less frequent and severe, and the other infections are exceptional (Rovira et al. 2012).

However, autologous candidates who receive immunosuppressive agents (steroids, purine ana-

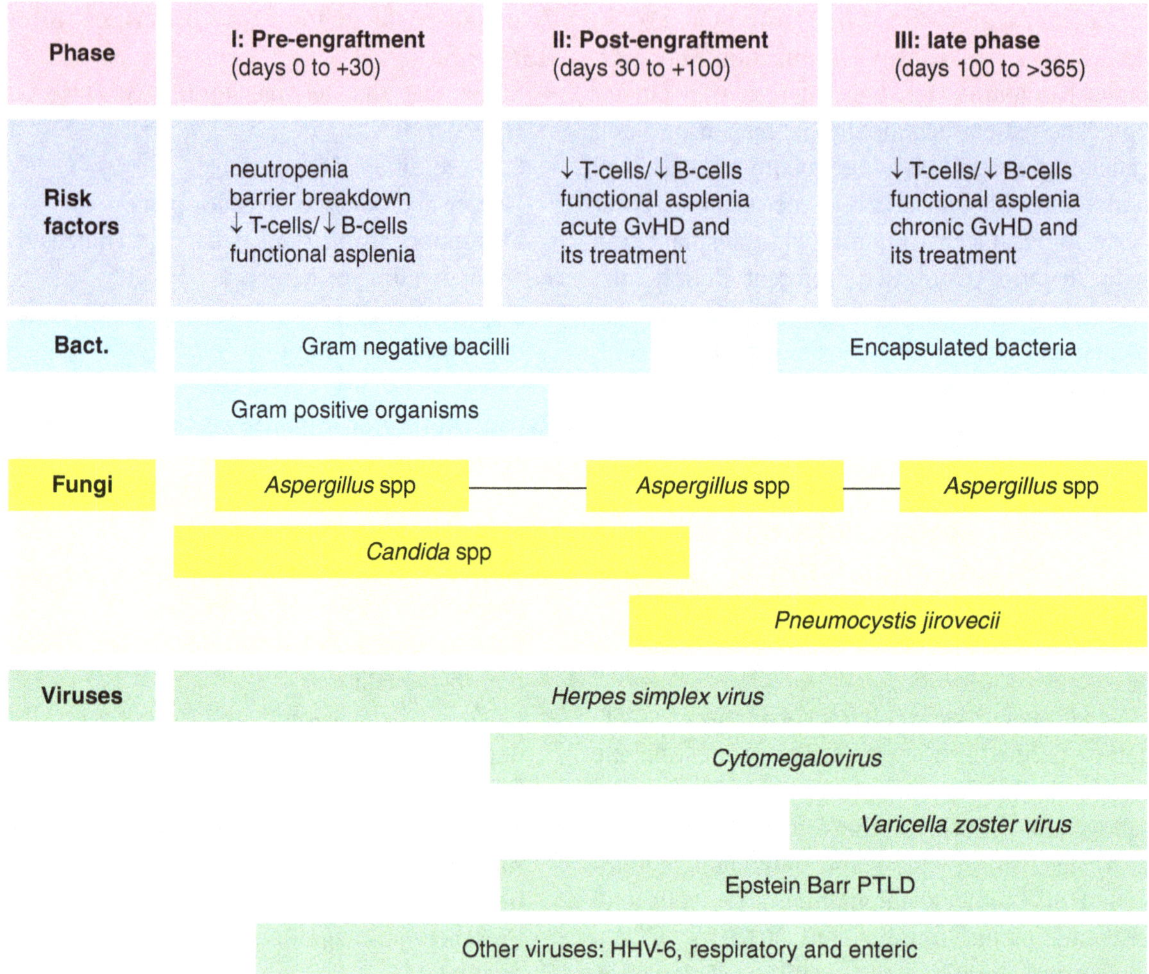

Fig. 7.2 Chronology of predominant infections after HSCT (Adapted from [1] and granted permission from (EBMT Handbook 2012))

logues or monoclonal antibodies such as rituximab or alemtuzumab) or with severe hypogammaglobulinaemia prior to the auto-HSCT run the same risk of developing infections as those patients undergoing allogeneic SCT.

In the past two decades, RIC-HSCT has been used increasingly worldwide (Rovira et al. 2012). Infections related to neutropenia and mucositis are less common with this modality of HSCT than after conventional HSCT. However, viral and fungal infections occurring in the intermediate and late period are comparable because the incidence and severity of GvHD are similar to that observed in myeloablative HSCT. Additionally, RIC-HSCT is usually used in older patients, who are usually in poorer general condition with or without the presence of comorbidities; for all these reasons, the infection-related mortality has not decreased in this setting (Rovira et al. 2012; Masszi and Mank 2012).

7.3.2 Reverse Barrier Nursing and Protective Isolation

Infections are a major cause of morbidity and mortality in allogeneic transplantation (Parody et al. 2006). Therefore, it is crucial to have a skilled nursing team to assess, prevent, detect and treat infections.

Delays in diagnosing an infection that results from a depressed inflammatory response may lead to increased susceptibility to a broad range of potentially life-threatening organisms. For this reason, in addition to antimicrobial prophylaxis, there are other important strategies to prevent infections, for example, building a multi-professional network team specialized in infection control measures (Masszi and Mank 2012).

7.3.2.1 Protective Isolation and Cleaning

The large number of patients considered at risk requires an evaluation of all proposals of protective systems, in relation to the effectiveness, applicability and cost benefit (Pizzo 1981).

The Centres for Disease Control and Prevention (CDC) has published in 2007 very specific recommendations regarding precautions to be taken in haematopoietic stem cell transplant.

(HSCT) reported and updated in 2009.

The CDC recommends a protective isolation for patients who are undergoing allogeneic HSCT. The indications are the use of single room and the use of filtered air entering through a central or portable high-efficiency filter (HEPA), capable of removing 99.97% of $\geq 0,3$ uM in diameter particles.

For autologous HSCT, there is no specific indication other than the reference to "standard" precautions (as shown in Table 7.2) for each interaction with the patient. Protection with lab

Table 7.2 Standard precautions of infection control (https://www.dhs.wisconsin.gov/ic/precautions.htm)

Standard precautions	Standard precautions are a set of infection control practices used to prevent transmission of diseases that can be acquired by contact with blood, body fluids, non-intact skin (including rashes) and mucous membranes. These measures are to be used when providing care to all individuals, whether or not they appear infectious or symptomatic
Hand hygiene	Hand hygiene refers to both washing with plain or antibacterial soap and water and to the use of alcohol gel to decontaminate hands. When hands are not visibly soiled, alcohol gel is the preferred method of hand hygiene when providing healthcare to clients
Personal protective equipment (PPE)	PPE includes items such as gloves, gowns, masks, respirators and eyewear protectors used to create barriers that protect the skin, clothing, mucous membranes and the respiratory tract from infectious agents PPE is used as a last resort when work practices and engineering controls alone cannot eliminate worker exposure The items selected for use depend on the type of interaction a public health worker will have with a client and the likely modes of disease transmission Wear gloves when touching blood, body fluids, non-intact skin, mucous membranes and contaminated items. Gloves must always be worn during activities involving vascular access, such as performing phlebotomies Wear a surgical mask and goggles or face shield if there is a reasonable chance that a splash or spray of blood or body fluids may occur to the eyes, mouth or nose Wear a gown if skin or clothing is likely to be exposed to blood or body fluids remove PPE immediately after use and wash hands. It is important to remove PPE in the proper order to prevent contamination of skin or clothing
Needle stick and sharp injury prevention	Safe handling of needles and other sharp devices is a component of standard precautions that are implemented to prevent healthcare worker exposure to blood-borne pathogens. The Needlestick Safety and Prevention Act (link is external) mandates the use of sharps with engineered safety devices when suitable devices exit
Cleaning and disinfection	Client care areas, common waiting areas and other areas where clients may have potentially contaminated surfaces or objects that are frequently touched by staff and clients (doorknobs, sinks, toilets other surfaces and items in close proximity to clients) should be cleaned routinely with EPA-registered disinfectants, following the manufacturer's instructions for amount, dilution and contact time

(continued)

Table 7.2 (continued)

Respiratory hygiene (cough etiquette)	Clients in waiting rooms or other common areas can spread infections to others in the same area or to local public health agency staff. Measures to avoid spread of respiratory secretions should be promoted to help prevent respiratory disease transmission. Elements of respiratory hygiene and cough etiquette include: Covering the nose/mouth with a tissue when coughing or sneezing or using the crook of the elbow to contain respiratory droplets Using tissues to contain respiratory secretions and discarding in the nearest waste receptacle after use Performing hand hygiene (handwashing with non-antimicrobial soap and water, alcohol-based hand rub or antiseptic handwash) immediately after contact with respiratory secretions and contaminated objects/materials Asking clients with signs and symptoms of respiratory illness to wear a surgical mask whilst waiting in common areas or placing them immediately in examination rooms or areas away from others. Provide tissues and no-touch receptacles for used tissue disposal Spacing seating in waiting areas at least three feet apart to minimize close contact among persons in those areas Supplies such as tissues, wastebaskets, alcohol gel and surgical masks should be provided in waiting and other common areas in local public health agencies. Place cough etiquette signs (link is external) where the general public can see them
Waste disposal	
Safe injection practices	Outbreaks of hepatitis B and hepatitis C infections in US ambulatory care facilities have prompted the need to re-emphasize safe injection practices. All healthcare personnel who give injections should strictly adhere to the CDC recommendations

coat, gloves and mask is not indicated in the absence of suspected or confirmed infection of patients (Tomblyn et al. 2010). The effectiveness of specific precautions in preventing infections in patients undergoing autologous HSCT has not been evaluated but must follow the standard precautions for every patient contact.

Some centres use additional protection in an effort to reduce the risk of infection, but there are insufficient data to recommend such behaviours (Tomblyn et al. 2010). Consistent with the organization of the department, it would be advisable to hospitalize the patient in a single room with attached bathroom, in order to give them greater comfort. The ventilation system should ensure at least 12 air changes per hour; a direct flow area of the room must have the way out on the opposite side with respect to that of entry. The optimum ambient air quality can be obtained without using the expensive laminar flow. The rooms, housing highly immunocompromised patients, need to be placed under positive pressure to prevent the entry into the room of airborne pathogens in the hallway or in adjacent spaces. In the rooms it is forbidden to keep fresh flowers and/or dried and potted plants (Tomblyn et al. 2010). Although it

is unlikely that exposure to plants causes invasive fungal infections in patients undergoing HSCT, it is recommended that plants and dried or fresh flowers do not enter the room during hospitalization (conditioning phase included) because of the *Aspergillus sp.*, isolated from soil of ornamental plants and flowers. In addition it was found a high proportion of gram-negative bacteria in the water of the cut flower vase (*Pseudomonas*) (Tomblyn et al. 2010).

For the patient hospitalized in a protective environment, exits from the room should be restricted just for the execution of diagnostic tests and for a short period. If a construction site is present nearby the hospital, it is indicated to use a filter mask (N95) to prevent inhalation of spores. There are no recommendations regarding use of the mask with filter in the absence of the construction work (Tomblyn et al. 2010).

7.3.2.2 Handwashing

The most important point in the prevention of infections in hospitalized patients, being in protective isolation, remains handwashing. Hand hygiene is a key element of the standard precautions for all types of patients (Tomblyn et al. 2010).

All staff and visitors must wash their hands before entering the patient's room in order to reduce the risk of cross infection.

Hand hygiene should be performed before touching the patient, before a clean/aseptic procedure, after body fluid exposure risk (blood, body fluids or excretions, mucous membranes, non-intact skin or dressing), after touching a patient and after touching patient's surrounding (WHO "My five moments for hand hygiene" 2009). It is also advisable not to wear false nails or extensions during direct contact with the patient and maintain the natural nails short. Even if there is still an unsolved problem, many studies have shown that the skin below the rings is more colonized than that without; rings and dirty jewelry can host microorganisms.

Furthermore hand hygiene cannot be done in a perfect way if you wear bulky rings. The experts' recommendation is strongly discouraging the use of rings during assistance (WHO guidelines 2009).

Nurses have an important role in educating the family, patient and visitors to an effective handwashing (as shown in Fig. 7.2) and to provide all relevant information to reduce the risk of contracting infections.

Some transplant centres display cartoons near the sinks at the entrance of the hospital room, where they describe the handwashing procedure step by step and how it needs to be performed (WHO guidelines 2009).

7.3.2.3 Environmental Cleaning

The environmental cleaning plays an important role in the prevention of nosocomial infections, particularly in patients with haematological cancers and diseases undergoing transplantation of haematopoietic stem cells. The cleaning staff must be well prepared and needs to be informed and trained, with particular attention to the problems of immunosuppressed patients. It is preferable to assign stable staff to the division, in order to ensure a continuity of service. The hospital room must be cleaned more than once a day, with special dust control, which must be removed by damp.

The light fixtures and outdoor grills of ventilation vents and all horizontal surfaces should be cleaned with pre-moistened disposable cloths with a disinfectant FDA and Environmental Protection Agency approved. The design and selection of the furniture of a transplant program should be focused in creating and maintaining an environment: free of dust and the floors and finishes should be brushable, waterproof, easy to disinfect and antistatic (Tomblyn et al. 2010).

To verify that hospital rooms are at effective reduced environmental load, periodic monitoring of the environments must be guaranteed.

7.3.2.4 Management of Linen

All linen should be changed daily and pillows and mattresses should have protective coatings. During the hospital stay for the patient undergoing HSCT, it is enough to wash clothes and linens at high temperatures in a washing machine (Tomblyn et al. 2010).

7.3.2.5 Access to Low Environmental Loading Department

Each centre has its own policy on the number of visitors allowed and the frequency of visits. However, all centres are in agreement in pointing out that they cannot come into contact with the patient when cooled or suffering from other infections, rashes, eyes' infections, nausea and/or vomiting or recent exposure to exanthematous diseases such as chickenpox or measles (Tomblyn et al. 2010).

7.3.2.6 Personal Hygiene

Personal hygiene is a key aspect for the patient undergoing HSCT. It represents the most effective way to reduce infections caused by endogenous organisms. The interview with the patient and his family is a very important moment and must be programmed before HSCT. The nurse must be able to define when, how and which are the major needs for the patient. It is important to explain the importance of personal hygiene and its role in preventing infections. Several centres are supported by audio-visual media and information booklets to reinforce the provided infor-

Table 7.3 Recommendations for personal hygiene, Carreras 2006, CDC 2007

When	How	What
Take a shower every day using mild liquid soap in dispensers Thorough intimate hygiene must be performed after each evacuation, especially in case of diarrhoea	Patients are advised to gently rub the skin and dry it accurately especially at the level of the armpits and groin, where the body microorganisms can proliferate if they find a moist environment	Do not use sponges or knobs (only if disposable) For teeth cleaning, it is recommended to use synthetic brushes with soft bristles
Towels need to be replaced every day	The material for the toilet must be new and in closed packs For dry and peeling skin, it may be useful to apply moisturizer on the body	During the hospitalization period, the following products should not be used: Soaps, perfumes, deodorants and aftershave containing alcohol, cotton sticks for ear cleaning (patient should clean the external pinna with soap and water only), lipsticks
Patients should be advised to cut the nails of the hands and feet before admission, as, during aplasia, they are more susceptible to infections and bleeding. Also keeping short nails facilitates good hand hygiene. Enamel or false nails should be removed	Thorough personal hygiene will allow the patient to evaluate daily the state of his/her skin and promptly notify the physician and nursing staff of any changes such as erythema, desquamation, haematomas	For men an electric razor is recommended; razor blades and scissors are forbidden due to their increased bleeding risk

mation. The nurse, giving precise indications, must be able to explain with thoughtfulness and sensitivity how incident personal hygiene is on the individual's intimate and personal sphere.

Table 7.3 shows recommendations of panel expert and of CDC (Carreras 2006; CDC 2007).

7.3.2.7 Oral and Gastrointestinal Mucositis

Oral and gastrointestinal mucositis caused by high-dose chemotherapy and/or radiation continues to be an important clinical problem.

Incidence of WHO grade 3 or 4 oral mucositis can be as high as 75% in patients undergoing HSCT, depending on the intensity of the conditioning regimen used and the prophylactic use of methotrexate to prevent graft versus host disease. Management of oral and gastrointestinal mucositis is one of the main challenges during the period of aplasia, with risk of sepsis related to degree of mucosal barrier breakdown and depth of marrow suppression (Peterson et al. 2015).

Oral care is an important aspect in the control of infections in transplant patients (Quinn et al. 2008). In order to improve oral care in patients undergoing chemotherapy/HSCT, it is useful to build a multi-professional team including medical, dental and nursing, nutrition, physical therapy and counselling providers. Training and continuing education programs will ensure that the knowledge will spread to an extensive community of healthcare providers, which can make a positive impact on patients' healthcare (Sharon Elad et al. 2014). All treatment strategies aimed to improve mouth care are dependent on four key principles: accurate assessment of the oral cavity, individualized plan of care, timely preventive measures and correct treatment initiation (Quinn et al. 2008).

7.3.2.8 Central Venous Devices

The use of central venous catheters (CVC) is linked to the need to infuse complex therapies for a long time, having available a valid and secure access. Generally the choice of the most appropriate catheter is shared by a multidisciplinary team taking into account the patient's compliance and the therapeutic process which he/she will face. The goals of care, for the CVC management, must aim to ensure prevention of infections and maintenance of the patency. This is feasible if the device is managed by competent healthcare workers and if the process is based on continuous improvement of performance (RCN 2010; INS 2011; CDC 2011).

The most important recommendations concerning the prevention of CVC-related bloodstream infections are:

- Hand hygiene and maximum barrier precaution.
- Appropriate choice of insertion site and catheter material.
- Plan an echo-guided insertion when possible, for both centrally and peripherally inserted central lines.
- Use of 2% chlorhexidine for skin antisepsis for continuous and discontinuous antisepsis of the exit site.
- Use of sutureless devices (StatLock) for fixing the catheter, wherever possible.
- Use of appropriate dressing.
- Removing the venous catheter when no longer necessary.
- Assessment → inspection (visual and palpation) of the exit site should be performed daily.
- Proper handling of parenteral solutions.
- Proper management of infusive lines.
- Education of the patients on the need to inform the nurse if changes at the level of the CVC are noticed.

7.3.2.9 Low Bacterial Diet

The low bacterial diet (LBD), also known as neutropenic diet or low microbial diet, is a diet aimed at reducing the ingestion of bacterial and fungal contaminants excluding it from foods such as fresh fruits and vegetables, raw eggs, raw meat and fish, unpasteurized dairy products, ice and yogurt that will be excluded from any type of diet or raw food containing probiotics. The consumption of fruits with thick skin, if peeled and washed, in accordance with good hygienic practices has low probability to be contaminated (Todd et al. 1999).

For decades, the concept of a neutropenic diet or diet containing food with low levels of bacteria (LBD) has implied a strict limitation of foods allowed for consumption, as a presumptive means of reducing the risk of infection in cancer patients.

The rationale was to limit the introduction of potentially harmful bacteria into the gastrointestinal tract by the restriction of certain foods that might harbour those organisms (Fox and Freifeld 2012).

However, there is no clear evidence that the use of a low bacterial diet (LBD) actually decreases the number of infections. It is clear from numerous surveys of current practice that the majority of hospitals place neutropenic patients on a restricted diet (Mank et al. 2008).

Many studies have limitations and conclude that there are no differences in terms of infectious episodes and survival when comparing a normal to a neutropenic diet (Van Tiel et al. 2007; Gardner et al. 2008; Trifilio et al. 2012).

In a randomized study of 153 patients with acute myeloid leukaemia undergoing induction therapy, no difference in terms of infectious episodes and survival was reported between patients prescribed with a LBD and those put on a normal diet. The conclusion was that the LBD has not prevented major infections or death (Gardner et al. 2008).

Notably, a study on the use of a non-neutropenic diet showed an increase in satisfaction for the meal from a 42.9% to a maximum of 75%. The feedback of the team was positive (Tarr and Allen 2013).

Patients who are prescribed a neutropenic diet may have a poor nutritional status and often need counselling and nutritional support (Murray and Pindoria 2009).

A study conducted in Brazil shows how dietary restrictions can lead to a deficiency of vitamin C (Galati et al. 2013).

A retrospective study in 2012 of 726 patients undergoing HCT showed that the rate of acute grade II–IV GI GvHD was higher in the neutropenic diet (ND) group, although the difference between the groups did not reach statistical significance. An association between GvHD and ND has not been reported previously. Almost one-half of the patients in the ND group who subsequently developed GvHD had a previous *C. difficile* infection, and non-relapse mortality was very high in this group. Nutritional support guidelines for patients with GI GvHD, which are also on common sense, include a low microbial diet (Trifilio et al. 2012).

The study results are in line with preclinical experiments conducted on mice where the presence of a mixed intestinal flora (e.g. Lactobacillus rhamnosus GG) would be able to decrease the proliferation of the most virulent bacterial species and of the system that immunomodulate what is in their intestine (Docampo et al. 2015).

A more liberal diet could bring benefits in terms of palatability, cholesterol reducing, use of parenteral nutrition and an improvement in quality of life.

The LBD, usually poorer from a nutritional point of view and less attractive compared to a normal diet, may be an unnecessary burden on patients who already have difficulties with eating. The studies reviewed do not support significant results on the effectiveness or ineffectiveness of the LDB, and many useful results still do not encourage the use of LBD.

7.3.2.10 Psychological Support

Protective isolation can have significant psychological effects on the patient. Patients are encouraged to personalize their rooms with family pictures. Some may have computer access and are able to maintain communication with family members and friends in this way. However, the length of time spent in isolation does lead to many patients having feelings of anxiety, fear for the future, concerns about the family and worry about whether engraftment will occur (Brown 2010). The need for regular monitoring of blood is a constant reminder of the patient's situation. Loss of body image as a result of weight loss or scars, sexuality issues and concerns about employment may preoccupy a patient (Gruber et al. 2003). Nurses should be aware of the potential effect that both, the transplant and the isolation, can have on patients. Spending time with the patient and offering him or her an opportunity to talk about concerns can be helpful. Providing information, education and advice may reduce the negative psychological effects of isolation (Brown 2010). However it should be considered for selected categories of patients the possibility

of an early discharge after transplantation to provide a more comfortable environment for patients and their family.

Increasing implementation of ambulatory treatment has the potential to decrease patient exposure to multidrug-resistant organisms in the hospital and to provide patients with the possibility to spend the neutropenic phase at home and to facilitate more admissions to the haematology ward (Mank et al. 2015).

7.3.2.11 Health Education at Discharge

Discharging is much desired by the patient, but it is the "most difficult time" in the course of treatment. Patient and family will have to face everyday life far from a safe hospital environment. In fact, in the hospital, the continued support of the multidisciplinary team makes them feel protected; in hospital, doctors, nurses and other professionals are always present to clarify doubts, give advice and also try to reduce anxiety and fears. Being aware of the risks of infection means that going home can be stressful (Brown 2010).

Nurses should spend time with the patient, identify and explore any concerns before discharge. In some cases, the patient may become overdependent on nursing staff, and this may need to be addressed. Allogeneic transplant patients have a high risk of readmission as a result of infection, and it is critical that discharge planning provides patients with the understanding and information on how best to minimize the risk of infection (Grant et al. 2005).

A checklist of information, which patients should receive on discharge, is provided in Table 7.4.

Patients should be advised to continue their oral care routine. It is very important.

reiterating to patients when handwashing should be carried out, particularly:

- Before eating
- Before and after meal preparation
- Before and after handling pets
- After sneezing or coughing
- Before taking oral tablets

Table 7.4 Discharge checklist for patients following allogeneic stem cell transplantation (Brown 2010 modified)

Discharge checklist for patients following allogeneic stem cell transplantation
Patients should avoid contact with people who have respiratory illnesses
Care should be taken when around schoolchildren, as there is a risk of exposure to sick children
Patients should be advised to stop smoking and avoid smoky areas for the first few months following transplantation
Patients should avoid communal swimming pools in the early weeks of discharge
It is advisable to avoid house cleaning, which will disturb dust
When considering travel, patients should seek advice regarding travel vaccinations, particularly if they would need live vaccines
It is essential that patients continue to take their medication and attend all follow-up outpatient appointments

- After touching soiled linen
- After going outdoors

(Brown 2010).

The patient will require a great deal of information before and at discharge, and this would include information on follow-up treatment.

7.4 Respiratory Infections

As recent research suggests, pulmonary complications are a leading cause of post-transplant complications and death in HSCT recipients (Alsharif 2009; Roychowdhury et al. 2005). Post-transplant pulmonary complications are classified as either infectious or noninfectious. The rate of complications is significantly lower for autologous transplant recipients than for allogeneic transplant recipients. This is because of the absent risk of GvHD in autologous transplants, the infrequent use of immunosuppressive medications such as ciclosporin or tacrolimus and the absence of radiation therapy in the preconditioning regimen (Ho et al. 2001; Kotloff et al. 2004). Methods that healthcare professionals can use to improve patient outcomes in autologous and allogeneic recipients include raising clinical awareness, improving diagnostics, shortening time to medical intervention and continuing multidisciplinary research (Stephens et al. 2013). The spectrum of pulmonary complications for transplant recipients will continue to change, due in part to rapid advances in supportive care, the increasing age of transplant recipients, new antiviral and antifungal agents and an increasing use of prophylactic broad-spectrum antibiotics post-transplant (Sharma et al. 2005). The real key, however, to decreasing morbidity and mortality in adult and paediatric HSCT patient populations remains in effective diagnostic techniques (Stephens et al. 2013).

Pulmonary infections are the largest cause of post-HSCT infective morbidity and have been reported in most recipients, carrying a mortality rate of 20% (Cooke et al. 2008; Zuccotti et al. 2005). The principal cause of infection is the severe immunocompromised status of the patients from the disease process (malignant or non-malignant), conditioning regimens (non-myeloablative and myeloablative) and immunosuppressive prophylaxis to prevent and treat GvHD. A CT study by Escuissato et al. (2005) found that viral infections (51%) were the most common in post-transplant recipients, followed by bacterial infections (23%), fungal infection (19%) and protozoal infections (less than 1%). In 5% of the cases examined, patients had two or more infectious agents concurrently.

7.4.1 Typical Onset of Pulmonary Complications Following Stem Cell Transplantation

Table 7.5.

7.4.2 Diagnostics

Diagnostic techniques for pulmonary disease in HSCT patients are similar to that for non-

Table 7.5 Typical onset of pulmonary complications following stem cell transplantation divided into three stages based on information from Antin and Raley (2009) Camus and Costabel (2005), Coomes et al. (2010), Polovich et al. (2009), and Soubani and Pandya (2010)

Day 0 to day 30	
Infections related to conditioning regimen and neutropenia	Pulmonary oedema
	Pleural effusion
	Transfusion-related acute lung injury
	Idiopathic pneumonia syndrome
	Engraftment syndrome
	Diffuse alveolar haemorrhage
	Aspergillosis
	Candidaemia (*Candida* sepsis) and candidiasis (general *Candida* infections)
	Respiratory viruses – Respiratory syncytial virus, parainfluenza, influenza
	Bacteraemias of gastrointestinal origin
	Infections of central venous catheter origin
	Acute respiratory distress syndrome (ARDS)
	Chemotherapy-associated pulmonary toxicity
Day 31 to day 100	
Classic opportunistic infections	Pulmonary veno-occlusive disease (due to hepatic sinusoidal obstructive Syndrome)
	Diffuse alveolar haemorrhage
	Cytomegalovirus
	Aspergillosis
	Pneumocystis carinii pneumonia
	Respiratory viruses – Respiratory syncytial virus, parainfluenza, influenza
	Toxoplasmosis
	ARDS
	Idiopathic pneumonia syndrome
	Chemotherapy-associated pulmonary toxicity
Greater than day 100	
Infections from encapsulated organisms	Aspergillosis
	Respiratory viruses – Respiratory syncytial virus, parainfluenza, influenza
	Varicella zoster virus
	Cytomegalovirus
	Pneumocystis carinii pneumonia
	Post-transplant lymphoproliferative disorder
	Pneumonia
	ARDS
	Bronchiolitis obliterans
	Bronchiolitis obliterans organizing pneumonia
	Chemotherapy-associated pulmonary toxicity

transplant patients. Chest radiograph (X-ray) and thoracic computed tomography (CT) scan remain the most popular and less invasive options. CT scans are particularly useful when compared with two-dimensional X-rays because they can expose acute and chronic changes in the lung parenchyma. Respiratory CT scans involve taking pictures of cross-sections of lung tissue using high special-frequency reconstruction during inhalation and exhalation (Stephens et al. 2013).

Changes such as nodules, "white out" and a "glassy" appearance signal the physician and radiology staff to consider additional diagnostics (Truong et al. 2010). This could include collecting sputum samples, bronchoscopy with or without bronchoalveolar lavage (BAL), open lung biopsy and needle biopsy (Kaplan et al. 2011; Truong et al. 2010).

Sputum samples can be collected by nurses, physicians or respiratory therapists according to transplant program protocols. Respiratory virus detection is highly dependent on the type of sample collected, the time of collection after the onset of clinical symptoms, the age of the patient and the transport and storage of the sample prior to testing. Several different upper respiratory tract specimens are applicable for testing, including nasopharyngeal (NP) washes, NP aspirates and NP swabs placed in virus transport media (Specter 2009; Storch 2000). Expectorations in the early morning or after a respiratory procedure can be the easiest for the patient to produce because of the natural accumulation of secretions at these times. About 15 ml of sputum is usually required for adequate laboratory analysis, and a recent study suggested that the sputum must reach the laboratory within a few hours from expectoration (Murray et al. 2010). Sputum can also be collected during a bronchoscopy. In some cases, broncholveolar lavage (BAL) will be performed during the bronchoscopy. BAL involves the flushing of fluid (usually a sterile normal saline solution) into a localized area of the lower respiratory tract and then immediately suctioning the fluid up the bronchoscope and into a sterile specimen container. BAL allows for the detection and characterization of several respiratory pathogens, including viral, fungal and bacterial agents, and is considered a major diagnostic mechanism for *Pneumocystis carinii* (now called *Pneumocystis jirovecii*) pneumonia (PCP) (Forslöw et al. 2010). In patients with focal pulmonary lesions, aspergillosis or pulmonary GvHD, fine-needle aspiration biopsy is considered the first-line diagnostic method (Gupta et al. 2010).

7.4.3 Bacterial Infections

These most commonly occur in the first month but can occur at any time. Both gram-negative and gram-positive organisms can cause pneumonia, the most common being *Escherichia coli*, *Klebsiella*, *Pseudomonas*, *Enterobacter*, *Acinetobacter*, *Staphylococcus aureus*, coagulase-negative *Staphylococcus*, *Streptococcus pneumoniae*, *Streptococcus viridans* and *Enterococcus*. One also needs to recognize the risk of *Mycoplasma* and Chlamydia infections, although the common use of fluoroquinolones will empirically treat these organisms. Other causes of late pneumonia that should not be missed include *Nocardia*, *Listeria* and *Actinomyces*.

7.4.4 Viral Causes of Pneumonia

These include CMV, herpes simplex virus (HSV), varicella zoster virus (VZV), adenovirus, respiratory syncytial virus (RSV), influenza, parainfluenza type III, herpesvirus-6 (HHV6), metapneumovirus and a variety of other respiratory pathogens. Non-CMV viral infections may occur earlier than 30 days or later in the transplant course. CMV typically occurs after 30 days. Early detection of CMV and advances in treatment have reduced disease and mortality associated with CMV disease. VZV can lead to pneumonia with or without classic vesicular rash. HSV/VZV prophylaxis should be initiated with the conditioning regimen and continue for 1 year or until the patient is off all immunosuppressant agents and CD4 numbers have been restored. Community-acquired viral infections can be lethal, especially parainfluenza type III. Since, with the exception of influenza, there is no effective therapy, the best approach is prevention through isolation.

Diagnosis of Viral Pathogens
Diagnosis is based on fever, cough, signs and symptoms of URI, nasal washing, viral swabs or PCR.

7.4.5 Fungal Pulmonary Infections

Invasive fungal diseases are a major obstacle to patients after transplant and are a major cause of pulmonary-related mortality (Ji et al. 2011). *Aspergillus* is the most common and most virulent fungal cause of pneumonia following HSCT

(Blaes et al. 2009; Wilson et al. 2009). Other fungal respiratory infections in post-HSCT patients, particularly those receiving myeloablative conditioning, include *Malassezia*, *Zygomycetes* and *Candida* species (Wilson et al. 2009). Over the past decade, several new antifungal medications have demonstrated increased success, showing improved remission rates and thereby decreasing morbidity.

Diagnosis
- Fever, pleuritic chest discomfort, dyspnoea.
- Imaging shows nodules or cavitating infiltrates.
- The classic "halo sign" may be seen on chest CT, but imaging may not be helpful.
- A BAL may be useful.
- Galactomannan and beta-glucan testing may be helpful but are not always informative.

Pneumocystis jirovecii Pneumonia

Risk of *Pneumocystis jirovecii* pneumonia (PCP) starts at around day +30.

Effectively administered prophylaxis eliminates PCP.

Diagnosis
- Fever, cough, ± hypoxemia.
- Positive BAL. CXR – bilateral ground-glass infiltrates.
- Beta-glucan is typically detectable.
- A history of noncompliance with prophylaxis medication should be elicited.

Typically involves the brain, heart and lung.

Biopsy sample has Giemsa stain to confirm diagnosis.

7.4.6 Mycobacteria

Testing with purified protein derivative (PPD) is often not helpful after allogeneic stem cell transplantation because of depressed delayed-type hypersensitivity reactions. Therefore a skin reaction with PPD will likely not occur.

Diagnosis
Cultured sputum sample/BAL various indirect assays such as Quantiferon gold are helpful.

7.4.7 Nursing Implications

All patients undergoing HSCT are at risk for pulmonary complications. Bedside nurses are the most likely to observe subtle changes in the patient's condition, and for this reason it is critical that nursing staff working with the HSCT population be highly trained in oncology and critical care interventions. Prompt reporting of symptoms can ensure proper and timely medical intervention and facilitate improved patient outcomes. This has been found particularly true in identifying GvHD, with clinical nurses at the forefront of identifying and reporting suspicious symptoms to the healthcare team (Mattson 2007). Nurses take a central role in patient and family education regarding the course of treatment, complications and other key pieces of the HSCT process, including caring for a central line (Stephens et al. 2013). By educating patients on what to expect after transplant with regard to troubling symptoms, nurses ensure patient participation in identifying developing complications early and improving HSCT outcomes. A thorough assessment can assist the nursing staff in detecting changes indicative of developing complications. Vital signs, including the rate and quality of respirations, and oximetry should be performed per program protocols, usually every 4 h and more frequently for patients at risk for pulmonary insufficiency. Taking the patient's temperature every 4 h or as necessary is another critical respiratory intervention, as most post-HSCT complications are infectious in nature (Stephens et al. 2013). Nurses are crucial in assessing patients for symptoms of bacterial infection and should perform routine laboratory tests as necessary. Regarding pulmonary infections, nurses should closely monitor patients for symptoms of progressing respiratory disease, such as decreased auscultation of air sounds in the lungs, increasing fevers and appearance of a productive cough with coloured sputum. Antibiotics should start as soon as possible in these patients. A nursing study of neutropenic patients in the early HSCT phase showed that commencement of antibiotics within 1 h of the onset of infectious symptoms can significantly reduce infectious complications, including sepsis

(Hyman 2005). The recent addition of monoclonal antibodies (MoAbs) to GvHD prophylaxis protocols has been met with mixed results. For example, a study using infliximab did not lead to lower rates of GvHD but did suggest higher rates of bacterial or fungal pulmonary infection in patients who participated in the study (Hamadani et al. 2008). It is important that patients in the post-transplant period are encouraged to pace their activity with their level of ability. Coughing and deep breathing exercises accompanying the regular use of an incentive spirometer constitute critical ways to open deep alveolar tissue and encourage pulmonary toileting on patients prone to fatigue and malaise and whose blood counts are very low (Stephens et al. 2013).

7.5 BMT Settings, Infections and Infection Control for Paediatric Patients

Be Aware

In Primary Immunodeficiency Patients.

Immunization with live viral or bacterial vaccines is a known hazard to patients with serious immunodeficiencies (Shearer et al. 2014).

They have no protective immune response and therefore are at risk of developing the disease itself (Marciano et al. 2014).

Avoid immunization with live Bacillus Calmette-Guerin (BCG), rotavirus vaccine or live poliovirus since they can cause persistent and disseminated infection (Shearer et al. 2014; Rivers and Gaspar 2015).

Patients with SCID that received BCG vaccine prior to diagnosis will need to start antituberculosis treatment (Rivers and Gaspar 2015).

Patients who received BCG vaccine prior to diagnosis will need to start anti-tuberculosis treatment.

BCGitis

If BCG vaccine is given to infants with severe primary immune deficiencies, they will develop BCGitis. It is characterized by local erythema and purulent regional lymph node enlargement.

BCG-osis.

The more severe form is disseminated infection that could be fatal. It involves distant lymph nodes, bone, liver and spleen.

Shrot et al. (2016).

References

Almyroudis NG, Osawa R, Samonis G, Wetzler M, Wang ES, McCarthy PL, Segal BH. Discontinuation of systematic surveillance and contact precautions for *Vancomycin-Resistant Enterococcus* (VRE) and its impact on the incidence of VRE *faecium* bacteremia in patients with hematologic malignancies. Infect Control Hosp Epidemiol. 2016;37(4):398–403.

Alsharif M. Time trends in fungal infections as a cause of death in hematopoietic stem cell transplant recipients: An autopsy study. Am J Clin Pathol. 2009;132:746–55.

Antin JH, Raley DY. Manual of stem cell and bone marrow transplantation. New York, NY: Cambridge University Press; 2009.

ASHM. Nurses and hepatitis C. Darlinghurst: ASHM; 2012. http://www.aph.gov.au/DocumentStore.ashx?id= 4799afa2-cddb-46cd-a393-f23719622ef8 &subId=303939

Bettinger D, Schorb E, Huzly D, Panning M, Schmitt-Graeff A, Kurz P, Bertz H, Finke J, Brass V, Thimme R, Hasselblatt P. Chronic hepatitis E virus infection following allogenic hematopoietic stem cell transplantation: an important differential diagnosis for graft versus host disease. Ann Hematol. 2015;94:359–60.

Blaes A, Cavert W, Morrison V. Malassezia: Is it a pulmonary pathogen in the stem cell transplant population? Transpl Infect Dis. 2009;11:313–7.

Boeckh M, Kim HW, Flowers MF, Meyers JD, Bowden RA. Long-term acyclovir for prevention of varicella zoster virus disease after allogeneic hematopoietic cell transplantation—a randomized double-blind placebo-controlled study. Blood. 2006;107(5):1800–5.

Boeckh M. The challenge of respiratory virus infections in hematopoietic cell transplant recipients. Br J Haematol. 2008;143:455–67.

Brown M. Nursing care of patients undergoing allogeneic stem cell transplantation. Nurs Stand. 2010;25(11):47–56.

Camus P, Costabel U. Drug-induced respiratory disease in patients with hematological diseases. Semin Respir Crit Care Med. 2005;26:458–81.

Carreras E. Preventing exposure to moulds. Clin Microbiol Infect. 2006;12(Suppl 7):77–83.

Castro ND, Neuville S, Sarfati C, Ribaud P, Derouin F, Gluckman E, Sociè G, Molina JM. Occurrence of *Pneumocystis jiroveci* pneumonia after allogeneic stem cell transplantation: a 6-year retrospective study. Bone Marrow Transplant. 2005;36:879–83.

Castro CG, Ganc AJ, Ganc RL, Petroli MS, Hamerschlack N. Fecal microbiota transplant after hematopoietic SCT: report of a successful case. Bone Marrow Transplant. 2015;50:145.

Chakrabarti S, Mautner V, Osman H, Collingham KE, Fegan CD, Klapper PE, Moss PAH, Milligan D. Adenovirus infections following allogeneic stem cell transplantation: incidence and outcome in relation to graft manipulation, immunosuppression, and immune recovery. Blood. 2002;100(5):1619–27.

Chen CS, Boeckh M, Seidel K, Clark JG, Kansu E, Madtes DK, Wagner JL, Witherspoon RP, Anasetti C, Appelbaum FR, Bensinger WI, Deeg HJ, Martin PJ, Sanders JE, Storb R, Storek J, Wade J, Siadak M, Flowers MED, Sullivan KM. Incidence, risk factors, and mortality from pneumonia developing late after hematopoietic stem cell transplantation. Bone Marrow Transplant. 2003;32:515–22.

Cidofovir SmPC. http://emc.medicines.org.uk/emc/industry/default.asp?page=displaydoc.asp&documentid=1585. Accessed 2017.

Cohen J. Epstein Barr virus lymphoproliferative disease associated with acquired immunodeficiency (review). Medicine. 1991;70:137.

Cohen CC, Cohen B, Shang J. Effectiveness of contact precautions against multidrug-resistant organism transmission in acute care: a systematic review of the literature. J Hosp Inf. 2015;90:275–84.

Cooke KR, Jannin A, Ho V. The contribution of endothelial activation and injury to end-organ toxicity following allogeneic hematopoietic stem cell transplantation. Biol Blood Marrow Transplant. 2008;14(Suppl. 1):23–32.

Coomes S.M, Hubbard L.L, Moore B.B. Impaired pulmonary immunity post-bone marrow transplant. Immunologic Research. Advance online publication. 2010.

Dalton HR, Saunders M, Woolson KL. Hepatitis E virus in developed countries: one of the most successful zoonotic viral diseases in human history? J Virus Erad. 2015;1(1):23–9.

De Keukeleire S, Reynders M. Hepatitis E: an underdiagnosed, emerging infection in nonendemic regions. J Clin Transl Hepatol. 2015;3:288–91.

Deeg J, Socie G. Malignancies after haematopoietic stem cell transplantation: many questions, some answers. Blood. 1998;91(6):1833–44.

Docampo MD, Auletta JJ, Jenq RR. Emerging influence of the intestinal microbiota during allogenic hematopoietic cell transplantation: control the gut and the body will follow. Review ASBMT. 2015;21(8):1360–6.

Dougherty L, Bravery K, Gabriel J, et al. Standard for infusion therapy. 2010; Royal College of Nursing. INFUSION NURSING STANDARDS OF PRACTICE Developed by Infusion Nurses Society REVISED 2011.

Dubberke ER, Riddle DJ. *Clostridium difficile* in solid organ transplantation recipients. Am J Transplant. 2009;9(4):S35–40.

Dykewicz CA, Kaplan JE. Guidelines for preventing opportunistic infections among haematopoietic stem cell transplant recipients. MMWR Recomm Rep. 2000;49(RR-10):1–125.

Elad S, Raber-Durlacher J, Michael T. Brennan, Deborah P. Saunders, Arno P. Mank, Yehuda Zadik, Barry Quinn, Joel B. Epstein, Nicole M.A. Blijlevens, Tuomas Waltimo, Jakob R. Passweg, M. Elvira P. Correa, Göran Dahllöf, Karin U. E. Garming-Legert, Richard M. Logan, Carin M. J. Potting, Michael Y. Shapira, Yoshihiko Soga, Jacqui Stringer, Monique A. Stokman, Samuel Vokurka, Elisabeth Wallhult, Noam Yarom, Siri Beier Jensen. Basic oral care for hematology–oncology patients and hematopoietic stem cell transplantation recipients: a position paper from the joint task force of the Multinational Association of Supportive Care in Cancer/International Society of Oral Oncology (MASCC/ISOO) and the European Society for Blood and Marrow Transplantation (EBMT). 2014.

Escuissato D, Emerson G, Marchiori E, de Melo Rocha G, Inoue C, Pasquini R, Muller N. Pulmonary infections after bone marrow transplantation: High-resolution CT findings in 111 patients. Am J Roentgenol. 2005;185:608–15.

Forslöw UU, Remberger M, Nordlander AA, Mattsson JJ. The clinical importance of bronchoalveolar lavage in allogeneic SCT patients with pneumonia. Bone Marrow Transplant. 2010;45:945–50.

Foscarnet SmPC. http://emc.medicines.org.uk/emc/industry/default.asp?page=displaydoc.asp&documentid=174. Accessed 2017.

Fox N, Freifeld AG. The neutropenic diet reviewed: moving toward a safe food handling approach. Oncology (Williston Park). 2012;26(572–575):580, 582 passim

Galati PC, Lataro RC, Souza VM, de Martins ECP, Chiarello PG. Microbiological profile and nutritional quality of raw foods for neutropenia patients under hospital care. Rev Bras Hematol Hemoter. 2013;35(2):94–8.

Ganciclovir SmPC. http://emc.medicines.org.uk/emc/assets/c/html/displaydoc.asp?documentid=3497. Accessed 2017.

Gardner A, Mattiuzzi G, Faderl S, Borthakur G, Garcia-Manero G, Pierce S, Brandt M, Estey E. Randomized comparison of cooked and noncooked diets in patients undergoing remission induction therapy for acute myeloid leukemia. J Clin Oncol. 2008;26:5684–8.

Garzoni C. Multiply resistant gram-positive bacteria *Methicillin-Resistant, Vancomycin-Intermediate and Vancomycin-Resistant Staphylococcus aureus* (MRSA,

VISA, VRSA) in solid organ transplant recipients. Am J Transplant. 2009;9(4):S41–9.

Gea-Banacloch J, Masur H, Arns da Cuhna C, Chiller T, Kirchoff L, Shaw P, Tomblyn M, Cordonnier C. Regionally limited or rare infections: prevention after hematopoietic cell transplantation. Bone Marrow Transplant. 2009;44:489–94.

Girmenia C, Rossolini GM, Piciocchi A, Beryainia A, Pisapia G, Pastore D, Sica S, Severino A, Cudillo L, Ciceri F, Scime R, Lombardi L, Viscoli C, Rambaldi A. Infections by carbapenem-resistant *Klebsiella pneumoniae* in SCT recipients: a nationwide retroscpective survey from Italy. Bone Marrow Transplant. 2015;50:282–8.

Grant M, Cooke L, Bhatia S, Forman S. Discharge and unscheduled readmissions of adult patients undergoing hematopoietic stem cell transplantation: implications for developing nursin interventions. Oncol Nurs Forum. 2005;32(1):E1–8.

Gratwohl A, Brand R, Frassoni F, Rocha V, Niederwieser D, Reusser P, Einsele H, Cordonnier C. Cause of death after allogeneic haematopoietic stem cell transplantation (HSCT) in early leukaemias: an EBMT analysis of lethal infectious complications and changes over calendar time. Bone Marrow Transplant. 2005;36:757–69.

Gruber U, Fegg M, Buchmann M, Kolb HJ, Hiddemann W. The long-term psychological effects of haematopoetic stem cell transplantation. Eur J Cancer Care. 2003;12(3):249–56.

Gu SL, Chen YB, Lv T, Zhang XW, Wei ZQ, Shen P, Li LJ. Risk factors, outcomes and epidemiology associated with *Clostridium difficile* infection in patients with haematological malignancies in a tertiary care hospital in China. J Med Microbiol. 2015;64:209–2016.

Gupta S, Mahipal A. Fatal pulmonary toxicity after a single dose of cyclophosphamide. Pharmacotherapy. 2007;27:616–8.

Hamadani M, Hofmeister CC, Jansak B, Phillips G, Elder P, Blum W, et al. Addition of infliximab to standard acute graft-versus-host disease prophylaxis following allogeneic peripheral blood cell transplantation. Biol Blood Marrow Transplant. 2008;14:783–9.

Heslop H. How I treat EBV lymphoproliferation. Blood. 2009;114:4002–8.

Ho V, Weller E, Lee S. Prognostic factors for early severe pulmonary complications after hematopoietic stem cell transplantation. Biol Blood Marrow Transplant. 2001;7:223–9.

https://www.cdc.gov/mmwr/preview/mmwrhtml/rr4910a1.htm. Retrieved on 10 Sep 2016.

Hyman J. Neutropenic patients-Are they receiving their antibioticson time? Nursing Monograph. 2005. 15–18.

Ihendyane N, Sparrelid E, Wretlind B, Remberger M, Andersson J, Ljungman P, Ringden O, Henriques Normark B, Allen U, Low DE, Norrby-Teglund A. Viridans streptococcal septicaemia in neutropaenic patients: role of proinflammatory cytokines. Bone Marrow Transplant. 2004;33(1):79–95.

Ji Y, Xu LP, Liu DH, Chen YH, Han W, Zhang XH, Huang XJ. Positive results of serum galactomannan assays and pulmonary computed tomography predict the higher response rate of empirical antifungal therapy in patients undergoing allogeneic hematopoietic stem cell transplantation. Biol Blood Marrow Transplant. 2011;17:759–64.

Kamar N, Dalton HR, Abravanel F, Izopet J. Hepatitis E virus infection. Clin Microbiol Rev. 2014;1(27):116–38.

Kamboj M, Sepkowitz K. Healthcare-associated infections in transplant recipients. In: Jarvis WR, editor. Bennett & Brachman's hospital infections. 6th ed. Philadelphia: Wolters Kluwer Lippincott Williams & Wilkins; 2014. p. 707–8.

Kamboj M, Xiao K, Kaltsas A, Huang YT, Sun J, Chung D, Wu S, Sheahan A, Sepkowitz K, Jakubowski AA, Papanicolaou G. *Clostridium difficile* infection after allogeneic hematopoietic stem cell transplant: strain diversity and outcomes associated with NAP-1/027. Biol Blood Marrow Transplant. 2014;20(10):1626–33.

Kanda Y, Mineishi S, Saito T, Saito A, Yamada S, Ohnishi M, Chizuka A, Niiya H, Suenaga K, Nakai K, Takeuchi T, Makimoto A, Tanosaki R, Kami M, Tanaka Y, Fujita S, Watanabe T, Kobayashi Y, Tobinai K, Takaue Y. Long-term low-dose acyclovir against varicella-zoster virus reactivation after allogeneic hematopoietic stem cell transplantation. Bone Marrow Transplant. 2001;28:689–92.

Kaplan R, Bashoura L, Shannon VR, Dickey BF, Stover DE. Noninfectious lung infiltrates that may be confused with pneumonia in the cancer patient. In: Safdar A, editor. Principles and practice of cancer infectious diseases; 2011. p. 153–65.

Kotloff R, Ahya V, Crawford S. Pulmonary complications of solid organ and hematopoietic stem cell transplantation. Am J Respir Crit Care. 2004;170:22–48.

Kuriyama T, Kawano N, Yamashita K, Ueda A. Successful treatment of rituximab-resistant Epstein-Barr virus-associated post-transplant lymphoproliferative disorder using R-CHOP. J Clin Exp Haem. 2014;54(2):149–53.

Kyvernitakis A, Mahale P, Popat UR, Jiang Y, Horsy J, Champlin RE, Torres HA. Hepatitis C virus infection in patients undergoing hematopoietic cell transplantation in the era of direct-acting antiviral agents. Biol Blood Marrow Transplant. 2016;22:717–22.

La Rosa AM, Champlin RE, Gajewski N, Giralt S, Rolston KV, Raad I, Jacobson K, Kontoyiannis D, Elting L, Whimbey E. Adenovirus infections in adult recipients of blood and marrow transplants. Clin Infect Dis. 2001;32:871–6.

Landelle C, Pagani L, Harbarth S. Is patient isolation the single most important measure to prevent the spread of multidrug-resistant pathogens? Virulence. 2013;4(2):163–71.

Landgren O, Gilbert ES, Rizzo JD, Sociè G, Banks PM, Sobocinski KA, Horowitz MM, Jaffe ES, Kingma DW, Travis LP, Flowers ME, Martin PJ, Deeg H, Curtis

RE. Risk factors for lymphoproliferative disorders after allogeneic hematopoietic cell transplantation. Blood. 2009;113:4992–5001.

Lau GKK, Strasser SI, McDonald GB. Hepatitis virus infections in patients with cancer. In: Wingard JR, Bowden RA, editors. Management of Infection in oncology patients. London: Martin Dunitz; 2003. p. 322–3.

Lin M, Weinstein R, Hayden MK. Multidrug-resistant organisms: epidemiology and control. In: Jarvis WR, editor. Bennett & Brachman's hospital infections. 6th ed. Philadelphia: Wolters Kluwer Lippincott Williams & Wilkins; 2014. p. 198–9.

Lindemann M, Koldehoff M, Fiedler M, Schumann A, Ottinger HD, Heinemann FM, Roggendorf M, Horn PA, Belen DW. Control of hepatitis B virus infection in hematopoietic stem cell (HSC) recipients after receiving grafts from vaccinated donors. Bone Marrow Transplant. 2016;51:428–31.

Ljungman P, Wang FZ, Clark DA, Emery VC, Remberger M, Ringden O, Linde A. High levels of human herpesvirus 6 DNA in peripheral blood leucocytes are correlated to platelet engraftment and disease in allogeneic stem cell transplant patients. Br J Haematol. 2000;111:774–81.

Ljungman P, Ribaud P, Eyrich M, Matthes-Martin S, Einsele H, Bleakley M, Machaczka M, Bierings M, Bosi A, Gratecos N, Cordonnier C. Cidofovir for adenovirus infections after allogeneic hematopoietic stem cell transplantation: a survey by the infectious diseases working Party of the European Group for blood and marrow transplantation. Bone Marrow Transplant. 2003;31:481–6.

Locasciulli A, Montante B, Morelli E, Gulino V, Proia A, Pinazzi MB. Hepatitis B and C in hematopoietic stem cell transplant. Med J Hemat Infect Dis. 2009;1:3.

Mackall C, Fry T, Gress R, Peggs K, Storek J, Toubert A. Background to hematopoietic cell transplantation, including post transplant immune recovery. Bone Marrow Transplant. 2009;44:457–62.

Mank AP, Davies M, for the EBMT-NG. Examining low bacterial dietary practice: a European survey on low bacterial food. Eur J Oncol Nurs. 2008;12:342–8.

Mank APM, Charlot Schoonenberg, Kim Bleeker, Susanne Heijmenberg, Koen de Heer, Marinus H. J. van Oers & Marie José Kersten. Early discharge after high dose chemotherapy is safe and feasible: a prospective evaluation of 6 years of home care. Leukemia & Lymphoma ISSN: 1042-8194 (Print) 1029–2403 (Online). 2015 Journal homepage: http://www.tandfonline.com/loi/ilal20

Marano G, Vaglio S, Pupella S, Facco G, Bianchi M, Calizzani G, Candura F, Catalano L, Farina B, Lanzoni M, Piccinini V, Liumbruno GM, Grazzini G. Hepatitis E: an old infection with new implications. Blood Transfus. 2015;13:6–20.

Marciano BE, Huang CY, Joshi G, Rezaei N, Carvalho BC, Allwood Z, Ikinciogullari A, Reda SM, Gennery A, Thon V, Espinosa-Rosales F, Al-Herz W, Porras O, Shcherbina A, Szaflarska A, Kiliç Ş, Franco JL, Gómez Raccio AC, Roxo P Jr, Esteves I, Galal N, Grumach AS, Al-Tamemi S, Yildiran A, Orellana JC, Yamada M, Morio T, Liberatore D, Ohtsuka Y, Lau YL, Nishikomori R, Torres-Lozano C, Mazzucchelli JT, Vilela MM, Tavares FS, Cunha L, Pinto JA, Espinosa-Padilla SE, Hernandez-Nieto L, Elfeky RA, Ariga T, Toshio H, Dogu F, Cipe F, Formankova R, Nuñez-Nuñez ME, Bezrodnik L, Marques JG, Pereira MI, Listello V, Slatter MA, Nademi Z, Kowalczyk D, Fleisher TA, Davies G, Neven B, Rosenzweig SD. BCG vaccination in patients with severe combined immunodeficiency: complications, risks, and vaccination policies. J Allergy Clin Immunol. 2014;133(4):1134–41.

Masszi T., Mank AP. Chapter 10. Haematopoietic stem cell transplantation – Handbook EBMT supportvive care page. 2012. 157–159.

Mattson M. Graft-versus-host disease: Review and nursing implications. Clin J Oncol Nurs. 2007;11:325–8.

Meijer E, Bolland GJ, Verdonck LF. Prevention of cytomegalovirus disease in recipients of allogeneic stem cell transplants. Clin Microbiolol Rev. 2003;16:647–57.

Murray SM, Pindoria S. Nutrition support for bone marrow transplant patients. Cochrane Database Syst Rev. 2009;

Murray MP, Doherty CJ, Govan JR, Hill AT. Do processing time and storage of sputum influence quantitative bacteriology in bronchiectasis? J Med Microbiol. 2010;59:829–33.

Nakasone H, Kurosawa S, Yakushijin K, Taniguchi S, Murata M, Ikegame K, Kobayashi T, Eto T, Miyamura K, Sakamaki H, Morishima Y, Nagamura T, Suzuki R, Fukuda T. Impact of hepatitis C virus infection on clinical outcome in recipients after allogeneic hematopoietic cell transplantation. Am J Hematol. 2013;88:477–84.

Neemann K, Eichele DD, Smith PW, Bociek R, Akhtari M, Freifield A. Fecal microbiota transplantation for fulminant Clostridium difficile infection in an allogeneic stem cell transplant patient. Transpl Infect Dis. 2012;14(6):E161–5.

Ogata M, Fukuda T, Teshima T. Human herpesvirus-6 encephalitis after allogeneic hematopoietic cell transplantation: what we do and do not know. Bone Marrow Transplant. 2015;50:1030–6.

O'Grady NP, Alexander M, Burns LA, et al. Guidelines for the prevention of intravascular catheter-related infections. Centers for Disease Control and Prevention 2011. http://www.cdc.gov/hicpac/pdf/guidelines/bsiguidelines-2011.pdf. Retrieved 11/09/2016.

Oliver NT. Severe hepatitis C reactivation as an early complication of hematopoietic cell transplantation. Bone Marrow Transplant. 2016; 1-3 published online 18 July 2016; exact reference: Bone Marrow Transplantation 2017;52:138–140.

Parker A, Bowles K, Bradley AJ, Emery V, Featherstone C, Gupte G, Marcus R, Parameshwar J, Ramsay A, Newstead C On behalf of the Haemato-oncology Task Force of the British Committee for Standards in Haematology and British Transplantation Society. Management of post-transplant lymphoproliferative disorder in adult solid organ transplant recipients – BCSH and BTS guidelines. Br J Haematol. 2010;149:693–705.

Parody R, Martino R, Rovira M, Vazquez L, Vázquez MJ, De la Cámara R, Blazquez C, Fernández-Avilés F, Carreras E, Salavert M, Jarque I, Martín C, Martínez F, López J, Torres A, Sierra J, Sanz GF, Infectious/Non-infectious Complications Subcommittee of the Grupo Español de Trasplante Hematopoyético (GETH. Severe infections after unrelated donor allogeneic hematopoietic stem cell transplantation in adults: comparison of cord blood transplantation with peripheral blood and bone marrow transplantation. Biol Blood Marrow Transplant. 2006;12:734–48.

Pattullo V. Prevention of hepatitis B reactivation in the setting of immunosuppression. Clin Mol Hepatol. 2016;22:219–37.

Peterson DE, Boers-Doets CB, Bensadoun RJ, Herrstedt J on behalf of the ESMO Guidelines Committee. Management of oral and gastrointestinal mucosal injury: ESMO clinical practice guidelines for diagnosis, treatment, and follow-up. Ann Oncol. 2015;26(Supplement 5):v139–51.

Pizzo PA. The value of protective isolation in preventing nosocomial infections in high risk patients. Am J Med. 1981;70(3):631–7.

Polovich M, Whitford JM, Olsen M. Chemotherapy and biotherapy guidelines and recommendations for practice. 3rd ed. Pittsburgh, PA: Oncology Nursing Society; 2009.

Quinn B, Potting C, Stone R, Blijlevens NM, Fliedner M, Marquiles A, Sharp L. Guidance for the assessment of oral mucositis in adult chemotherapy, radiotherapy and haematopoietic stem cell transplant patients. Eur J Cancer. 2008;44(1):61–72.

Rasch L, Kapp M, Einsele H, Mielke S. EBV-induced post-transplant lymphoproliferative disorders: a persisting challenge in allogeneic haematopoietic SCT. Bone Marrow Transplant. 2014;49:163–7.

Rivers L, Gaspar HB. Severe combined immunodeficiency: recent developments and guidance on clinical management. Arch Dis Child. 2015;100:667–72.

Robin M, Marque-Juillet S, Scieux C, Peffault de Latour R, Ferry C, Rocha V, Molina J, Bergeron A, Devergie A, Gluckman E, Ribaud P, Socié G. Disseminated adenovirus infections after allogeneic hematopoietic stem cell transplantation: incidence, risk factors and outcome. Haematologica. 2007;92:1254–7.

Rovira M., Mensa J., Carreras E.. Chapter 10. Haematopoietic stem cell transplantation – Handbook EBMT, infections after HSCT. 2012, 197–200.

Royal College of Nursing. Standards for infusion therapy. 3rd ed. 2010. https://www.rcn.org.uk/professional-development/publications/pub-005704. Retrieved 15/09/2016.

Roychowdhury M, Pambuccian S, Aslan D, Jessurun J, Rose A, Manivel J. Pulmonary complications after bone marrow transplantation: An autopsy study from a large transplantation center. Archives of Pathology and. Lab Med. 2005;129:366–71.

Sharma S, Nadrous H, Peters S, Tefferi A, Litzow M, Aubry M, Afessa B. Complications in adult blood and marrow transplant recipients. Chest. 2005;128:1385–92.

Shearer WT, Fleischer TA, Buckley RH, Ballas Z, Ballow M, Blease M, Bonilla F, Comley M, Cunningham C, Filipovich A, Fuleihan R, Gelfand E, Hernandez-Trujillo V, Holland S, Hong R, Lederman H, Malech h MS, Notarangelo L, Ochs H, Orange J, Puck J, Routes J, Stiehm E, Sullivan K, Torgerson T, Winkelstein J. Recommendations for live viral and bacterial vaccines in immunodeficient patients and their close contacts medical advisory Committee of the Immune Deficiency Foundation. J Allergy Clin Immunol. 2014;133:961–6.

Shrot S, Barkai G, Ben-Shlush A, Soudack M. BCGitis and BCGosis in children with primary immunodeficiency — imaging characteristics. Pediatr Radiol. 2016;46:237. https://doi.org/10.1007/s00247-015-3464-z.

Siegel JD, Rhinehart E, Jackson M, Chiarello L. Health Care Infection Control Practices Advisory Committee. Guideline for Isolation Precautions: Preventing Transmission of Infectious Agents in Healthcare Settings 2007;35(10 Suppl 2):S65-164.

Soubani AO, Pandya CM. The spectrum of noninfectious pulmonary complications following hematopoietic stem cell transplantation. Hematol Oncol Stem Cell Ther. 2010;3:143–57.

Specter S. Clinical virology manual. 4th ed; 2009.

Steer CB, Szer J, Sasadeusz J, Matthews JP, Beresford JA, Grig A. Varicella-zoster infection after allogeneic bone marrow transplantation: incidence, risk factors and prevention with low-dose aciclovir and ganciclovir. Bone Marrow Transplant. 2000;25:657–64.

Stephens Jennifer M.L. Hematopoietic stem cell transplantation. A manual for nursing practice. ONCOLOGY NURSING SOCIETY Edited by Susan A. Ezzone, MS, RN, CNP, AOCNP® Oncology Nursing Society Pittsburgh, PA; 2nd ed. 2013.

Storch GA. Essentials of diagnostic virology. 1st ed; 2000.

Styczynski J, Einsele H, Gil L, Ljungman P. Outcome of treatment of Epstein-Barr virus-related post-transplant lymphoproliferative disorder in haematopoietic stem cell recipients: a comprehensive review of reported cases. Transpl Infect Dis. 2009;11:383–92.

Swerdlow AJ, Webber SA, Chadburn A, Ferry JA. WHO classification of tumours of haematopoietic and lymphoid tissues. 4th ed. Lyon: World Health Organisation Press; 2008.

Tacconelli E, Cataldo MA, Dancer SJ, De Angelis G, Falcone M, Frank U, Kahlmeter G, Pan A, Petrosillo N, Rodriguez-Bano J, Singh N, Venditti M, Yokoe DS, Cookson B. ESCMID guidelines for the management of the infection control measures to reduce transmission of multidrug-resistant gram-negative bacteria in hospitalized patients. Clin Microbiol Infect. 2014;20:1–55.

Tarr S, Allen DH. Evidence does not support the use of a neutropenic diet. Clinical journal oncology. Nursing. 2013;13(6):617–8.

Thomas CFJ, Limper AH. Pneumocystis Pneumonia. N Engl J Med. 2004;350:2487–98.

Thomson KJ, Har DP, Banerjee L, Ward KN, Peggs KS, Mackinnon S. The effect of low-dose aciclovir on reactivation of varicella zoster virus after allogeneic haemopoietic stem cell transplantation. Bone Marrow Transplant. 2005;35:1065–9.

Todd J, Schmidt M, Christian J, Williams R. The low-bacteria diet for immunocompromised patients reasonable prudence or clinical superstition? Cancer Pract. 1999;7(4):205–7.

Tofas P, Skiada A, Angelopoulou M, Sipsas N, Pavlopoulou I, Tsaousi S, Pagoni M, Kotsopoulou M, Perlorentzou S, Antoniadou A, Pirounaki M, Skoutelis A, Daikos GL. Carbapenemase-producing Klebsiella pneumonia bloodstream infection in neutropenic patients with haematological malignancies or aplastic anaemia: analysis of 50 cases. Int J Antibicrob Agents. 2016;47:335–9.

Tomblyn M, Chiller T, Einsele H, Gress R, Sepkowitz K, Storek J, Wingard JR, Young JH, Boechk M. Guidelines for preventing infectious complications among Haematopoietic cell transplantation recipients: a global perspective. Biol Blood Marrow Transplant. 2009;15:1143–238.

Tomblyn M, Chiller T, Einsele H, et al. Guidelines for preventing infectious complications among hematopoietic cell transplantation recipients: A global perspective. Biol Blood Marrow Transplant. 2010;15:1143–238.

Torres HA, Chong PP, Lima M, Friedman MS, Giralt S, Hammond SP, Kiel PJ, Masur H, McDonald GB, Wingard JR, Gambarin-Gelwen M. Hepatitis C virus infection among hematopoietic cell transplant donors and recipients: American Society for Blood and Marrow Transplantation Task Fore Recommendations. Biol Blood Marrow Transplant. 2015;21:1870–82.

Trifilio S, Helenowski I, Giel M, Gobel B, Greenberg D, Mehta J. Questioning the role of a neutropenic diet following Hematopoetic stem cell transplantation. Biol Blood Marrow Transplant. 2012;18(9):1385–90.

Trubiano JA, Worth LJ, Thursky KA, Slavin MA. The prevention and management of infections due to multidrug resistant organisms in haematology patients. Br J Clin Pharmacol. 2013;79(2):195–207.

Truong MT, Sabloff BS, Ko JP. Multidetector CT of solitary pulmonary nodules. Radiol Clin North Am. 2010;48:141–55.

Tzouvelekis LS, Markogiannakis A, Psichogiou M, Tassios PT, Daikos GL. Carbapenemases in *Klebsiella pneumoniae* and other Enterobacteriaceae: an evolving crisis of global dimensions. Clin Microbiol Re. 2012;25(4):682–707.

Ullmann AJ, Schmidt-Hieber M, Bertz H, Heinz WJ, Kiehl M, Kruger W, Mousset S, Neuburger S, Neumann S, Penack O, Silling G, Vehreschild JJ, Einsele H, Maschmeyer G. Infectious diseases in allogenic haematopoietic stem cell transplantation: prevention and prophylaxis strategy guidelines 2016. Ann Hematol. 2016;95:1435–55.

Valganciclovir SmPC. http://emc.medicines.org.uk/emc/assets/c/html/displaydoc.asp?documentid=9315. Accessed 2017.

Van Tiel F, Harbers MM, Terporten PH, van Boxtel RT, Kessels AG, Voss GB, Schouten HC. Normal hospital and low- bacterial diet in patients with cytopenia after intensive chemotherapy for hematological malignancy: a study of safety. Ann Oncol. 2007;18(6):1080–4.

Weston D. *Clostridium difficile*. In: Fundamentals of infection prevention and control. Theory and practice. 2nd ed. Chichester: Wiley; 2013. p. 332–9.

WHO guidelines on hand hygiene in health care: a summary. 2009.

Wilson D, Drew R, Perfect J. Antifungal therapy for invasive fungal diseases in allogeneic stem cell transplant recipients: An update. Mycopathologia. 2009;168:313–27.

Zaia J, Baden L, Boeckh MJ, Chakrabarti S, Einsele H, Ljungman P, McDonald GB, Hirsch H. Viral disease prevention after hematopoietic cell transplantation. Bone Marrow Transplant. 2009;44:471–82.

Zerr DM, Corey L, Kim HW, Huang M, Nguy L, Boeckh M. Clinical outcomes of human herpesvirus 6 reactivation after hematopoietic stem cell transplantation. Clin Infect Dis. 2005;40(7):932–40.Zuccotti G, Strasfeld L, Weinstock DM. New agents for the prevention of opportunistic infections in haematopoietic stem cell transplant recipients. Expert Opin Pharmacother. 2005;6:1669–79.

Transplantation Through the Generations

8

Alberto Castagna, Lisa Mcmonagle,
Corien Eeltink, and Sarah Liptrott

8.1 Transplanting the Child

Abstract *Biologically, a child* is a human being
between the *stages of birth and puberty. The legal
definition of child generally refers to a minor, otherwise known as a person younger than the age of
majority* (*Oxford University Press* (Accessed 5th
January 2013)).

A. Castagna
Paediatric Hemato-Oncology and HSC Transplant
Nurse at Paediatric Hematology-Oncology and
HSCT Unit, Ospedale Donna e Bambino – Azienda
Ospedaliera Universitaria Integrata (AOUI) Verona,
Verona, Italy
e-mail: alberto.castagna@aovr.veneto.it

L. Mcmonagle, BSc (Hons), MSc, RN
Teenage Cancer Trust Advanced Nurse Practitioner
for Teenagers and Young Adults, University College,
London, United Kingdom
e-mail: lisa-marie.mcmonagle@nhs.net

C. Eeltink (✉)
Department of Hematology, Cancer Center
Amsterdam/ VU University Medical Center,
Amsterdam, The Netherlands
e-mail: c.eeltink@vumc.nl

S. Liptrott
Division of Haemato-oncology, European Institute
of Oncology, Milan, Italy
e-mail: sarah.liptrott@ieo.it

The ability to cure children with cancer has radi-
cally improved over the recent decades. Today,
more than 80% of children with cancer are cured
of their disease (Franklin 2014). This incredible
achievement is one of the greatest triumphs in the
history of medicine and is the result of numerous
factors, including developments in paediatric
haematopoietic stem cell transplantation (HSCT).
Treatment advances for the sick child have been
accomplished in various cancer treatments
including chemotherapy, surgery, radiotherapy
and HSCT. Whilst these therapies have vastly
improved outcomes in childhood cancers, there
remains scope for further improvement.

Keywords HSCT • Paediatric

8.1.1 The Role of EBMT in Paediatric HSCT

Changes in HSCT approaches are responsible for
progress in this particular area. The role and status
of transplantation have evolved. It is no longer considered a salvage therapy for patients in desperate
circumstances but is now the treatment of choice
for many diseases. The history of paediatric HSCT
in Europe began in Poland in 1949 (Raszek-
Rosenbusch), with therapeutic transfusion of bone
marrow in children with leukaemia and other blood
diseases. Subsequent developments in paediatric
HSCT were driven on by the creation in 1974, of

© EBMT and the Author(s) 2018
M. Kenyon, A. Babic (eds.), *The European Blood and Marrow Transplantation Textbook for Nurses,*
https://doi.org/10.1007/978-3-319-50026-3_8

the European Society for Blood and Marrow Transplantation (EBMT). The goal of the society remains to promote all aspects associated with HSCT. Since the launch of the EBMT Society in 1974, several working parties were established, and in 1995, the Board of the EBMT founded the Paediatric Diseases Working Party (PDWP). Shortly after, the registry of the EBMT began to analyse transplant outcomes in children and adolescents increasing our understanding which in turn informed changes and developments in the field. The continuous progressions and evolution of paediatric HSCT in Europe have been resulted in the establishment of HSCT as a standard therapeutic procedure in paediatric haemato-oncology.

The number of children and adolescents undergoing HCST has been steadily increasing since the 1980s. It is clear that close national and international collaboration between HSCT units helps to resolve common difficulties with this complex treatment. The scale of collaboration within the EBMT members is underpinned by the EBMT survey of Passweg et al. (2016) reporting more than 40,000 HSCT per year in 680 centres from 49 countries in Europe and affiliated countries. The report described:

- Transplant rates
- Indications
- Donor type
- Stem cell source
- Conditioning MAC and RIC
- Donor lymphocyte infusions

This report enables us to observe trends and changes in HSCT practice over time. The paper reported 4400 paediatric transplants in 2014 of which almost 75% are allogeneic. A family member donated cells in 53% of these (70% HLA-identical, 29% non-HLA-identical, 1% syngeneic) and 47% of unrelated donor (Table 8.1).

The high proportion of allogeneic transplants in paediatrics is largely due to the characteristics of paediatric diseases that are amenable to transplantation such as haemoglobinopathies, immune deficiencies, immune dysregulation and metabolic diseases.

Furthermore, in paediatric allogeneic transplantation, the leading indication is ALL (26%), followed by primary immune deficiencies (16%) and then AML (14%). Conversely, in the paediatric autologous transplant, the major indications are neuroblastoma (35%), other solid tumours (31%) and lymphoma (15%).

The 2012 EBMT report notes that more paediatric patients receive BM stem cells than PBSC, irrespective of donor type (Passweg et al. 2014).

8.1.2 Child Growth and Development

It is important to know and understand the developmental stages of infants and children because appreciation of the ages, stages, common milestones and abilities allows nurses to relate to the children and their relatives appropriately. The knowledge of the normal growth and development equips the nurses to identify any developmental delay. Growth and development are a single process which begins during pregnancy and continues throughout childhood and into adolescence. Growth is a change in the body size and structure, whilst development is a change in the body function.

Table 8.1 Number of paediatric haematopoietic SCTs in Europe in 2014 by donor type

'Paediatric centres'	227	Combined adult-paediatric centre	118		
		Paediatric only centre	109		
Number of transplants	4400	Allogeneic	3279		
		Autologous	1121		
Donor type	3279	Family member	1729	HLA-identical	1224
				Non-HLA-id	501
				Syngeneic	4
		Unrelated donor	1550		

8.1.2.1 Child Growth

Child growth refers to progressive structural and physiological changes in the size of a child body. Physical growth includes gaining full height and appropriate weight and increasing in size of all organs. The measurements of weight, length, head circumference, body composition and tooth eruption aid assessment of normal and standard physical growth (Mona 2015).

8.1.2.2 Child Development

Child development concerns a child's ability to undertake more complex processes as they mature. Child development is subdivided into specific areas:

- Motor
- Language
- Cognitive
- Behavioural and emotional

8.1.3 The Child and the Experience of Disease

The child is aware of the condition and often the severity of their disease whatever his age (Badon and Cesaro 2015). This consciousness derives primarily from their perception of the body and wellness state changes but also communicative and relational aspects.

8.1.3.1 Hospitalisation

The child is sensitive to the experience of disconnection that disease imposes. The disease acts as a breaking event in the life of the child and alters the way the body is considered and treated. Hospitalisation changes the physical and relational environment and modifies the emotional climate and the usual style of education.

During the hospitalisation, the child's world is changed; for instance, they are relieved of responsibilities, and many rules disappear or are replaced. They become the target of therapeutic measures, sometimes with little consideration for privacy or confidentiality, and the child becomes separated from their world. If this disconnect remains within the child's limits of tolerance, it is absorbed into their normal development. However, if this disconnect exceeds their tolerance, it results in a traumatic experience and becomes in itself a source of anxiety and distress (Badon and Cesaro 2015).

8.1.3.2 Disease Awareness

A child's disease awareness is determined by the child's own level of cognitive function and experience. These factors impact upon a child's ability to understand the meaning and significance of what is happening. The reactions that a child may exhibit will be governed by:

- Age and stage of intellectual development
- Previous experiences
- Quality of relationships established with reference figures
- Psycho-emotional structure

8.1.3.3 Emotional Reactions to Hospitalisation

The child often does not have the ability to understand the causes and the logic of the events that lead suddenly to being excluded from their family environment, separated from significant figures and entrusted to the care of strangers. The child will tend to experience hospitalisation with a sense of danger that derives primarily from the inability to understand and control the absent parent (Badon and Cesaro 2015).

8.1.4 Patient, Caregiver and Sibling Donor Experience HSCT

HSCT is usually an elective, planned treatment. Children who suffer from malignant disease and undergo- transplantation often have experienced previous treatments and hospitalisations for treatment of complications such as fever, pain, mucositis, nausea and vomiting as well as periods of isolation. HSCT is an intensive treatment process and offers the chance of a cure, but at the same time it can generate a range of feelings including fear, isolation and depression. The skills of the child to address the emotional and psychosocial aspects of transplantation depend on their age, development phase, cognitive level, individual personality and type of psychological support. The hospitalised child receives important support from their family. Parents are invited to actively participate in the care of their child, and during the period of transplant, a parent or a close family member usually stays with the child for the duration of hospitalisation. The experience of HSCT should not hinder the psychosocial growth of the child and may even aid the promotion of development and self-esteem. Nurses have a principal role in providing emotional support to the child and the family caregiver and can assist the child in understanding their condition and overcoming negative emotions.

8.1.4.1 The Paediatric Patient Experience of HSCT

Paediatric patients undergoing HSCT can experience numerous psychological reactions during hospitalisation and recovery:

- Anxiety
- Depression
- Behavioural issues
- Psychosocial issues (adherence, self-esteem, social competence)
- Post-traumatic stress reactions (Packman et al. 2010)

Many of these concerns arise from lengthy hospitalisations away from home, school and friends, isolation and an uncertain future. These factors contribute to high levels of emotion at admission and are reported to escalate until 1 week post HSCT (Phipps et al. 2002). The paediatric HSCT patient can experience multiple hospitalisations, which can occasionally last up to 1 year or longer depending on the severity of the complications. HSCT and its immediate and late consequences have substantial impact on the child's physical, emotional, cognitive, and social well-being and consequently severely compromise the child's quality of life (QoL).

QoL

QoL is potentially affected during all stages of HSCT, including pre-transplant, during the acute post-HSCT time and during isolation and reintegration to life outside the hospital. Pre-transplant predictors of QoL include family functioning and individual resources. It is reported that during hospitalisation, children undergoing HSCT present low baseline levels of QoL. However, QoL improves as early at some months post-HSCT and returns to baseline within some years from HSCT (Tremodala et al. 2009).

Cognitive Impact

The effect of HSCT on cognitive abilities may differ depending on age at HSCT and conditioning regimens, TBI containing regimes versus non-TBI. The younger the child is at HSCT, the higher the risk for deficits in intelligence quotient, academic achievement, fine motor skills and memory. The child with good cognitive developmental level at the time of HSCT can be at lower risk for cognitive deterioration (Barrera et al. 2007).

Mental Health and Emotional Concerns

Many paediatric HSCT patients demonstrate stable psychosocial adjustment or return to baseline functioning 1 to 2 years after HSCT. However, psychiatric morbidity in HSCT survivors is reported in some studies as higher than in the general population and appears to correlate with lower educational level and shorter post-HSCT period. Furthermore, shorter time post-HSCT, higher numbers of major infections, high symptomatology score and low educational level are predictive factors of higher psychosocial distress (Tremolada et al. 2009).

Such psychosocial distress is not unique to the immediate post-transplant period. There are concerns later post-HSCT as well. At 1-year post-HSCT when many survivors return to school, they function at a lower academic level than what is expected for their age. They can be described by peers as absent from school more, less likely to be chosen as a best friend, less athletic and less attractive, and those who experience extensive periods of isolation may demonstrate development decline in socialisation and communication (Packman et al. 2010). There is a further possibility of long-term emotional and social-behavioural problems.

Depression and Anxiety

Depression and anxiety in an ill child can result in disability and morbidity and are associated with psychiatric illness (Chang 2012). Children undergoing HSCT are a high-risk group for developing these problems (Manookian et al. 2014). Contributing factors include:

- Intense medical treatments
- Single room isolation
- Parental concern
- Uncertainty and loss of control

Almost all children report some difficulties during the transplant process such as loneliness, sense of fear and worsening depressive and isolation symptoms (Packman et al. 2010).

- *Intense Medical Treatments*

The HSCT in the child can be associated with medical and psychosocial stressor. The main medical stressors identified to the child are medical interventions and treatment side effects. At the same time the psychosocial stressors can be recognise as missing home or social isolation. Therefore, the HCST can evoke in the child feelings of nervousness, sadness and anger.

- *Isolation*

It is widely recognised that physical isolation could contribute to increased depressive symptoms during hospitalisation with factors such as strict isolation and specialist care due to decreased immune functioning potential stressors. During this time, their main concerns are separation from their family members, or even from their toys or possessions, inability to attend school or participate in normal social activities. The common experience of all these children is the feeling of loneliness. Reactions include depression, anger, frustration and attempts to 'overcontrol' their life, food and hygiene. The isolation period can be perceived as a loss of freedom and control and an intrusion on privacy. If isolation is extended, due to problems related to HSCT, children can report declines in social competence and self-esteem (Packman et al. 2010).

It is important for the child to benefit from sibling support. This can increase tolerance of difficult conditions encountered during the HSCT and aid progress and recovery. During this time, they can develop deep sibling friendships, fed by a desire to be more helpful especially when the ill sibling feels lonely. When stem cells are donated by one a sibling, the ill child experiences more positive feelings about him/her (Manookian et al. 2014).

- *Parental Concern*

There is a close relationship between the child's adaptation to HSCT and the parent's psychological health and comfort (Asadi et al. 2011).

- *Uncertainty and Loss of Control*

Transplantation should be viewed as a chance of hope for a healthy future and long-lasting happiness for the child. If he/she maintains this positive attitude being hopeful about his/her recovery, the child can have a positive response from the treatment and overcoming complications (Manookian et al. 2014).

Support and Fostering Healthy Coping Strategies

As expected, most children experience a sense of fear during their HSCT process. This feeling can be related to a lack of information or understanding regarding his/her condition and conditioning and transplantation process. Providing clear and understandable answers to the child's questions about the illness, treatment and prognosis can help them feel reassured and more relaxed. Information seeking is an important coping strategy for children undergoing to HSCT. Developmental status and psychological state should be considered to enable appropriate communication and provision of information.

Coping strategies used to address a perceived medical or psychosocial stressor may change over time depending on personal factors and context. The child can use several different coping strategies which are often categorised:

- Approach (i.e. information seeking)
- Avoidance (i.e. distraction or distancing)
- Problem-focused (i.e. problem solving)
- Emotion-focused (i.e. seeking emotional support)

Additionally, Bingen et al. (2012) observed wishful thinking, distraction, cognitive restructuring and social support being used both pre- and post-HSCT.

Social Support

Social support is the individual's perception of positive regard from relationships with others, the feelings to being loved, being part of a group, reassurance of self-worth and reliable alliance with others (Barrera et al. 2007). Social support is reported to be the most efficacious, for a child undergoing a HSCT, whether this is from family, friends, teachers, classmates and medical, nursing and psychosocial providers. It is both instrumental and emotional and may be provided directly to the child in the form of hospital visits or via telecommunication (e.g. video calls, phone conversation or texting, online social networking sites and e-mailing). Higher or more positively perceived social support has been identified to be associated with positive adjustment, lower distress and higher self-esteem in paediatric patients undergoing HCST (Barrera et al. 2007).

8.1.4.2 The Parent Experience of HSCT

Asadi et al. (2011) reported in a qualitative study the *Parents' Experiences of their Children Bone Marrow Transplantation*. The experience of HSCT is an unfamiliar, frightening, worrying and stressful experience for the parents of the child undergoing this treatment. Child-centred reasons include:

- Severity of the disease
- Uncertain prognosis
- Complications and risks
- Isolation of patients
- Long hospitalisation period

Parent-centred reasons include:
- Family and financial pressures
- Feelings of guilt

- Loneliness
- Hopelessness
- Fear of disease recurrence
- Transplant centre relocation
- Living in two separate households
- Commuting between home and transplant centre
- Other family member's and carer's responsibilities
- Work-related changes
- Lengthy hospital stays
- Parental informed consent for the HSCT procedure
- Medication compliance
- HSCT-related complications

During HSCT, parents develop high expectation about a successful outcome and are afraid of possible failure. The child's condition can cause parental distress, anxiety and depression. Physical, emotional and cognitive exhaustion or burnout in parents may adversely affect their ability to meet the needs of their child. They could be in extreme crisis and be unable to care for their children or perform traditional parental roles and consequently have feeling of hopelessness, concern and guilt. Parental psychological reactions may in turn negatively affect the child. The psychological load on parents continues when the child is discharged from the ward. Burnout in mothers and fathers is associated with the child's number and severity of late effects up to 5 years after HSCT (Norberg et al. 2014). It is recommended that parents of child that underwent HSCT should be followed up and receive specialist psychological support, particularly for those whose child suffers from late effects.

Common coping strategy amongst families is use of social support. Parents' interactions with their support network can alleviate stress and enable parents to adapt. Some parents feel that communication with family members of other patients aids in acquiring information and in sharing of experiences and helped to take control of their emotions to reduce fear and become adaptive (Badon and Cesaro 2015). Caregivers also attempt to cope by actively participating, engaging in and asking questions pertaining to their child's medical illness and the procedures involved in helping them. Parents who received cognitive-behavioural stress inoculation training in a group format had lower anxiety scores and higher positive self-statement scores (Packman et al. 2010). They can also increase their coping strategies by interacting with other families who share the same problem.

Creating a Therapeutic Alliance

Parents and the healthcare team need to unite to form a therapeutic alliance. Parents should be integrated into the multidisciplinary healthcare team as appropriate. The healthcare team's explanations regarding the transplant process can help them to better understand their conditions and, consequently, can alleviate parental anxiety and fear of uncertainty and help to further reducing their emotional burden.

8.1.4.3 Sibling Donor Experience in HSCT

Matched sibling donors are often preferred over unrelated donors due to decreased risk of complications. Most family members find the experience of donation as beneficial, despite some concerns about the donation process itself (Pentz et al. 2014). Sibling donors actively participate in the effort to achieve cure for their sick sibling. They have a dual role; as family members they experience the difficulties of a life-threatening illness of one of their siblings. As donors they are exposed to an invasive medical procedure which adds anxiety, stress and uncertainty and places them in a complex situation (Munzenberger et al. 1999; Williams et al. 2003). When a close relationship exists between siblings, one can more safely assume that the donation will be of psychological benefit to the donor (Vogel 2011). However, sibling donors are at risk of developing emotional disturbances such as post-traumatic stress reactions, anxiety and low self-esteem and can potentially lead to the development of long-term distress responses (Packman et al. 2010). Attention should be paid to the possibility of these issues. During the pre-transplant workup, potential donors may experience anxiety and fear about the processes used to determine donor eligibility as well as during the donation process itself (Bauk and Andrews 2013). Although

matched siblings may feel content and proud that they are able to be a donor, the unmatched siblings may feel inadequate or rejected and uninvolved in the transplant process. Once HLA typing has confirmed a sibling match, the workup for most haematopoietic stem cell donors involves determining both the risks to the recipient and the risks to the donor. It is also important to consider that these various tests may be overwhelming to the paediatric donor, and the importance of explaining their necessity cannot be understated. The workup process may have a significant impact on the family. In 2010 the American Academy of Pediatrics published a policy statement on children as haematopoietic stem cell donors. Children may ethically serve as donors if five criteria are fulfilled: 1. There is no medically equivalent histocompatible adult relative who is willing and able to donate; 2. there is a strong personal and emotionally positive relationship between the donor and recipient; 3. there is a reasonable likelihood that the recipient will benefit; 4. the clinical, emotional and psychosocial risks to the donor are minimised and are reasonable in relation to the benefits expected to accrue to the donor and to the recipient; and 5. parental permission and, when appropriate, child assent are obtained. It is also recommended that the donor child will have a donor advocate or some similar mechanism, with expertise in paediatric development that should be appointed for all individuals who have not reached the age of majority (Committee of Bioethics 2010).

The HSCT process can enhance family closeness, improved relationships with the unwell sibling and create a sense of pride and happiness about donating (Vogel 2011). Wiener et al. (2007) found that younger donors focus more on the pain of the donation and tend to experience low self-esteem, anxiety, and depression. Conversely older sibling donors report lower levels of anxiety probably because they arc able to think more globally about the donation process.

Studies of physical aspects and the safety of stem cell collection in paediatric sibling concluded that it is a safe procedure even in young children (Pulsipher et al. 2005; Styczynski et al. 2012). There are potential physiological risks and side effects of donation with the most common being pain, fatigue and transient changes in the white blood count, haemoglobin and platelet values. In the immediate days following the donation, staff must closely assess the donor for evidence of bleeding, infection and other acute complications of the donation procedure. Feeling responsible for the transplant outcome is of notable concern for sibling donors. Maladjustment and poor coping in sibling donors may be attributed in part to a lack of information about the transplant process (Wiener et al. 2007).

The nurse can have a significant role in decreasing the sibling donor's stress and anxiety about the impending donation. Providing accurate and age-appropriate information about the impending procedure, the nurse may also help the child prepare for the experience and adapt to it more rapidly. This information increases the predictability of frightening medical procedures, thereby increasing the probability of a less stressful experience and a more rapid recovery. The nurse can also create opportunities to express emotion, concerns and questions in order to manage anxiety and guilt, involve parents in the donor's preparation and follow-up to ensure family's communication during HSCT and organise a tour of the hospital and an introduction to staff.

8.1.5 Centred Nursing Care of Patients and Caregiver's Undergoing HSCT

Psychological and emotional aspects of the paediatric experience are complex and intricate. Health workers who take care of the sick child should be the privileged listeners of the child and be receptive to the child's point of view creating opportunities to talk.

8.1.5.1 The Relationship Between Nurse, Caregiver and Child

The approach of the paediatric team is strongly characterised by interpersonal and communication methods that are centred on empathic understanding, smiling, patience and gentleness. The relationship between nurses and children, but especially amongst nurses and parents, is difficult to summarise. However, this triangulation involves many mechanisms, roles and functions and impact on different aspects of personality and character.

8.1.5.2 Nursing Involvements in Care of Children Undergoing HSCT

Communication with the Child Undergoing HSCT
To employ an effective communication, professionals need to improve their listening and observation skills and exercise the ability to transmit ideas and feelings to others.

Information and Reassurance
It is through age-appropriate dialogue that healthcare professionals can explain to the sick child the sense of what is happening, the need for frightening interventions, recognition and meaning of fears. The child must know that they will never be left alone and nothing will happen that was not first controlled or decided by someone else in whom they are confident (Manookian et al. 2014).

The opportunity for the child to be properly informed allows them to become aware of what is happening to him in his life, to have greater familiarity with hostile hospital setting and be able to work together in their treatment path. Communication about the transplant process between the care staff, child and family can be further complicated by the different opinions with respect to what it is to be explained to the sick child. In general, it is preferred to adopt an attitude that respects the will of the parents, but this can lead to difficulties when it is the child themselves asking or looking for other information. The information, however, allows a reduction of the perception of pain, an increase in the child's compliance and a general improvement of the quality of life in the hospital (Badon and Cesaro 2015). The child who reports more free expression of emotion in their family in turn experiences lower levels of distress throughout the transplant period. Openness and honesty in communication in the family environment can encourage the emotional well-being of child and further promote their resiliency after the HSCT procedure is complete (Packman et al. 2010).

Listening

The ability to listen allows us to establish constructive relations. A real attitude to listening implies the attention, interest, tolerance, understanding and acceptance of the other. All of these are necessary preconditions for the establishment of an open relationship in which it is easier for the child to express and give information about himself. It is useful to encourage the patient to express themselves freely because, in addition to containing their distress, it is possible for the nurse to better understand the organisation of their personality and the defences put into place to cope with the situation (Badon and Cesaro 2015).

Psychological Support Service

Psychological support services are well developed and considered the standard of care in paediatric HSCT settings. Psychological support is configured, therefore, as the accompaniment's relationship of an entire family system in all phases of the transplant path. The presence of psychologist with the child who undergoes HSCT:

- Enables meaningful relationships to develop
- Facilitates understanding the illness of the child in all its complexity
- Makes request for help, expressed or implied, in view of practical difficulties, organisational, relational and emotional that may arise.

The intervention must be thought according to age, and even if the parent is always present in the isolation room, one can try to find some private moments between patient and psychologist. The attention to psychological and psychopathological aspects is not realised only through specialised interventions, but it must be realised every day by all staff members. Even the nursing staff, if trained, may perform work in the role of counsellor or coach (Barrera et al. 2007).

8.2 Transplantation Through the Ages: Teenage and Young Adults (TYA)

Abstract During the ages of 13–24, a person will undergoes perhaps the most rapid and formative changes of their life. The journey of transitioning from child to adult can be severely impacted when undergoing hospital treatment such as a haematopoietic stem cell transplant (HSCT) and complicates an already turbulent time. TYA patients present health professionals with a unique set of challenges, and it is important that care settings are designed to address and respond to the particular needs of young people and their families.

8.2.1 Introduction

A cancer diagnosis in young people is rare, with over 14000 15–24-year-olds diagnosed across Europe yearly (Stark et al. 2016). It is a growing number; the incidence of cancer in this group has increased by 50% in the past 30 years (Grinyer 2007). In response to this, guidance such as that published by the National Institute for Health and Care Excellence (NICE) aims to shape services and care to the needs of the TYA patient, which spans the ages of 13–24 years old (National Institute for Health and Clinical Excellence 2014). This is in response to research suggesting that this age group were receiving inadequate care when being treated in the paediatric or older adult setting as they have their own particular needs (Whiteson (2003). Patients undergoing HSCT require long-term clinical care beyond the acute phase of transplant and will be in regular contact with transplant clinicians and the multidisciplinary team (MDT) for a significant amount of time after bone marrow recovery and discharge from inpatient care. Care must be delivered within age-appropriate surroundings by health professionals experienced in caring for this group.

8.2.2 Special Indications for HSCT in TYA (AYA)

The most common indication for HSCT in the TYA age group is in the treatment of malignant haematological diseases lymphoma and acute leukaemia (Transplant 2015). Patients with non-Hodgkin's lymphoma, acute lymphoblastic leukaemia or acute myeloid leukaemia HSCT will be considered if high-risk, refractory or relapsed disease. In the case of Hodgkin's lymphoma, guidelines for teenagers indicate avoiding HSCT in the case of successful complete remission (CR) following first line of chemotherapy as chemotherapy alone usually yields successful long-term outcomes. However, once a patient requires second- or third-line treatment, the need for HSCT becomes more important (Transplant 2015). Standard recommendations are for an autologous transplant following successful CR after second-line treatment. Failure to obtain remission at this stage opens up the possibility of allograft, but this would require further discussions with local MDT. Full-intensity allografts are more routinely used in the younger adult patients as opposed to the older population as they tend to not have comorbidities associated with getting older, e.g. heart disease, and as such can tolerate stronger conditioning.

A small number of HSCTs are carried out every year for solid tumours. According to British Society for Bone Marrow Transplant (BSBMT) data, there were 162 transplants carried out on solid tumour patients of any age in 2015 within the UK, all of which were autografts (BSBMT 2015). The most common solid tumours for which HSCT is indicated includes neuroblastoma, germ cell and Ewing's sarcoma with clinicians using transplants to increase dose intensity (Gratwohl et al. 2004).

8.2.3 Considerations for Care

8.2.3.1 Risk-Taking Behaviour and Non-compliance

Becoming a teenager can herald a time of risk-taking behaviours as adolescents push the boundaries of their growing independence. At a time when peers are being afforded greater freedoms, often a cancer diagnosis re-establishes the dependency relationship between the young person and their family. Smoking, drinking alcohol, use of recreational drugs and engaging in unsafe sexual practices can allow the young person to regain some control, as can determining how compliant they choose to be with treatment. In the context of HSCT, indulging in unsafe behaviours can increase the risk of organ toxicity and infections. Failing to comply with supportive medications such as anti-infectives and immunosuppressives increases the morbidity and mortality rate of HSCT. As teenagers often focus on short-term outcomes if the effects of non-compliance are not immediately obvious, this can reinforce the behaviour. Similarly if there have been immediate side effects to therapy, e.g. nausea and weight gain, the patient may be less likely to adhere to medical advice. Patients who are compliant to treatment are almost three times more likely to have a better outcome than those who are not (Taddeo et al. 2008).

Gender, socio-economic status and ethnicity do not have an impact on whether a patient adheres to care (Kondryn et al. 2011). Depression and lowered self-esteem can increase rate of non-compliance, as can the perception of the illness severity. The relationship between the patient and their family can impact on how compliant a young person is with family conflict increasing the risk of non-adherence. Young patients who are treated in specialist young adult ward are more likely to be compliant compared to those who are treated in an adult cancer unit, further supporting the development of clinical areas dedicated to the care of the adolescent and young adult. This will be discussed further in the chapter.

Health professionals should be aware of the signs of non-compliance and facilitate an open and honest conversation with the patient. Confidentiality should be respected although in the instances where risky behaviour is disclosed, patients should be made aware if it is necessary to inform other members of the team. Healthy lifestyle choices should be promoted but within a non-judgemental environment. It is important that young patients are aware of appropriate boundaries whilst in hospital and local conduct, and operational policies must support staff in challenging risk-taking behaviours within the care environment (Smith et al. 2012).

8.2.3.2 Fertility

Fertility has been covered elsewhere in other chapters, but there are challenges unique to this age group which will be addressed in this section. Total body irradiation (TBI) and high-dose conditioning chemotherapy are highly likely to cause infertility. As often the type of transplant for the TYA patient is a full-intensity approach, this makes the risk of infertility a likely side effect of HSCT. If applicable, patients must be advised about the options of fertility preservation as part of transplant workup and given the opportunity to explore fertility preservations options although the urgency of the transplant may make this difficult.

In a study of TYA patients by Smith et al. (2007), fertility counselling was only provided to 36% undergoing treatment for cancer. Barriers to communication include a mutual awkwardness between the TYA patient and health professional when it comes to the topic of fertility. Clinicians can employ a jocular approach to young patients and find it difficult to broach sensitive topics (Quinn et al. 2009). Patients can feel confused and frightened about the potential effects of cancer treatment, or they are unable to envisage how fertility issues will impact them in the future (Smith et al. 2012).

For post-pubertal males, fertility preservation can be achieved through obtaining a sperm sample. Prior to attending fertility sessions, it should be clearly explained that the sample is obtained through masturbation, so they are prepared for the process. Sperm banking can potentially be an embarrassing process. Failing to bank a sample can leave the young person feeling disappointed and let-down, and it should be reinforced that not all attempts at sperm banking are successful.

Female fertility preservation is a more complex process. Ovarian stimulation and oocyte collection may be considered, but currently such methods have yielded limited success. Embryo collection can be difficult in this age group as they are unlikely to be ready to consider their current partners as a potential lifelong spouse (Levine and Stern 2010). Furthermore there is the added issue of time as it can take 2–4 weeks to harvest reproductive material from females. However female patients should partake in a full discussion about fertility preservation and be offered the opportunity to be referred to fertility experts as part of HSCT workup.

Discussions about fertility preservation should take place as early as possible, and parents should be included in order to support the teenager in their decision-making. Psychological input should be offered, as infertility can be one of the most impacting aspects of long-term survivorship, and there are many cultural, religious and social stigmas attached to being unable to bear a child. Although a difficult topic, in a study by Saito et al. (2005), young male patients indicated that the process of sperm banking was a positive one as they found it gave them some hope in the cancer journey, even if the sperm was never used.

8.2.3.3 Impact of Treatment on the Family Unit

Healthcare professionals looking after the TYA population must also care for the family unit and approach care holistically. During the ages of 13–24, young people undergo many developments in relation to the family unit. They may still be dependent on their parents, or they themselves may have their own children and responsibilities. Care needs to be adapted accordingly.

With TYA patients who are parents, often children will be babies and preschoolers. Moore and Rauch (2006) described what parents can expect from this age group in the context of a cancer diagnosis; even with age-appropriate explanation, under 5s will have little awareness of the diagnosis and aims associated with HSCT. What they will be aware of is the absence of a parent, stress in the household and changes to their routine. Rather than understand that these are caused by illness, the child may believe that they are somehow responsible for the absence. Parents may also recognise regression in the child's behaviour, such as bed-wetting in previously toilet-trained children.

Parents of HSCT patients can find their relationship health with their partners placed under considerable strain. In Long and Marsland (2011) the authors noted that the needs of the parents were put on hold to prioritise the needs of the TYA patient. In the case of hospitalisation, parental separation places even further strain as there is a decrease in communication, interaction and closeness between spouses. Reaction to the treatment process varies according to gender. Males try to withhold emotion to remain strong for their families, leaving them feeling quite isolated. To their partners they can be perceived as cold and uncaring. Differences in approach can cause emotional distance and feelings of loneliness. However in some partnerships, going through the experience of having a child with cancer can make the partnership stronger, with spouses being viewed as the main source of support.

There has been limited research on the effects of HSCT on the siblings of the recipient. One of the few studies performed by Pot-Mees and Zeitlin (1987) found that siblings developed new behavioural problems during and after their brother or sister's HSCT. The respondents described feelings of post-traumatic stress disorder, anxiety and low self-esteem as their family model was perceived as 'abnormal' and 'interrupted'. Parents and health professionals should include the sibling in discussions about their brother or sister, provide them with choices and create a safe hospital environment to help them adjust to the HSCT experience (Wilkins and Woodgate 2007).

Unlike other areas of medicine, family members may be directly involved in the treatment of HSCT patients by becoming the stem cell donors and as such a second patient. Siblings are usually the first option for a stem cell source. This can create an ethical dilemma for parents and healthcare staff, especially if the potential donor is a minor. What if the child refuses? What are the limitations of parental decision? What are the consequences for the child who refuses to donate? The Human Tissue Authority provides guidance on consenting a minor for stem cell collection in their 2015 guidelines (Human Tissue Authority 2015).

There is a significant potential for psychological impact on those siblings who undergo HLA tissue typing, regardless of whether they actually turn out to be a match or not. In MacLeod et al. (2003) siblings reported feeling as if they had 'no choice' about being tested and donating if matched. Reluctance was often not because they did not want to help but rather the fear of the procedure. In the case of siblings who were not matched, they described feelings of relief but also guilt. If they were matched but the sibling died, donors felt angry and blamed themselves, especially in the context of graft failure or graft-versus-host disease. By comparison, siblings in Wiener et al. (2008) found that the process of donating harboured an increase closeness between themselves and their siblings and their parents. Being able to help gave them a sense of pride. Response to the process does seem to be linked to whether the transplant was successful or not. A further family stem cell source is the parent. In the case of failing to find a suitable donor through siblings or the register, often parents will make a motivated stem cell donor. However, as in the case of the sibling, parents can also be left with profound feelings of guilt if the transplant fails (Barfield and Kodish 2006).

Health professionals have a duty to care for the family as a unit. Through the use of multidisciplinary team meetings, staff should be aware of family dynamics. Healthcare professionals should guide patients and their families on appropriate open communication though needs will vary depending on the family. For patients who are parents of young children, they should reassure the child that mum or dad's absence is not their fault and that they have done nothing wrong. Donors, whether siblings or parents, should be involved in the HSCT process from the start, and the complex variables associated with transplant success be carefully explored. Members of the MDT, such as psychologists, youth support workers, school teachers, social workers etc. should be involved early in the journey with patient consent. Creating a family-friendly space in the clinical environment can encourage children and siblings to visit. Key workers should be aware of support networks and resources locally to refer or signpost as appropriate.

Case Study
A 14-year-old girl was treated in a TYA unit for acute lymphoblastic leukaemia. From an early point in treatment, it was clear that disease was high risk due to existing cytogenetics and poor response at reassessment. She was placed on UKALL 2011 Regimen C but experienced complications including methotrexate encephalopathy and drug reactions to asparaginase and the alternative, erwinase. Treatment was suboptimal. The clinical team decided to test her brother and sister to plan for a sibling allograft when a repeat bone marrow showed a significant amount of minimal residual disease after 6 months of treatment. Her sister was found to be a 10/10 HLA match. However her mother struggled greatly with the fact that her 'healthy' child would be put through procedures, especially as she was only 10 years old. The younger child was clear on her intention to help her sister but did experience distress when subjected to blood tests. This exacerbated the inner turmoil felt by her mother as she worried about the eventual bone marrow harvest and openly discussed refusing consent for the procedure in front of her 14-year-old daughter, despite knowing that finding an alternative stem cell source was unlikely as the patient was from a complex ethnic background. With the help of the available psychological team and activity coordinators at the paediatric and TYA centre the patient, her sibling, mother and family received separate counselling, and the resulting harvest was successful.

8.2.3.4 Body Image

Side effects of drugs used in the HSCT process can cause significant physical changes to a patient's appearance. This is not exclusive to the TYA patient but can be more psychologically harmful as they are at an age where physical appearance is central to their world and when feeling different from peers can have a negative impact on self-esteem (Smith et al. 2012). Issues such as weight gain and alopecia can have a psychological impact which is greater compared to the older adults. Appearance concerns amongst TYA cancer patients have been linked to lower self-esteem, depression, anxiety, feelings of loneliness and suicidality and decreased treatment compliance (Fan and Eiser 2009).

Weight loss is an inevitable part of the acute and recovery phase of HSCT as patients struggle with the gastrointestinal side effects of treatment. For female patients, weight loss can alarmingly seem like a positive aspect of treatment in line with societies' perceptions of what is attractive. The opposite is true of male patients. It is becoming more normal for young males to try to obtain a muscular physic through careful gym and diet regimens. Often newly diagnosed young males are bulky with little body fat. Anecdotally the biggest struggle they tend to have is with muscle wasting aspect of HSCT, in the context of fatigue, poor appetite and reduced exercise tolerance. Research into this area with the TYA population is limited although a study by Rodgers et al. (2010) interviewed TYA patients on their experiences of nutrition post-HSCT. Participants described abnormal appetites until day 50 post-HSCT, by which point they were able to manage a small amount of food. Progress continued, with stark improvement in feeling hungry by day +100. Participants were able to correlate the link between improved eating habits and appetite with returning to their 'normal selves', advising future patients to have some control over what they cat and portion size rather than being forced into eating by parents and health professionals.

Weight and hair gain is something that not everyone associates with chemotherapy. Often media depictions of cancer patients include gaunt, cachexic figures with alopecia. For patients receiving high-dose steroids, for example, in the treatment of graft-versus-host disease, a typical side effect includes development of facial swelling, known as 'moon face' and unwanted facial hair. This can drastically alter appearance and be devastating for a young person. This can also lead them to become non-compliant to the treatment with poor consequences for their treatment success.

Alopecia is a common and well-known side effect of chemotherapy and usually one of the first things TYA patients ask about when discussing treatment. Hair is often very much tied into identity, and the idea of losing it can make some teenagers refuse treatment when the idea is initially discussed. Youth support workers and nurse specialists are excellent at helping to organise a replacement before hair loss starts to occur (usually 2 weeks after the start of chemotherapy). There are wigs made of real hair which can often be difficult to identify next to the real thing. However a lot of hair replacement focuses on females, with male patients finding options to be limited.

Conditioning regimens containing TBI can impact on the growth of patients who are treated at a young age, i.e. prepubertal (Leiper 1995). This is due to the radiation administered to the hypothalamic-pituitary axis and the resting reduction to the growth hormone. Replacement therapy can aid to reduce further loss of height, but cannot reverse loss. Clinicians need to carefully monitor growth of patients to ensure early intervention (Lowis 2000).

8.2.3.5 Impact on Life

Approximately 60% of children and adolescents who are long-term survivors of HSCT experience late effects, both of the physical and psychological nature (Forinder and Posse 2008). Fertility and growth issues have been covered already in this chapter, and organ toxicity associated with HSCT is written about in other sections of this book. There are other ways that HSCT impacts of life which are unique challenges to the TYA patient.

For the adolescent and young adult, peers are an important feature of life. However patients of this age undergoing a HSCT experience social isolation from their friends and community. This is not only due to physical absence from school, university and work but also a difficulty on the part of the healthy young person to understand and empathise with the experiences of their unwell friend (Thomas et al. 2006). From the perspective of the survivor of a HSCT, they can find it difficult to relate to their peers after what they have been through. In interviews with Forinder and Posse (2008), TYA HSCT patients felt they had a different perspective on life, with material things and physical appearance not being as important as they once were. That said, subjects were conscious of their change in appearance and upset at looking different to those in their social network.

The relationship between the parents and the unwell adolescent is difficult to navigate. Necessary increased dependency is at odds with the need for autonomy that is typical at this age. This can lead to direct conflict between the two parties, especially once the TYA patient has completed the acute phase of the transplant. A sharp difference of priorities can exist between parent and patient (Grinyer 2009). Research also suggests that TYA patients may not have fully developed executive function due to regression and cognitive development delay which adds to the tension between the parent and patient relationship (Kaufman 2006).

Survivorship is a growing area of research as outcomes from cancer treatment improves. Health professionals and researchers recognise that completion of cancer treatment is the start of a difficult journey of adjustment and transition. Clinical staff need to consider the fall out of treatment, and patients should be aware that they can and should continue to access support. Treatment within dedicated TYA clinical areas can help patients to access peer support which is tailored more to their development needs.

8.2.4 Teenager as a Child vs. Adult

Under 18s present legal challenges for healthcare professionals as the young person must be assessed on their ability to make appropriate decisions about their care on an individual basis. In the following section, issues of consent, confidentiality and guardian roles are discussed. Much of this part will discuss current legislation within the UK. Health professionals should refer to local legislation for further clarity.

8.2.4.1 Consenting for Treatment

Informed consent is a cornerstone of medical practice. Violation of this has legal implications for clinicians but more importantly jeopardises the ethical rights of the patient (Bayer et al. 2011). In order to satisfy the principles of informed consent, it must be given freely and with full comprehension. Patients must be provided with adequate information in understandable terms. Treatment options should be reviewed, and a discussion about the risks, benefits and alternatives to the proposed treatment should take place and be documented. Signing of a consent form is symbolic, representing completion of the consenting process.

Informed consent is a relatively straightforward process when concerning over 18s as long as the individual has capacity. In the UK, patients between 16 and 18 can consent for treatment but may not be able to refuse treatment in the case of saving their lives or preventing serious harm. Under 16s may legally consent if they meet certain criteria of being Gillick competent. This principle is based on a case in the 1980s where Victoria Gillick took her local authority to court to prevent them from providing contraception to her children without her knowledge (Wheeler 2006). The high court determined that minors under 16 have the potential to independently consent to treatment if deemed competent to do so. However it is a good practice to involve the young person's family in the process. In the case of under 18s who are deemed Gillick competent but refusing treatment, it is possible for the decision to be overturned where it will lead to death or serious injury (Department of Health 2009).

In the case where a minor cannot independently consent and parental involvement is required, the Oviedo Convention recommends the use of the term 'authorisation' rather than 'consenting on behalf of a child' as the former relates to the concept of a third authority, i.e. the parent, and is slightly different from informed consent. As informed consent is an expression of personal choice, it can only relate to the person being treated. Authorising treatment is acknowledging that it is in the best interests of the child. Furthermore the Oviedo Convention requires that the opinion of the minor must still be taken into consideration. Thus the decision-making process involves three parties: the clinicians, the person with parental responsibility and the child undergoing treatment (Nicolussi 2015). According to the Children Act 2004, parental responsibility extends to the child's parents if married at the time of conception or birth, the child's father if not married to the mother but who features on the birth certificate or the child's legally appointed guardian or a local authority who has been granted a care order in respect of the child.

Scenarios where there are disputes between parties involved in treatment decisions are rare but do occur. This can be between patients and their parents, between health professionals and the family or between parents to provide more common instances. A well-known example is when parents who are Jehovah's Witnesses refuse blood transfusions on behalf of their child. Cultural beliefs should be respected, but bone marrow failure can be a life-threatening complication of HSCT. In instances such as this, which can be pre-empted, plans should be made about how to deal with the complication before it arises, i.e. the use of erythropoietin as an alternative. Unfortunately not every eventuality can be considered, and advice may need to be sought through legal channels which will provide protection to the patient, family and the health professionals concerned.

8.2.4.2 Communication

Regardless of whether a minor is able to consent, they should still be encouraged to participate in discussions about their care, and if they choose to attend consultations, information should be directed at them. Healthcare professionals should give the same time and respect to young people as they would do to adult patients. Information should be provided using language that is understandable, giving all involved parties the opportunity to ask questions. Discussions should be truthful and open, with consideration given to confidentiality. The information provided should be appropriate to the age of the young person and include a discussion about:

- Their illness and proposed treatment
- The purpose of investigations and treatments and what they involve
- Benefits and risks, including of not having treatment
- Who will be responsible for their care
- Their right to ask for a second opinion or retract consent if deemed capable (GMC 2007)

If is justifiable to keep the above information from the young person if you think that it will cause them serious harm (this does not include concerns about upsetting them) or if the patient asks you not to tell them, preferring to leave someone else to make the decision for them.

Often guardians and young people can struggle to have honest discussions together as they are afraid of upsetting each other especially in the context of sensitive subjects. It should be made clear to the young person that they can have consultations on their own. A chaperone may be appropriate, although this could deter the young person from having a frank discussion.

8.2.4.3 Confidentiality

Respecting confidentiality is important in harbouring good relations with young people, making them feel confident about seeking care and advice. If required to share information with parents or other health professionals, the young person should be made aware and agree. If they refuse, there are still circumstances where information should be disclosed including where it would be in the public's best interest, when it is in the best interests of the young person when they lack capacity and when disclosure is required by law. Examples include if the information would help prevent or prosecute in the case of a serious crime (usually against the young person)

and if the patient is engaging in activities that might put them at risk, e.g. serious addiction and self-harming.

8.2.5 TYA Cancer Care in Europe: A General Review

Across Europe, cancer is the second cause of death amongst 15–24-year-olds (Gatta et al. 2009). Despite this, the services for this population remain in the developing stage in comparison to that of children or older adults. This is a strive for change, and an example of this is the European Network for Cancer Research in Children and Adolescents (ENCCA) programme which aims to share knowledge and services across the continent. Stark et al. (2016) summarised the work across individual countries and set out guidelines with collaborative aims to:

- Not necessarily have agreed age cut-offs set across Europe; rather treat according to the needs of their population.
- Provide an age-appropriate environment for TYA patients to complete their care, with services tailored to the needs of the patient and family.
- Have an active relationship between paediatric and adult oncologists or a dedicated TYA team, including specialist health professionals such as nurses, social workers, psychologists, teachers and activity coordinators.
- Have a fertility preservation programme.
- Have a transition programme for those moving from child to TYA services and TYA to older adult care.
- Have clinical trials available to the TYA population in varying tumour groups.

Stark et al. (2016) also summarised progress of individual countries in regard to TYA care:

The UK pioneered the TYA model back in the 1990s through collaboration between the Teenage Cancer Trust (TCT) and National Health Service (NHS). As such the pathway swell is defined. All TYA patients with a cancer diagnosis must be discussed at a TYA MDT, and those between 13 and 19 must be treated in a dedicated TYA centre. The service undergoes yearly peer review, and lead clinicians are at the forefront of specialist networks. There is a separate TYA clinical studies group with the aim of including the availability of trials to this patient group. TYA health professionals have their own UK professional membership organisation which provides peer support and sharing of information between services. There are 25 TYA centres across the county, and development of such services is discussed in detail in the next section.

In Germany there is separate infrastructure for paediatric and adult cancer patients with a strict age barrier of 18 years separating them. The majority of adolescent care is performed within paediatric oncology. However practice is changing and a collaborative approach is happening, with some centres creating TYA-specific MDT programmes.

In Italy the Committee on Adolescents was formed by the Associazione Italiana Ematologia Oncologia Pediatrica in 2010 to ensure TYA cancer patients have prompt, adequate and fair access to the best care. Since then two TYA units have been opened. A national task force dedicated to teenagers and young adults with cancer was set up in 2013 to push the agenda for TYA care further.

In France research by Desandes et al. (2012) showed that 82% of 15–18-year-olds with cancer were treated in an adult environment and few were enrolling clinical trials. This prompted the initiation of an improvement plan. Since then eight TYA units and three specialist centres have been opened with dedicated teams; improvements have been made to the inclusion of TYA patients in clinical trial, and a specific psychosocial programme has been initiated. The Institut de France planned to create localised care pathways and has started a national association to focus on cancer care for patients between 15 and 25 years old.

In Spain in 2011 the Adolescents with Cancer Committee was set up by the Spanish Society of Paediatric Haematology; however, a survey in 2014 showed that over 14-year-olds were still generally being treated in adult care settings (Lassaletta et al. 2013). TYA oncologists and patients have founded the charity 'Spanish Association of Adolescents and Young Adults with Cancer' to create support for young people with cancer and push the TYA agenda.

In Denmark a TYA project started by nurses commenced in 2000 at Aarhus University. A national initiative is also being planned to bring together the collective view of young patients, to create TYA-focused unit and to specialise treatment.

In 2013 in the Netherland health professionals started a national TYA project dedicated to the care of 18–35-year-olds and focused on quality of life, late effects and fertility.

In Portugal that is no national project yet, but in Lisbon a project has commenced to create a TYA unit for patients aged between 16 and 25. In other countries, e.g. Belgium, Bulgaria, Czech Republic, Ireland, Greece, Hungary, Lithuania, Norway, Poland, Romania, Slovenia and Sweden, there is no national project yet, but there are some local projects occurring.

8.2.6 Development of TYA Cancer Units: The UK Experience

It was first recognised that young UK patients had specific needs in the 1950s with the publication of the Platt Report (Ministry of Health 1959). Publication of the Calman-Hine report in 1995 particularly acknowledged the issues faced by young cancer patients. Treating 13–18-year-olds in the same units as toddlers or over 18s with the elderly fails to provide care that meets their needs. The UK has been at the forefront of developing TYA-specific treatment areas; however, age-appropriate care is still not available to all.

The Teenage Cancer Trust charity was set up over 10 years ago to act as support and advocate for young people facing cancer. Alongside other charity organisations internationally including CanTeen Australia, CanTeen New Zealand, LIVESTRONG and SeventyK, they created the International Charter of Rights for Young People with Cancer which states that young people with cancer should:

- Receive education about cancer and its prevention
- Be taken seriously when seeking medical attention to ensure that they receive the earliest possible diagnosis and referral for a suspected cancer
- Have access to suitable qualified health professionals with significant experience in treating patients with cancer in this age group
- Access to suitable clinical trials
- Receive age-appropriate support
- Empowered in making decisions
- Fertility preservation
- Access to specialised treatment and services in age-appropriate facilities
- Financial support
- Long-term survivorship support

The Teenage Cancer Trust was set up over a decade ago and works in partnership with the National Health Service to open inpatient and outpatient cancer units, providing education, specialist staff and annual meetings to raise awareness of the issues associated with caring for this age group. In 1990 they opened the first dedicated unit at the Middlesex Hospital in London and currently have 28 units operating across the UK. Other European countries have followed with the Institut Gustave-Roussy in Paris opening in 2003 (Whelan 2003). Development of TYA-dedicated units is down predominantly to initiatives in response to local needs rather than a general coordinated health policy. As a consequence there is great variation in the provision of services for TYA patients with cancer across the UK. In 2005 the National Institute for Health and Care Excellence (NICE) published recommendations for health professionals treating teenager and young adults with cancer. Amongst the guideline was advice about where young people should be treated; under 18s should be treated in a principle treatments centre, and those 19 and over should be offered a choice about where they go. Principle treatment centres are designed to offer expert medical care, an age-appropriate environment, psychosocial support and access to a multidisciplinary team.

During the development stage of a new unit, often patients will be asked for their opinion and input into the facilities and design. Use of the internet is important in this age group as a means of staying in touch with normality whilst an inpatient, so facilities should be provided. Patients should have access to appropriate equipment including game consoles, music, pool tables etc. Designated recreational areas can provide a space for patients to socialise and relax away from their hospital beds. This can also encourage peer support as patients interact in communal spaces. Support for the young person can be gained by having somebody staying with them, and clinical areas should be able to accommodate. This is often possible in paediatric and teenage settings but can be difficult to provide in adult units.

The ethos of TYA care is to approach holistically. This is achieved by presenting each new patient at weekly TYA and site-specific MDTs. During TYA MDTs, health professionals from across the service attend to participate in discussions about new patients and their planned treatments. All TYA patients, irrespective of place of treatment, should be discussed at a TYA MDT to ensure that they have the opportunity to receive the correct support. According to (Smith et al. 2012) barriers to setting up a TYA MDTs, including time constraints, perceived duplication and resources. However uses of MDTs are thought to improve clinical trial recruitment, outcomes and multi-agency working.

Due to duration of follow-up post-HSCT, patients may be required to transition as they pass landmark birthdays. This should be a planned process that addresses the needs of TYA patients with chronic health problems as they move from child-centred care to the TYA setting or TYA care to the adult health system. This can be a difficult time for patients and their families as they leave behind the team that has moved them through the acute phase of the HSCT process and with whom they have built up a strong bond. Planning may take a number of months and should be approached sensitively. The process can be helped by patients visiting the new units and good communication between all parties.

8.2.7 Summary

- TYA cancer patients include those aged between 13 and 24 years old.
- Often HSCT indications in this age group are for malignancies including refractory or relapsed leukaemia and lymphoma.
- There are unique challenges facing this age group when diagnosed and undergoing treatment.
- One significant challenge is the impact that a cancer diagnosis has on the family unit especially in the younger siblings providing the stem cell.
- Even when considered a minor, patients do still need to be assessed for competence and afforded the same respect as adult patients.
- Partnership between the NHS and charities such as the Teenage Cancer Trust can provide an age-appropriate environment for patients and their families.
- There is still much work to be done across Europe to ensure each patient is getting care that is responsive to their needs.

8.3 Transplanting the Adult and the Older Adult: Nursing Considerations

Abstract Older people are usually identified by their chronological age, and persons aged 65 years or over are often referred to as 'elderly' (WHO 2010). The median age at diagnosis of patients with acute myeloid leukaemia (AML), myelodysplastic syndromes (MDS), chronic lymphatic leukaemia (CLL), multiple myeloma (MM) and non-Hodgkin's lymphoma (NHL) is over 65 years old (Eichhorst et al. 2011; NCI 20003; Palumbo and Anderson 2011; Sekeres 2010; Smith et al. 2011; Siegel et al. 2015). Most of these haematological diseases are not curable unless an allogeneic or autologous haematopoietic cell transplantation can be performed.

Currently the indications for and subsequently the use of haematopoietic cell transplantation as a treatment option in older adults with haemato-logical malignancies are increasing, yet the majority of our experience is with patients under the age of 65.

Older patients however represent a very heterogeneous group with respect to overall health status; some individuals stay fit, whilst others are frail or become fragile suddenly.

In order to help healthcare professionals decide on the best treatment option for their older patients, geriatric assessment (GA) (Extermann et al. 2005) can identify unknown medical, functional, cognitive and social issues, making it possible to plan early interventions. Although GA still requires prospective validation in larger cohorts, this assessment is able to predict survival and toxicities and to detect unknown geriatric problems.

A substantial percentage of older adults have more difficulties processing and remembering information than younger ones. It is important to make sure that also older adults understand their disease, the prognosis and the treatment plan to make an informed decision. Therefore, it is essential to assess cognitive functioning and in case of mild cognitive impairment that the information is tailored to reflect the individual's needs.

Most healthcare professionals working in haematology settings are not trained in geriatrics. The aim of this section is to describe GA, to provide information about the increasing prevalence of certain risk factors (impaired cognitive function, medication non-adherence) and how patient information can be adjusted to the needs of older patients.

Keywords Older patients • Fragile • Geriatric problems • Geriatric assessment • Patient information

8.3.1 Differences Between Older and Younger Patients

The incidence of acute myeloid leukaemia (AML), myelodysplastic syndromes (MDS), chronic lymphatic leukaemia (CLL), multiple myeloma (MM) and non-Hodgkin's lymphoma

(NHL) increases with age, with the majority of patients being over 65 years of age (Eichhorst et al. 2011; NCI 20003, Palumbo and Anderson 2011; Sekeres 2010; Smith et al. 2011; Siegel et al. 2015). Most of these haematological diseases are not curable unless the appropriate allogeneic and/or autologous haematopoietic cell transplantation is performed.

Chronological age is becoming less of a barrier to reduced-intensity conditioning in allogeneic haematopoietic cell transplantation (HCT), and as a result, HCT in the older adult population is increasing. However the majority of experience with stem cell transplantation remains amongst younger adults.

Older age is still associated with:

- Pharmacokinetic and pharmacodynamic changes
- An increased risk of toxicities and infectious complications from chemotherapeutic agents
- An impaired immune system
- A high prevalence of comorbid conditions and an overall worse performance status

These factors may result in higher risks of non-relapse death after both autologous and allogeneic HCT (Artz and Chow, 2016; Mamdani et al. 2016).

Older patients represent a very heterogeneous group in terms of health and functioning; as whilst some individuals remain fit, others are frail or become fragile suddenly.

More than half of adults aged over 65 have three or more medical problems (Boyd et al. 2012) and may be taking multiple medications, making care more complex.

In older patients, therapeutic decisions are widely based on the patient's age, general health, the disease features, as well as the patient's personal wishes, and clinical judgement. However, even amongst older patients with a good performance status, geriatric impairments are reported (Extermann et al. 2005). In order to help healthcare professionals (HCP) work with patients and caregivers to decide on the best treatment option, GA can be used to objectively evaluate patients, identifying medical, functional, cognitive and social issues, making it possible to uncover potential problem areas and plan early interventions. Although GA still requires prospective validation in larger cohorts, and in the transplant setting (Elsawy and Sorror 2016), this assessment is able to predict survival and toxicities (Artz et al. 2006; Palumbo et al. 2015) and to detect unknown geriatric problems, making it possible to plan early interventions and to influence treatment decisions (Kenis et al. 2013).

8.3.2 Geriatric Assessment

GA strategies need to be implemented early on in the patient pathway in order to facilitate decision-making in relation to the optimal approach to treatment. It can assist in identifying patients most likely to benefit from standard induction and post-remission therapies, as well as in the consideration of performing a HCT. To determine the best treatment for the patient, GA is needed to systematically uncover medical, functional, cognitive and social issues, which may compromise the treatment. Table 8.2 provides an overview of domains and tools commonly used. Domains are assessed by means of commonly used tools to measure functional status, cognitive function, nutritional status, comorbidities, polypharmacy and socio-economic status. Some use this in combination with a short screening tool to detect vulnerability. An appropriately trained healthcare professional can perform the assessment, and in some cases this may be a nurse. GA instruments aid in identifying potential problems; however, when the problem is identified as being severe, a thorough assessment is needed to understand the cause. In order to optimise the outcomes of the older patient, a geriatric intervention or referral may be necessary, for example, to the geriatrician, dietician, physiotherapist, social worker or psychologist.

A full GA can be time-consuming and burdensome for HCP who are not trained in the evaluation of older adults. The use of more simplified screening tools like the Vulnerable Elders Survey (VES) (Saliba et al. 2001) and G8 screening tool (Soubeyran et al. 2011) (see Table 8.2) can be

Table 8.2 Comprehensive geriatric assessment domains and commonly used tools, and screening tools

Domain	Tools	Reference
Functional status	Performance Status (PS)	Karnofsky and Burchenal (1949), and Mor et al. (1984)
	Activities of Daily Living (ADL)	Mahoney and Barthel (1965)
	Instrumental Activities of daily Living (IADL)	Graf (2008)
	Self-reported number of falls	Peeters et al. (2010)
Comorbidities	hematopoietic cell transplantation comorbidity index (HCT-CI)	Sorror et al. (2005)
Polypharmacy	comprehensive drug review	
Geriatric syndromes	Mini mental State Examination (MMSE)	Folstein et al. (1975)
	Geriatric Depression Scale (GDS-15)	Almeida and Almeida (1999)
Nutrional status	Malnutrition Universal Screening Tool (MUST)	Stratton et al. (2004)
	Simplified Nutritional Assessment Questionnaire (SNAQ)	Kruizenga et al. (2005)
	Mini Nutrional Assessment Short Form (MNA)	Guigoz (2006)
Screening tool		
Vulnerable elders survey	Age	Saliba et al. (2001)
	Self-rated health	
	6 physical function limitations	
	5 IADL/ADL items	
G8 Screening tool	Appetite, Weight loss, BMI	Soubeyran et al. (2011)
	Mobility	
	Mood and cognition	
	Number medications	
	Patient-related health	
	Age categories	

employed in an initial appraisal, identifying those who would benefit most from a more detailed and complete GA.

8.3.2.1 Functional Status

An important determinant of frailty is functional status, including Karnofsky's performance status (PS) (Karnofsky and Burchenal 1949; Mor et al. 1984), the activities of daily living (ADL) (Mahoney and Barthel 1965) and the instrumental activities of daily living (IADL) (Graf 2008). The PS is utilised routinely in HCT and is a global estimate of the overall health of patients according to their doctor. The ADL measures the level of independence or dependence of patients and, in terms of limitations to self-care, mobility and being able to walk and continence status.

The IADL describes the more complex ADLs necessary for living in the community and assesses the competence in skills such as shop-ping, cooking and managing finances, which are required for independent living.

Evaluation of gait difficulty and self-reported number of falls may also be useful when looking at functional status. Problems may be caused by fatigue, muscle weakness, dizziness or neuropathies induced by cancer or its treatment and can cause significant mortality and morbidity.

8.3.2.2 Vision and Hearing Impairments

Many older adults have either a visual impairment, a hearing impairment, or both. There is evidence of an association between hearing impairment and cognitive decline amongst older adults (Valentijn et al. 2005). An evaluation of visual and hearing acuity of any patient should be undertaken during the physical assessment. Where possible, hearing and visual impairments should be corrected, so that elders can function better, promoting greater independence.

8.3.2.3 Comorbidity and Polypharmacy

Typical older adults have multiple comorbidities. For HCT, comorbidity can be assessed by using the haematopoietic cell transplantation comorbidity index (HCT-CI) introduced by Sorror et al. in 2005, as an evaluation of organ dysfunction for potential HCT recipients. The HCT-CI was developed from the historical Charlson comorbidity index (Charlson et al. 1987).

Due to existing comorbidities, the older patient is often taking multiple medications – each with their own side effects, interactions and contraindications. Polypharmacy, (defined as an excessive number of medication (≥ 5)), is sometimes further increased by medications which can be bought over the counter without prescription. Some of these medications may interact with prescribed cancer treatments or even supportive medications such as immunosuppressive agents that are used following HCT. A comprehensive drug review is strongly advised before initiating therapy and then regularly throughout the patients' treatment pathway to maintain accurate records of concomitant drugs and ensure avoidance of potentially inappropriate medications.

8.3.2.4 Cognitive Functioning

Although cognitive decline is acknowledged to increase with age, significant variability is noted amongst the older population (Greene and Adelman 2003). They define mild cognitive impairment as 'deficits in memory that do not impact on daily functioning'.

However, consequences of even mild cognitive impairment are significant because these patients may have more difficulty understanding the risks and benefits of treatment and also adhering to complex cancer treatment regimens. It should be remembered that a diagnosis of cognitive impairment does not necessarily mean that the patient is incapable of making decisions and consenting. Most patients are still able to understand the risks and benefits of treatment and of being involved in research. It is important that researchers do not automatically exclude patients with cognitive impairment from treatment but that every effort is made to ensure that patients are fully informed in order to be able to give their consent.

Assessment of cognitive function is included as a domain in GA. In addition, the Mini-Mental State Examination (MMSE) is widely used as a screener for cognitive impairment and for dementia in older persons (Folstein et al. 1975) .

8.3.2.5 Geriatric Syndromes

Geriatric syndromes include dementia, depression, delirium, osteoporosis, falls and fatigue. Specific geriatric syndromes can be assessed with instruments such as the MMSE and the geriatric depression scale (GDS-15) (Almeida and Almeida 1999). The MMSE assesses to which degree the person is alert, oriented and able to concentrate and perform complex mental tasks and affective functions and detects signs of dementia (Folstein et al. 1975; Sattar et al. 2014). The geriatric depression scale (GDS-15) searches for signs of depression (Sheikh and Yesavage 1986; Almeida and Almeida 1999). The presence of dementia and/or depression is associated with a negative impact on survival (Pallis et al. 2010).

8.3.2.6 Medication Adherence

During HCT it is imperative that patients adhere to the prescribed treatment. Non-adherence leads to poorer health outcomes, such as increased incidence of transplant-related morbidity and mortality, higher cancer recurrence rates and shorter survival (Puts et al. 2014).

Older age has not been identified as a risk factor for non-adherence, unless the older adult himself perceives insufficient social support. For older adults, certain factors are known to impact upon medication non-adherence. These include factors relating to the healthcare system and the treatment team:

- High cost of medication whilst patient income is low
- Incomplete insurance coverage
- Lack of coordinated care
- Individual factors such as misunderstanding of instructions, intentional choice of medication and non-adherence to accommodate the individuals' lifestyle and daily activities (Van Cleave et al. 2016)

Whilst there is no screening tool currently available for non-adherence in gero-oncological patients, there are several existing medication adherence scales available to assess patients' adherence to medication (Lam and Fresco 2015).

8.3.2.7 Nutritional Status

Nutritional deficiency and malnutrition are common in older adults. The presence of weight loss and/or anorexia points towards malnutrition, which increases vulnerability to illness. In order to determine nutritional status, screening instruments like the Malnutrition Universal Screening Tool (MUST) (Stratton et al. 2004) or Simplified Nutritional Assessment Questionnaire (SNAQ) (Kruizenga et al. 2005) are available. In all these screening instruments, unintentional weight loss in a short time is a fixed-item parameter to evaluate malnutrition. In order to diagnose malnutrition, the Mini Nutritional Assessment (MNA) (Guigoz 2006) can be used. The MNA assesses:

- Decline in food intake
- Weight loss, mobility
- Neuropsychological problems
- Body mass index
- Number of medications taken per day
- Patients' assessment of their health status compared with others their own age

A multidisciplinary approach to nutrition assessment, care planning, intervention and evaluation in HCT patients should be advocated where possible, with the involvement of healthcare professionals such as dieticians and nutrition specialist teams in collaboration with the medical and nursing team.

8.3.2.8 Socio-economic

Social support, persons' general living conditions as well as availability and adequacy of caregivers should be an integral part of GA. There are different types of support, such as:

- Everyday emotional support
- Emotional support with problems
- Appreciation support
- Practical support
- Social companionship
- Informative support

Everyone needs everyday support in a certain way. The type and amount of support needed will depend on the individual and also the phase of the illness and treatment. Consideration should also be given to the well-being of the caregiver as the quality of life and quality of care of the patient also depend upon this factor.

8.3.2.9 Decision-Making

Older persons may have grown up in a healthcare culture where decision-making was more paternalistic. As a result, this may either lead to lower requests for information by the patient or to a risk of poor overall communication. For most young patients, the decision and desire to be transplanted are often clear. For older patients however, the decision is often far less obvious, and the choice to proceed to HCT is a complex one (Randall et al. 2016). Patients might think they are 'too old' for HCT or be concerned whether they can find an available caregiver and whether they have enough money for extra costs incurred or that it will impair their quality of life (Randall et al. 2016). Medical information about the general process and outcomes of the transplant, donor sources, medications, timelines, and risks and benefits of the procedure are usually provided after induction therapy has been successful. However, older people have more difficulties processing and remembering information than younger ones (Posma et al. 2009), and cognition may have been affected further by the chemotherapy that has been given (Williams et al. 2016). It is important, therefore, to provide education about HCT, which is gradual and repeated during induction and, afterwards, presented using plain language, empowering the older patient to make the decision about transplant (Randall et al. 2016). In order to improve the patients' ability to actively participate in the decision-making process and increase treatment adherence, a step-by-step approach should be considered (Posma et al. 2009) and narrowed down to what is meaningful to make a decision (D'Souza et al. 2015, Posma et al. 2009). Regarding risks and general knowledge of medical procedures, written information, multimedia interventions, extended discussions and test/feedback techniques can improve the patients' understanding (Schenker et al. 2011). Particular attention should be paid to implementing interventions that are accessible to patients with limited literacy and/or limited vision. These groups are at increased risk for poor comprehension.

References

Transplanting the Child

Asadi M, Manookian A, Nasrabadi AN. Parent' experiences of their children bone marrow transplantation: a qualitative study. Int J Hema Oncol Stemm Cell Res (IJOSCR). 2011;

Badon P, Cesaro S. Assistenza infermieristica in pediatria. In: CEA, editor. 2nd ed. CEA; 2015

Barrera M, Andrews GS, Burners D, Atenafu E. Age differences in perceived social support by paediatric haematopoietic progenitor cell transplant patients: a longitudinal study. Child Care Health Dev. 2007;34(1):19–24.

Bauk K, Andrews A. The pediatric sibling donor experience in hematopoietic stem cell transplant: an integrative review of the literature. J Pediatr Nurs. 2013;28:235–42.

Bingen K, Kent MW, Rodday AM, Ratichek SJ, Kupst MJ, Parsons SK. Children's coping with hematopoietic stem cell transplant stressors: results from the journeys to recovery study. J Child Health Care. 2012;41(2):145–61.

Chang G, Recklitis SJ, Recklitis C, Syrjala K, Patel SK, Harris L, Rodday AM, Tighiouart H, Parsons SK. Children's psychological distress during pediatric HSCT: parent and child perspectives. Pediatr Blood Cancer. 2012;58:289–96.

Committee on Bioethics Children as Hematopoietic Stem Cell Donors. Pediatrics. 2010;125:392; originally published online 25 Jan 2010.

Manookian A, Nikbakht Nasrabadi A, Asadi M. Children's lived experiences of hematopoietic stem cell transplantation. Nurs Health Sci. 2014;16:314–20.

Munzenberger N, Fortanier C, Macquart-Moulin G, Faucher C, Novakovitch G, Maraninchi D, et al. Psychosocial aspects of haematopoietic stem cell donation for allogeneic transplantation: how family donors cope with this experience. Psychooncology. 1999;8(1):55–63.

Mona M. 2015 link: http://nursingexercise.com/child-growth-development-overview.

Norberg L, Mellgren K, Winiarksi J, Forinder U. Relationship between problems related to child late effects and parent burnout after pediatric hematopoietic stem cell transplantation. Pediatr Transplant. 2014;18:302–9.

Packman W, Weber S, Wallace J, Bugescu N. Psychological effects of hematopoietic SCT on pediatric patients, siblings and parents: a review. Bone Marrow Transplant. 2010;45:1134–46.

Passweg JR, Baldomero H, Peters C, Gaspar HB, Cesaro S, Dreger P, Duarte RF, Falkenburg JHF, Farge-Bancel D, Gennery A, Halter J, Kröger N, Lanza F, Marsh J, Mohty M, Sureda A, Velardi A, Madrigal A, for the European Society for Blood and Marrow Transplantation (EBMT). Hematopoietic SCT in Europe: data and trends in 2012 with special consideration of pediatric transplantation. Bone Marrow Transplant. 2014:1–7.

Passweg JR, Baldomero H, Bader P, Bonini C, Cesaro S, Dreger P, Duarte RF, Dufour C, Kuball J, Farge-Bancel D, Gennery A, Kröger N, Lanza F, Nagler A, Sureda A, Mohty M, for the European Society for Blood and Marrow Transplantation (EBMT). Hematopoietic stem cell transplantation in Europe 2014: more than 40000 transplants annually. Bone Marrow Transplant. 2016:1–7.

Pentz RD, Alderfer MA, Pelletier W, Stegenga K, Haight AE, Hendershot KA, et al. Unmet needs of siblings of pediatric stem cell transplant recipients. Pediatrics. 2014;133(5):e1156–62.

Phipps S, Dunavant M, Lensing S, Rai SN. Acute health related quality of life in children undergoing stem cell transplant: II. Medical and demographic determinants. Bone Marrow Transplant. 2002;29:435–42.

Pulsipher MA, Levine JE, Hayashi RJ, Chan KW, Anderson P, Duerst R, et al. Safety and efficacy of allogeneic PBSC collection in normal pediatric donors: the pediatric blood and marrow transplant consortium experience (PBMTC) 1996–2003. Bone Marrow Transplant. 2005;35(4):361–7.

Smith FO, Reaman GH, Racadio JM. Hematopoietic cell transplantation in children with cancer: Springer; 2014.

Styczynski J, Balduzzi A, Gil L, Labopin M, Hamladji RM, Marktel S, et al. Risk of complications during hematopoietic stem cell collection in pediatric sibling donors: a prospective European Group for Blood and Marrow Transplantation Pediatric Diseases Working Party study. Blood. 2012;119(12):2935–42.

Tremolada M, Bonichini S, Pillon M, Messina C, Carli M. Quality of life and psychosocial sequelae in children undergoing hematopoietic stem-cell transplantation: a review. Pediatr Transplant. 2009;12:955–70.

Vogel R. The management of the sibling hematopoietic stem cell transplant donor. J Pediatr Oncol Nurs. 2011;28(6):336–43.

Wiener LS, Steffen-Smith E, Fry T, Wayne A. Hematopoeitic stem cell donation in children: a review of the sibling donor experience. J Psychosoc Oncol. 2007;25(1):45–66.

Williams S, Green R, Morrison A, Watson D, Buchanan S. The psychosocial aspects of donating blood stem cells: the sibling donor perspective. J Clin Apher. 2003;18(1):1–9.

Transplantation Through the Ages: Teenage and Young Adults (TYA)

Barfield R, Kodish E. Ethical considerations in pediatric hematopoietic stem-cell transplantation. Pediatr Hematopoietic Stem Cell Transplant. 2006:251–70.

Bayer SR, Alper MM, Penzias AS. The Boston Ivf handbook of infertility: a practical guide for practitioners who care for infertile couples: CRC Press. Florida; 2011.

Department of Health. Reference guide to consent for examination or treatment. In: Doh, editors. London; 2009

Desandes E, Bonnay S, Berger C, Brugieres L, Demeocq F, Laurence V, Sommelet D, Tron I, Clavel J, Lacour B. Pathways of care for adolescent patients with cancer in france from 2006 to 2007. Pediatr Blood Cancer. 2012;58:924–9.

Fan S-Y, Eiser C. Body image of children and adolescents with cancer: a systematic review. Body Image. 2009;6:247–56.

Forinder U, Posse E. A life on hold': adolescents' experiences of stem cell transplantation in a long-term perspective. J Child Health Care. 2008;12:301–13.

Gatta G, Zigon G, Capocaccia R, Coebergh JW, Desandes E, Kaatsch P, Pastore G, Peris-Bonet R, Stiller CA. Survival of european children and young adults with cancer diagnosed 1995–2002. Eur J Cancer. 2009;45:992–1005.

GMC. 0-18 Years: guidance for all doctors. In: Council, G. M, editor. London; 2007.

Gratwohl A, Baldomero H, Demirer T, Rosti G, Dini G, Ladenstein R, Urbano-Ispizua A. Hematopoetic stem cell transplantation for solid tumors in Europe. Ann Oncol. 2004;15:653–60.

Grinyer A. Young people living with cancer: implications for policy and practice. London: Mcgraw-Hill Education; 2007.

Grinyer A. Contrasting parental perspectives with those of teenagers and young adults with cancer: comparing the findings from two qualitative studies. Eur J Oncol Nurs. 2009;13:200–6.

Human Tissue Authority. Guidance to bone marrow and peripheral blood stem cell transplant teams and accredited assessors: HTA; 2015.

Kaufman M. Role of adolescent development in the transition process. Prog Transplant. 2006;16:286–90.

Kondryn HJ, Edmondson CL, Hill J, Eden TOB. Treatment non-adherence in teenage and young adult patients with cancer. *Lancet Oncol*. 2011;12:100–8.

Lassaletta A, Andión M, Garrido-Colino C, Gutierrez-Carrasco I, Echebarria-Barona A, Almazán F, López-Ibor B, Ortega-Acosta MJ. The current situation of adolescents with cancer in pediatric hematology-oncology units in Spain. Results of a national survey. Anales De Pediatria (Barcelona, Spain : 2003). 2013;78:268.E1–7.

Leiper AD. Late effects of total body irradiation. Arch Dis Child. 1995;72:382–5.

Levine J, Stern CJ. Fertility preservation in adolescents and young adults with cancer. J Clin Oncol. 2010;28:4831–41.

Long KA, Marsland AL. Family adjustment to childhood cancer: a systematic review. Clin Child Fam Psychol Rev. 2011;14:57–88.

Lowis S. Malignant disease and the adolescent. J Royal College Physicians. 2000;34:27–31.

Macleod KD, Whitsett SF, Mash EJ, Pelletier W. Pediatric sibling donors of successful and unsuccessful hematopoietic stem cell transplants (HSCT): a qualitative study of their psychosocial experience. J Pediatr Psychol. 2003;28:223–30.

Ministry of Health. The welfare of children in hospital, Platt report. In: Office, H. M. S. S, editors. London; 1959.

Moore C, Rauch P. Addressing parenting concerns of bone marrow transplant patients: opening (and closing) pandora's box. Bone Marrow Transplant. 2006;38:775–82.

National Institute for Health and Clinical Excellence. Children and young people with cancer. London: Nice; 2014.

Nicolussi A. Informed consent and minors. Ital J Pediatr. 2015;41:1–1.

Pot-Mees CC, Zeitlin H. Psychosocial consequences of bone marrow transplantation in children: a preliminary communication. J Psychosoc Oncol. 1987;5:73–81.

Quinn GP, Vadaparampil ST, Group, F. P. R. Fertility preservation and adolescent/young adult cancer patients: physician communication challenges. J Adolesc Health. 2009;44:394–400.

Rodgers C, Young A, Hockenberry M, Binder B, Symes L. The meaning of adolescents' eating experiences during bone marrow transplant recovery. J Pediatr Oncol Nurs. 2010;27:65–72.

Saito K, Suzuki K, Iwasaki A, Yumura Y, Kubota Y. Sperm cryopreservation before cancer chemotherapy helps in the emotional battle against cancer. Cancer. 2005;104:521–4.

Smith S, Davies S, Wright D, Chapman C. The experiences of teenagers and young adults with cancer—results of 2004 conference survey. Eur J Oncol Nurs. 2007;11:362–8.

Smith S, Vogel CL, Waterhouse K, Pettitt N, Beddard L, Oldham J, Hubber D, Simon S, Siddall J. A blueprint of care for teenagers and young adults with cancer. Guidelines for Health Professionals: London; 2012.

Stark D, Bielack S, Brugieres L, Dirksen U, Duarte X, Dunn S, Erdelyi DJ, Grew T, Hjorth L, Jazbec J, Kabickova E, Konsoulova A, Kowalczyk JR, Lassaletta A, Laurence V, Lewis I, Monrabal A, Morgan S, Mountzios G, Olsen PR, Renard M, Saeter G, Van Der Graaf WT, Ferrari A. Teenagers and young adults with cancer in Europe: from national programmes to a European integrated coordinated project. Eur J Cancer Care. 2016;25:419–27.

Taddeo DM, Egedy MM, Frappier JYM. Adherence to treatment in adolescents: Paediatr Child Health. 2008;13(1):19–24.

Thomas D, Seymour J, O'brien T, Sawyer S, Ashley D. Adolescent and young adult cancer: a revolution in evolution? Intern Med J. 2006;36:302–7.

Transplant, B. S. B. M. Indications for HSCT in children – Uk Paediatric BMT Group 2015, UK: BSBMT; 2015.

Wheeler R. Gillick or fraser? A plea for consistency over competence in children. BMJ. 2006;332:807.

Whelan J. Where should teenagers with cancer be treated? Eur J Cancer. 2003;39:2573–8.

Whiteson M. The Teenage Cancer Trust—advocating a model for teenage cancer services. Eur J Cancer. 2003;39:2688–93.

Wiener LS, Steffen-Smith E, Battles HB, Wayne A, Love CP, Fry T. Sibling stem cell donor experiences at a single institution. Psychooncology. 2008;17:304–7.

Wilkins KL, Woodgate RL. Supporting siblings through the pediatric bone marrow transplant trajectory: perspectives of siblings of bone marrow transplant recipients. Cancer Nurs. 2007;30:E29–34.

Transplanting the Adult and the Older Adult: Nursing Considerations

Almeida OP, Almeida SA. Short versions of the geriatric depression scale: a study of their validity for the diagnosis of a major depressive episode according to ICD-10 and DSM-IV. Int J Geriatr Psychiatry. 1999;14(10):858–65.

Artz AS, Chow S. Hematopoietic cell transplantation in older adults: deciding or decision-making? Bone Marrow Transplant. 2016;51(5):643–4.

Artz AS, Pollyea DA, Kocherginsky M, Stock W, Rich E, Odenike O, Zimmerman T, Smith S, Godley L, Thirman M, Daugherty C, Extermann M, Larson R, van Besien K. Performance status and comorbidity predict transplant-related mortality after allogeneic hematopoietic cell transplantation. Biol Blood Marrow Transplant. 2006;12(9):954–64.

Boyd CM, McNabney MK, Brandt N, Correa-de-Araujuo R, Daniel M, Epplin J, Fried TR, Goldstein MK, Holmes HM, Ritchie CS, Shega JW. Guiding principles for the care of older adults with multimorbidity: an approach for clinicians: American Geriatrics Society expert panel on the care of older adults with multimorbidity. J Am Geriatr Soc. 2012;60(10):E1–E25.

Charlson ME, Pompei P, Ales KL, MacKenzie CR. A new method of classifying prognostic comorbidity in longitudinal studies: development and validation. J Chronic Dis. 1987;40:373–83.

D'Souza A, Pasquini M, Spellecy R. Is 'informed consent' an 'understood consent' in hematopoietic cell transplantation? Bone Marrow Transplant. 2015;50(1):10–4.

Elsawy M, Sorror ML. Up-to-date tools for risk assessment before allogeneic hematopoietic stem cell transplantation. Bone Marrow Transplant. 2016;51(10):1283–300.

Eichhorst B, Dreyling M, Robak T, Montserrat E, Hallek M. Chronic lymphocytic leukemia: ESMO Clinical Practice Guidelines for diagnosis, treatment and follow-up. Ann Oncol. 2011;22(Suppl 6):vi50–4.

Extermann M, Aapro M, Bernabei R, Cohen HJ, Droz JP, Lichtman S, Mor V, Monfardini S, Repetto L, Sørbye L, Topinkova E. Task Force on CGA of the International Society of Geriatric Oncology. Use of comprehensive geriatric assessment in older cancer patients: recommendations from the task force on CGA of the International Society of Geriatric Oncology (SIOG). Crit Rev Oncol Hematol. 2005;55(3):241–52.

Folstein MF, Folstein SE, McHugh PR. Mini-mental state: a practical method for grading the cognitive state of patients for the clinician. J Psychiatr Res. 1975;12:189–98.

Graf C. The Lawton instrumental activities of daily living scale. AJN. 2008;108(4):52–62.

Greene MG, Adelman RD. Physician-older patient communication about cancer. Patient Educ Couns. 2003;50(1):55–60.

Guigoz Y. The Mini Nutritional Assessment (MNA) review of the literature: what does it tell us? J Nutr Health Aging. 2006;10:466–87.

Karnofsky DA, Burchenal JH. The clinical evaluation of chemotherapeutic agents in cancer. In: MacLeod CM, editor. Evaluation of chemotherapeutic agents. New York: Columbia Univ Press; 1949. p. 191–205.

Kenis C, Bron D, Libert Y, Decoster L, Van Puyvelde K, Scalliet P, Cornette P, Pepersack T, Luce S, Langenaeken C, Rasschaert M, Allepaerts S, Van Rijswijk R, Milisen K, Flamaing J, Lobelle JP, Wildiers H. Relevance of a systematic geriatric screening and assessment in older patients with cancer: results of a prospective multicentric study. Ann Oncol. 2013;24(5):1306–12.

Kruizenga HM, Seidell JC, de Vet HC, Wierdsma NJ, van Bokhorst-de van der Schueren MA. Development and validation of a hospital screening tool for malnutrition: the Short Nutritional Assessment Questionnaire (SNAQ). Clin Nutr. 2005;24:75–82.

Lam WY, Fresco P. Medication adherence measures: an overview. Biomed Res Int. 2015:217047. Published online 11 Oct 2015. doi:https://doi.org/10.1155/2015/217047.

Mamdani H, Santos CD, Konig H. Treatment of acute myeloid leukemia in elderly patients-a therapeutic dilemma. J Am Med Dir Assoc. 2016;17(7):581–7.

Mahoney FI, Barthel DW. Functional evaluation: the Barthel Index. Md State Med J. 1965:1461–5.

Mor V, Laliberte L, Morris JN, Wiemann M. The Karnofsky performance status scale. Cancer. 1984:2002–7.

National Cancer Institute. MDS, median age 71 years, Sekeres MA. The epidemiology of myelodysplastic syndromes. Hematol Oncol Clin North Am 2010. 2003;24(2):287–94.

Pallis AG, Wedding U, Lacombe D, Soubeyran P, Wildiers H. Questionnaires and instruments for a multidimensional assessment of the older cancer patient: what clinicians need to know? Eur J Cancer. 2010;46:1019–25.

Palumbo A, Anderson K. Multiple myeloma. N Engl J Med. 2011;364:1046–60. https://doi.org/10.1056/NEJMra1011442.

Palumbo A, Bringhen S, Mateos MV, Larocca A, Facon T, Kumar SK, Offidani M, McCarthy P, Evangelista A, Lonial S, Zweegman S, Musto P, Terpos E, Belch A, Hajek R, Ludwig H, Stewart AK, Moreau P, Anderson K, Einsele H, Durie BG, Dimopoulos MA, Landgren O, San Miguel JF, Richardson P, Sonneveld P, Rajkumar SV. Geriatric assessment predicts survival and toxicities in elderly myeloma patients: an International Myeloma Working Group report. Blood. 2015;125(13):2068–74.

Posma ER, van Weert JC, Jansen J, Bensing JM. Older cancer patients' information and support needs surrounding treatment: an evaluation through the eyes of patients, relatives and professionals. BMC Nurs. 2009;8:1.

Puts MT, Tu HA, Tourangeau A, Howell D, Fitch M, Springall E, Alibhai SM. Factors influencing adherence to cancer treatment in older adults with cancer: a systematic review. Ann Oncol. 2014;25(3):564–77.

Randall J, Keven K, Atli T, Ustun C. Process of allogeneic hematopoietic cell transplantation decision making for older adults. Bone Marrow Transplant. 2016;51(5):623–8.

Saliba D, Elliott M, Rubenstein LZ, Solomon DH, Young RT, Kamberg CJ, Roth C, MacLean CH, Shekelle PG, Sloss EM, Wenger NS. The vulnerable elders survey: a tool for identifying vulnerable older people in the community. J Am Geriatr Soc. 2001;49:1691–9.

Sattar S, Alibhai SM, Wildiers H, Puts MT. How to implement a geriatric assessment in your clinical practice. Oncologist. 2014;19(10):1056–68.

Schenker Y, Fernandez A, Sudore R, Schillinger D. Interventions to improve patient comprehension in informed consent for medical and surgical procedures: a systematic review. Med Decis Making. 2011;31(1):151–73.

Sekeres MA. The epidemiology of myelodysplastic syndromes. Hematol Oncol Clin North Am. 2010;24(2):287–94.

Sheikh JA, Yesavage JA. Geriatric Depression Scale (GDS): recent findings and development of a shorter version. In: Brink TL, editor. Clinical gerontology: a guide to assessment and intervention. New York: Howarth Press; 1986.

Siegel RL, Miller KD, Jemal A. Cancer statistics, 2015. CA Cancer J Clin. 2015;65:5–29.

Smith A, Howell D, Patmore R, Jack A, Roman E. Br J Cancer. 2011;105(11):1684–92.

Sorror ML, Maris MB, Storb R, Baron F, Sandmaier BM, Maloney DG, Storer B. Hematopoietic cell transplantation (HCT)-specific comorbidity index: a new tool for risk assessment before allogeneic HCT. Blood. 2005;106(8):2912–9.

Soubeyran P, Bellera C, Goyard J, et al. Validation of the G8 screening tool in geriatric oncology: the ONCODAGE project. J Clin Oncol. 2011;29(Suppl):abstr 9001.

Stratton RJ, Hackston A, Longmore D, Dixon R, Price S, Stroud M, et al. Malnutrition in hospital outpatients and inpatients: prevalence, concurrent validity and ease of use of the "malnutrition universal screening tool" ("MUST") for adults. Br J Nutr. 2004;92(05):799–808.

Valentijn SA, van Boxtel MP, van Hooren SA, Bosma H, Beckers HJ, Ponds RW, Jolles J. Change in sensory functioning predicts change in cognitive functioning: results from a 6-year follow-up in the maastricht aging study. J Am Geriatr Soc. 2005;53(3):374–80.

Van Cleave JH, Kenis C, Sattar S, Jabloo VG, Ayala AP, Puts M. A research agenda for gero-oncology nursing. Semin Oncol Nurs. 2016 Feb;32(1):55–64.

Williams AM, Zent CS, Janelsins MC. What is known and unknown about chemotherapy-related cognitive impairment in patients with haematological malignancies and areas of needed research. Br J Haematol. 2016;174(6):835–46.

WHO. Definition of an older or elderly person. Geneva, Switzerland: World Health Organisation; 2010. Accessed 14 Apr 2017. http://www.who.int/healthinfo/survey/ageingdefnolder/en/index.html.

Early and Acute Complications and the Principles of HSCT Nursing Care

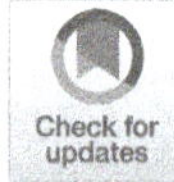

Elisabeth Wallhult and Barry Quinn

Abstract

Haematopoietic stem cell transplantation (HSCT) generally includes preparative or conditioning regimes containing chemotherapy and/or radiotherapy in high doses. These regimens, as well as other treatments before and after HSCT such as immunosuppressive drugs to prevent graft versus host disease (GvHD) (see Chap. 11), may affect the patient's organs and tissues and may cause both acute and long-term complications. In the evolving field of stem cell therapies, some complications that traditionally have been regarded as early complications are now, due to changes in preparative regimens and choice of stem cell source, sometimes seen later in the post-transplant out-patient setting. The complications covered in this chapter generally occur within 100 days post HSCT and are thus classified as early complications. Two of the most common early complications are oral complications/mucositis and sepsis. Some other relatively rare complications are also covered here: haemorrhagic cystitis (HC), endothelial damage (ED) syndromes including engraftment syndrome (ES), idiopathic pneumonia syndrome (IPS), diffuse alveolar haemorrhage (DAH), transplant-associated microangiopathy (TAM) and sinusoidal obstruction syndrome/veno-occlusive disease (SOS/VOD). For all complications, recommendations for prevention and principles for nursing care are presented since careful nursing monitoring, prompt intervention and care may have an influence on patients' morbidity and mortality.

E. Wallhult (✉)
Section of Hematology and Coagulation, Department of Medicine, Sahlgrenska University Hospital, Gothenburg, Sweden
e-mail: elisabeth.wallhult@vgregion.se

B. Quinn
Woking and Sam Beare Hospices, Surrey, UK
e-mail: b.quinn@wsbhospices.co.uk

© EBMT and the Author(s) 2018
M. Kenyon, A. Babic (eds.), *The European Blood and Marrow Transplantation Textbook for Nurses*,
https://doi.org/10.1007/978-3-319-50026-3_9

Keywords

Oral complications • Mucositis • Sepsis • Haemorrhagic cystitis SOS/VOD • Endothelial damage syndromes

9.1 Oral Care in Transplantation

9.1.1 Introduction

Mindful of the many developments in the field of HSCT aimed at improving survival and quality of life, the correct and consistent approach to managing oral care problems still remains a challenge in many transplant settings across Europe. There is much evidence to show that rather than taking a proactive approach to this aspect of care, many clinicians simply react to oral complications once they occur with a sometimes inconsistent and anecdotal approach.

Oral problems and damage may be temporary or permanent resulting in a significant health burden for the individual while making substantial demands on limited healthcare resources. However, oral complications are not always inevitable, and much can be done to reduce or minimise the severity of symptoms by taking a more proactive approach to this aspect of care. Working as a multidisciplinary team with the patient at the centre of care and treatment plan, the early detection of potential and actual problems and treatment can help to reduce oral problems and prevent interruptions to treatment while maximising patient safety and comfort (National Cancer Institute 2013).

9.1.2 Oral Mucositis (OM)

Oral mucositis (OM) has been defined by Rubenstein et al. (2004), Al-Dasoogi et al. (2013) and others as the inflammation of the mucosal membrane, characterised by ulceration, which may result in pain, swallowing difficulties and impairment of the ability to talk. The mucosal injury caused by OM provides an

Table 9.1 Oral complications of HSCT include

Oral mucositis	Xerostomia
Oral infections	Oral graft versus host disease
Ulceration	Trismus
Taste changes	Halitosis
Bleeding	Dry lips
Pain	Dental decay
Osteonecrosis	Fibrosis

Leading to difficulties in eating, sleeping and talking and a reduction in quality of life

opportunity for infection to flourish, and in particular putting the severely immunocompromised patient in the HSCT setting at risk of sepsis and septicaemia.

OM and oral problems in the HSCT setting (Table 9.1) can be expected to occur in as many as 68% of patients undergoing autologous HSCT and 98% of patients undergoing allogeneic HSCT (Filicko et al. 2003; Bhatt et al. 2010). With the increasing use of targeted drug therapies and approaches in the cancer and haematology setting, problems in the oral cavity will increase and become even more of a challenge (Quinn et al. 2015).

9.1.3 Key Principles of Treatment

All treatment strategies aimed at improving mouth care are dependent on four key principles: accurate assessment of the oral cavity, individualised plan of care, initiating timely preventative measures and correct treatment (Quinn et al. 2008). The assessment process should begin prior to HSCT by identifying all the patient risks most likely to increase oral damage. Each patient needs to be assessed in relation to the following risk factors that may put them at higher risk of oral complications during treatment:

- Pre-existing dental problems
- Prior treatment
- Older patients and females (at higher risk of oral damage)
- History of alcohol and/or tobacco use
- Poor nutrition and hydration
- Supportive feeding (nasogastric, PEG, RIG)
- Supportive therapies (opiates diuretics, sedatives, oxygen therapy – may cause dryness)

Patients about to commence HSCT should undergo dental assessment by a specialist (Elad et al. 2015). This is to establish general oral health status and identify and manage existing and/or potential source of infection, trauma or injury. Any identified dental problems should be corrected before starting treatment regimen. Some patients will need regular dental follow-up following treatment. A further baseline assessment of the oral mucosa should be taken as close to the administration of the first treatment dose as possible.

The oral cavity should be assessed by trained healthcare professionals using a recognised grading system to ensure accurate monitoring and record keeping. The tool chosen should contain both objective and subjective elements. The assessment should include changes to the oral mucosa, the presence or absence of pain and the patient's nutritional status (Quinn et al. 2008).

Assessments should be completed daily during HSCT and at regular intervals posttreatment to monitor for complications. Patients can be encouraged to assess their own mouth using a patient-reported tool and to report any changes they notice or experience to the transplant team.

9.1.4 Inspecting the Oral Cavity

- Clinical tools: good light source, gloves, tongue depressor and dry gauze
- Patient in convenient and comfortable position
- Use valid and reliable assessment instrument which is easy to interpret
- Oral sites to be evaluated (cheeks, lips, soft palate, floor of mouth, tongue)

9.1.5 Care of the Oral Cavity

Care of the oral cavity is central to helping to prevent and/or reduce oral complications during and after treatment. The oral care team in the HSCT setting includes dental professionals, dietician, nurse, doctor and pharmacist. The support provided by the team along with good communication and the patient at the centre of all care plans is central to maintaining patient's oral health.

All patients should be provided with clear instructions and encouraged to maintain good oral hygiene. Education should also include potential oral complications to enable patients to identify and report these early (Clarkson et al. 2011; Quinn et al. 2015). All patients should receive written information, as well as verbal instruction, about oral care as part of the prevention and treatment of oral changes.

Good nutrition is vital in helping to fight infection, maintain mucosal integrity, enhance mucosal tissue repair and reduce exacerbation of existing mucositis. Issues that may affect nutrition such as loss of appetite, taste changes and dysphagia should be addressed.

There are certain foods that can damage the oral mucosa; this may include rough, sharp and hard foods and should be avoided. Spicy, very salty and acidic foods may cause mucosal irritation but may be preferred or tolerated by some patients.

Brushing of teeth, gums and tongue should be performed two to four times a day preferably after meals and before going to bed (Peterson et al. 2015). Soft-bristled toothbrush (manual or electric) is recommended to prevent injury to the oral mucosa and must be rinsed thoroughly with water after each use. If the mouth is painful or patients cannot open their mouths fully, soft oral sponges may be used.

To prevent infections, the toothbrush should be stored with the brush head upwards and not soaked in disinfectant solution. These should also be monitored for evidence of fungal/bacterial colonisation. In order to protect the enamel, non-abrasive toothpaste containing mild fluoride (1000–1500 ppm) should be used.

Daily interdental cleaning with brushes may reduce plaque formation between the teeth (Sambunjak et al. 2011). However, the use of interdental cleaners should be used with caution for patients with thrombocytopenia or clotting disorders.

After each meal, dentures must be rinsed. Thorough cleaning by brushing with soap and water should be performed at least twice a day. Dentures should be cleaned, dried and stored in a closed container overnight (Duyck et al. 2013).

The goal of using mouthwashes may include oral hygiene, preventing/treating infection, moistening the oral cavity or providing pain relief. As a minimum to keep the mouth clean, bland gargles and rinses with water, normal saline (0.9% NaCl) and saltwater are recommended at least four times a day (Lalla et al. 2014; Quinn et al. 2015).

Some patients will require assistance; it may be necessary for healthcare professionals to perform/support oral care through rinsing with normal saline (0.9% NaCl) (Elad et al. 2015), with or without suction.

Lubricants, lip balm or lip cream may be used to moisten the lips.

Patients should maintain adequate hydration and drink water frequently to keep the mouth moist. Several factors could contribute to dryness such as oxygen therapy and supportive care medications (e.g. antidepressants, antihistamines, sedatives and opioids). To keep the oral mucosa moist, regular sipping or spraying water may help. Use of saline sprays and mouthwashes as well as use of saliva substitutes may be used. There is anecdotal evidence that fresh pineapple chunks may also help stimulate saliva but should be used with caution as their acidity could irritate the oral mucosa and affect the teeth (Lalla et al. 2014).

9.1.6 Prevention of Oral Mucositis

The choice of prevention regimens should be guided by evidence-based or expert opinion interventions, working with the individual patient and the potential risk of oral mucositis which may include the following (adapted Quinn et al. 2015).

- Educate and encourage self-reporting of any oral changes
- Good and regular oral hygiene including gargling to remove any unwanted debris
- Interdental cleaning
- Fluoride toothpaste/foam/gel/tray
- 0.9% sodium chloride/saltwater rinse
- Early nutritional intervention
- Cryotherapy/sucking ice chips during melphalan infusion
- Consider oral rinses (Caphosol®, Benzydamine®)
- Mucosal protectants/barrier rinses licenced to use as a preventative measure/reduce pain (Mugard®, Episil®)
- Anti-infective prophylaxis
- Palifermin
- Low-level laser therapy

9.1.7 Anti-infective Prophylaxis

While good oral hygiene is fundamental, antifungal and antiviral treatments will be prescribed to reduce infections in patients in the transplant setting. Patients should receive an antifungal agent given orally or intravenously. Antiviral prophylaxis should also be given. The choice of drug will be dependent on local policies/guidance.

9.1.8 Treatment of Oral Complications

All treatment plans should be based upon the grading of oral damage and patient reports; these may include the following.

9.1.8.1 Mild/Moderate Mucositis/Oral Complications

- Once oral damage develops, patients should be supported to continue oral care.
- Frequency of oral rinsing may be increased. The aim is to keep the oral surfaces clean and moist (Elad et al. 2014).
- Check for oral infections, swab and treat appropriately. Review of antifungal treatment,

local or systemic, should be administered if required (Watson et al. 2011).

- Dexamethasone containing gels may be used for aphthous lesions.
- Consider mucosal protectants (Quinn et al. 2015).
- Dietary requirements should be assessed and foods causing discomfort avoided.
- Swallowing problems, malnutrition and weight loss should be monitored and patients given support/advice. Adjustments to food consistency, methods of intake, food fortification and methods of intake should be assessed, support and education offered to patients. Use of supplement drinks, PEG, RIG or nasogastric feeding should be considered (Quinn et al. 2015).
- Fluid intake should be assessed and route of administration of pain relief continually monitored. General health problems should also be assessed (swallowing of tablets, decreased blood sugar levels and decreased blood pressure, decreased renal function leading to overdosing of substances).
- Patients will need adequate pain medication including topical and systemic analgesia such as paracetamol, codeine, morphine rinses, Benzydamine mouthwash, trimecaine and lidocaine. Patients should be offered education on use and possible side effects including numbness of the oral mucosa.

9.1.8.2 Severe Mucositis/Oral Complications

- Increase pain medication following patient needs
- Increase nutritional support
- Increase oral rinses and care

When oral damage progresses, closer monitoring and support for patients is required. An important aspect of care is to control the pain thereby helping the patient to continue food and fluid intake, communication and sleep.

For topical treatment the use of topical analgesics can be intensified. There is insufficient evidence that many products reduce the severity of mucositis but comfort can be provided for the

patient by some of these oral care products. Institutions can offer a range of mouthwashes selecting the most appropriate for the clinical situation and the patients trying out which one works best for them. Generally spoken, topical antibacterial substances are not recommended. The use of oral rinses, topical gels or films can be individually considered. Any with sufficient safety and positive experiences can be used: Caphosol®, Mugard®, Oralife®, Gelclair® and Episil® are just a few of them.

For systemic pain medication, it is useful to follow a step-by-step increase, with the aim of the patient becoming pain-free within 24 h. It can be helpful to monitor the efficacy of pain medication with pain assessment tools. Institutions should follow a standardised pattern of pain medication following the WHO recommendations where applicable.

In severe mucositis, the use of opiates with the optimal application route should be considered. The best route of application depends on many individual and setting factors and may be oral, subcutaneous, intravenous or transdermal with patches. Patients may require a combination of slow-release and fast-acting drugs. Patient controlled analgesia should be considered. Careful monitoring should include pain relief and any potential side effects, and including family members may prove helpful to obtain a wider view of how well the patient copes outside the treatment unit.

9.1.8.3 Treatment of Specific Oral Complications

Bleeding from OM

Continue mouth gargling. Tranexamic acid has been widely used in oral surgery, and gargling/swishing with tranexamic acid (500 mg) as a mouthwash may be worth considering (Watson et al. 2011).

Xerostomia (Dry Mouth)

As this may be due to or increased by concurrent mediation, a review of the patient's medications is needed and if possible adjustments made. Patients should be encouraged to increase sipping of fluids. Artificial saliva, viscous solutions and gels to protect and moisten the mucosa should be considered; patients should be counselled on correct application. In chronic radiotherapy-related xerostomia, pilocarpine should be used.

Trismus (Spasm of the Jaw Muscles)

This is a common side effect during and post high-dose radiotherapy. Patients should be given helpful exercises, and the team may consider mechanical devices to help alleviate the problem.

Graft Versus Host Disease (GvHD)

Oral damage may be a hallmark of graft versus host disease (GvHD) in patients following allogeneic stem cell transplantation, and the presence of lichenoid hyperkeratotic plaques (diagnostic sign), gingivitis, mucositis, erythema, pain, xerostomia and ulcers may indicate GvHD. Kuten-Shorrer et al. (2014) suggest that solutions of dexamethasone or other steroids are used as first-line treatment; second-line may include solutions of steroids in combination with other immunosuppressant drugs.

9.1.9   Posttreatment Care/ Follow-Up

Oral damage in the HSCT will require several weeks/months to heal, and patients need continuing support and care during this period. Advice and support by suitably qualified health professional should continue during this period. Support to manage side effects including pain and the gradual reduction of analgesia is extremely important.

Chronic side effects may include dental decay, trismus, fibrosis, lymphedema, chronic xerostomia and chronic pain and will require careful management. All patients should be individually assessed and appropriate care and treatment given. Follow-up care should be planned and supervised to address longer-term and late complications.

9.1.10 Conclusion

The principles presented here are intended as a support and in no way should replace clinical decision-making related to the particular patient and clinical situation. Depending on the severity of oral complications and the impact on the patient, the team will need to review the plan of care.

Acknowledgement   European Oral Care in Cancer Group (EOCC).

9.2   Sepsis and Principles of Care

9.2.1   Introduction

The increased risk of infections in patients undergoing haematopoietic stem cell transplantation (HSCT) is well known, and infection is a leading cause of morbidity and mortality. HSCT patients are particularly at risk, especially during the neutropenic period following the conditioning treatment. In HSCT patients, signs and symptoms of sepsis may be subtle and difficult to recognise due to neutropenia or other complications of the transplant procedure. Preventive measures should be applied, but vigilance and close monitoring of the patient, strong team collaboration and immediate action will allow for prompt and appropriate management of septic patients.

9.2.2   Definition of Sepsis

There are multiple definitions and clinical criteria for sepsis. The terms below are all terms for severe infection where bacteria may or may not be identified in blood cultures.

- Sepsis
- Severe sepsis
- Septicaemia
- Septic syndrome
- Septic shock

According to the Third International Consensus Definitions for Sepsis and Septic Shock (Sepsis-3) (Singer et al. 2016), sepsis can be defined as:

> A life-threatening condition caused by aberrant and dysregulated host response to infection. The pathobiology is still not completely known but the divergent infection response injures the body's own tissues and organs and causes organ dysfunction.

That is also what differentiates sepsis from infection in general. Septic shock is a subset of sepsis in which particularly profound circulatory, cellular and metabolic abnormalities are associated with a greater risk of mortality than with sepsis alone.

The table below has limited clinical diagnostic relevance but is a schematic description of the evolution from systemic inflammatory response system (SIRS) to septic shock (Table 9.2). It is worth noting that the symptoms of SIRS will not delineate between SIRS and sepsis itself, and since many of the signs and symptoms may be present in HSCT patients, an individual assessment, including other examinations as well, needs to be performed for the diagnosis of sepsis.

The consequence of the inflammatory response and evolution of sepsis is called the sepsis cascade and is illustrated in Fig. 9.1.

Table 9.2 Evolution from SIRS to septic shock

Term	Definition	Signs and symptoms
Systemic inflammatory response system (SIRS)	The body's response to different severe clinical insults, which may or may not be infection	Fever (>38 °C) or hypothermia (<36 °C) Pulse rate > 90 beats/min Respiratory rate > 20/min WBC >12 $\times10^9$/L or <4 $\times10^9$/L or >10% bands
Sepsis	Systemic inflammatory response caused by infection	SIRS symptoms Evidence of infection
Severe sepsis	Sepsis with hypoperfusion or acute organ dysfunction or hypotension	Sepsis with:Increased lactate level Mental changes, Saturation < 90% Decreased urine output Increased liver function tests levels Reduced platelet levels Abnormal coagulation parameters Systolic blood pressure < 90 mmHg
Septic shock	A subset of severe sepsis with hypotension despite adequate fluid resuscitation and with presence of perfusion abnormalities that may include lactic acidosis, oliguria or alteration of mental status	Severe sepsis with:Vasopressor requirement Serum lactate level > 2 mmol/L (>18 mg/dL) At least two of the following quick Sequential [sepsis-related] Organ Failure Assessment (qSOFA) clinical criteria: Respiratory rate of ≥22/min Altered mental status Systolic blood pressure ≤ 100 mm Hg

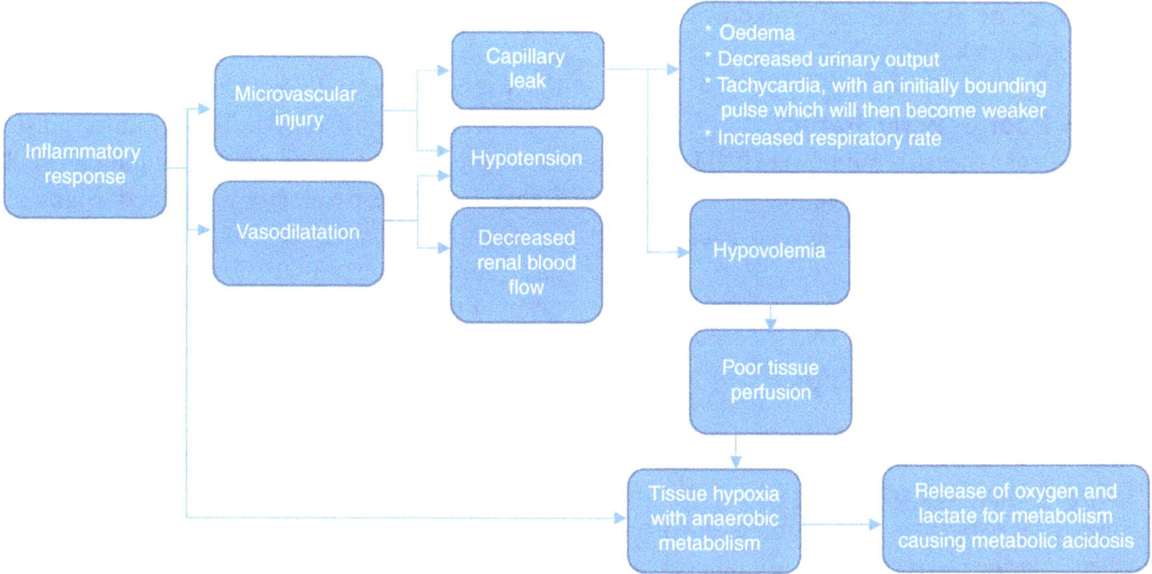

Fig. 9.1 The sepsis cascade starts with an inflammatory response that will cause microvascular injury, vasodilation and tissue hypoxia. The microvascular injury will lead to capillary leak resulting in oedema, decreased urinary output, tachycardia, with an initially bounding pulse which will then become weaker, and an increased respiratory rate. Hypotension is another symptom caused by both microvascular injury and vasodilation. The vasodilation will also cause decreased renal blood flow. The hypovolemia will cause poor tissue perfusion causing tissue hypoxia with anaerobic metabolism. In this process oxygen and lactate are released for metabolism and thus causing metabolic acidosis (E-learning package Sepsis and Sepsis Six http://sonet.nottingham.ac.uk/, 2017)

9.2.3 Risk Factors

In the early phase of HSCT, i.e. day 0 to day +100, the main risk factors for infections are (Rovira et al. 2012):

9.2.3.1 Neutropenia

A longer period of neutropenia can be expected in allogeneic than in autologous transplant. The stem cell source also affects the length of the neutropenic period where peripheral blood (PBSC) has an expected neutropenic phase of about 2 weeks, bone marrow (BM) 3 weeks and cord blood (CB) 4 weeks.

Myeloablative conditioning (MAC) treatment will cause a longer neutropenic phase than reduced intensity conditioning (RIC).

9.2.3.2 Barrier Breakdown

All kinds of barrier breakdown will increase the infection risk and mucositis occur in almost all transplant patients. Skin breakdown can be caused by, e.g. drugs and acute graft versus host disease (aGvHD). Indwelling catheters such as peripheral cannulas, central lines, urinary catheters and pyelostomy catheters are a potential port of entry for microorganisms into the blood stream.

9.2.3.3 Depressed T- and B-Cell Function

Allogeneic transplant is always followed by long-lasting immunodeficiency. Conditioning treatment may include T-cell depleting agents and even non-myeloablative regimens cause lymphodepletion with prolonged periods of immune incompetence. Donor type and degree of histocompatibility (human leukocyte antigen (HLA) match) are other factors that influence the time to immune reconstitution. Immunosuppression for GvHD prophylaxis is necessary in allogeneic HSCT and will delay immune reconstitution (Toubert 2012).

9.2.3.4 Presence of Acute Graft Versus Host Disease (aGvHD)

Need for immunosuppressive treatment will increase the risk for infections.

Mucosal or skin barrier breakdown further increases the risk.

9.2.3.5 Poor General Status

If the patient is not in remission at HSCT, there is a greater risk for infection and sepsis. Comorbidity, such as diabetes, is another risk factor.

9.2.4 Strategies for Sepsis Prevention

The most important action to prevent infections acquired by exogenous organisms is good hand hygiene performed correctly. All clinical staff should also wear a uniform that is clean and short sleeved. Protective isolation during the neutropenic phase is recommended, and the patient should not be in contact with any staff or visitors with symptoms of infection. For prevention of endogenous infections, oral hygiene and skin care to maintain the mucosal and skin barrier and use of prophylactic antibiotics are the most important actions. Correct handling of any indwelling catheters is also a key nursing responsibility in infection control.

Other areas where infections can be prevented are air and water quality, food hygiene and the environmental cleaning. Environmental cleaning includes medical equipment as well. For more detailed guidance on infection control, see Chap. 7.

Routine surveillance screening for infection by bacterial and/or fungal cultures, i.e. blood, urine, faeces, swabs from nasopharynx and central line insertion site and serum galactomannan blood test, may allow for earlier identification and implementation of therapy, although the benefit of such routines can be discussed (Nesher et al. 2014). Regular monitoring of blood tests such as full blood count, electrolytes, urea and/or creatinine and C-reactive protein (CRP) may assist in detecting any changes that could indicate infection.

Prophylactic antibiotics, e.g. fluoroquinolones, antifungal and antiviral medication, will be used in most HSCT patients, at least during the neutropenic phase.

9.2.5 Diagnosis and Management

Early recognition and treatment is vital for a successful outcome of sepsis. Temperature, pulse, blood pressure, respirations and saturation (vital signs) should be frequently monitored. Signs of infection are not always obvious, but if the patient has a temperature ≥38.0 °C, cultures should be taken, i.v. antibiotics and i.v. fluids started or increased and oxygen therapy initiated. The goal is always to *start antibiotic treatment within 1 h* from detection of fever (Swedish "Pro Sepsis" Programme Group Sepsis 2015). This is sometimes referred to as "the golden hour" (or "door to needle time" for patients admitted from outside the hospital) and is the most critical period in the patient's survival from sepsis.

Recognising sepsis can be a challenge in HSCT patients during the immediate posttransplant period where often a plethora of symptoms are present but also after discharge, in the outpatient setting, since some symptoms are rather unspecific. Other than fever, chills or rigouring, feeling unwell or different (without clear explanation), changes in behaviour or mental changes, feeling faint or changes in skin tone can indicate sepsis. An increased respiratory rate can be seen even if saturation is normal. An increased pulse and lowered blood pressure may be noted. Some patients may not develop fever, and hypothermia, i.e. <36 °C, can also be a sign of sepsis. If an outpatient with symptoms that could be sepsis-related reports a normal body temperature, it should be checked again in the clinic with a reliable thermometer and correct method. Diarrhoea and vomiting are frequently seen in sepsis but can easily be mistaken for gastroenteritis, mucositis or acute graft versus host disease (aGvHD). Diffuse or local pain, e.g. in the abdomen, is common. Falls are often secondary to sepsis particularly in elderly patients. Any of these indices need prompt and thorough assessment.

The concept of the *Sepsis Six* has been developed as a guide to prioritise interventions in patients where sepsis is suspected (Daniels et al. 2011).

1. Oxygen therapy
2. Blood cultures

3. I.v. antibiotics
4. Fluid resuscitation
5. Serum lactate
6. Assess urine output (may require catheterisation)

When sepsis is suspected, all cultures should be taken prior to commencing antimicrobials, if possible (Rhodes et al. 2017). Cultures should be taken from central lines, wounds, nasopharynx, urine and faeces. It is also sensible to consider peripheral i.v. cannulae as a possible source of infection. Despite conventional practice to collect blood cultures at a fever spike in order to increase the chances of detecting bacteraemia, there is so far no data to support this principle (Kee et al. 2016). Testing could include polymerase chain reaction (PCR) virology (e.g. for cytomegalovirus (CMV) or Epstein-Barr virus (EBV)) and screening for fungus (e.g. oral swab), depending on symptoms and suspected microbial agent. For the procedures for diagnosis of central line-associated bloodstream infections (CLABSI), please see Chap. 4. Laboratory tests should be taken to monitor electrolyte status, organ function, blood count and signs of infection.

A site of infection may not always be identified. If a source of infection is confirmed, or strongly suspected, applicable actions should be taken, e.g. wound care or removal of peripheral i.v. needle with signs of thrombophlebitis (Schorr et al. 2014).

Upon initiation of antimicrobial treatment, a broad-spectrum antibiotic is usually used. Depending on the results of the cultures performed, the chosen drug may need to be changed later.

Fever and infection will affect the blood count and frequently cause platelet consumption why transfusions may be necessary.

9.2.6 Nursing Considerations and Care

Early recognition and intervention are achieved by frequent monitoring of the patient's vital signs and general condition and paying attention to subtle changes that should be promptly reported.

As described above, immediate action is required at the first indication of sepsis. When treatment has been initiated, the patient must be continually monitored to determine the effect of treatment or worsening of the condition. This includes vital signs, fluid balance including weight and assessment of identified and/or potential infection sites (mouth, skin, any indwelling or tunnelled catheter, urine, stools, etc.), mental status, signs of bleeding, pain and general appearance and well-being.

Antibiotics should be delivered with strict adherence to the prescribed time schedule. Antipyretics should be avoided since they may mask fever but may under certain circumstances be used to alleviate patient discomfort and pain.

Laboratory tests results will guide the need for electrolyte replacement and blood product transfusion that may be ordered prophylactically or in case of bleeding. Cultures may need to be repeated to confirm infection and/or response to treatment. Oxygen should be administered as needed to ensure adequate saturation (i.e. $\geq 94\%$, or 88–92% for patients with chronic obstructive pulmonary disease (COPD) (Royal College of Physicians 2012)). If the patient's condition worsens and organ support such as assisted ventilation or haemodialysis is required, the patient may need to be prepared for transfer to the intensive care unit (ICU).

Extra psychological support is important for both the patient and family. Educating the patient and the carer about the condition and actions taken or planned will prevent unnecessary worrying and enable them to alert the staff about symptoms or changes. Information and education may also facilitate mental preparedness if the condition worsens and a higher level of care, ICU, is needed.

Patients with sepsis are likely to need additional nursing care such as assistance with oral care and personal hygiene. It is important to ensure that the patient's and caregivers' information, education and support needs are met. On discharge from the hospital, we need to ensure that the patient and their caregiver are aware of when, why and how to contact the clinic or hospital that they have a fever thermometer at home, know when to take their temperature and are aware of the level that constitutes a fever.

9.3 Haemorrhagic Cystitis

9.3.1 Introduction

Haemorrhagic cystitis (HC) is sometimes seen in haematopoietic stem cell transplantation (HSCT) patients and can on its own or by subsequent complications cause significant morbidity and even death.

9.3.2 Definition

According to NCI Dictionary of Cancer Terms, it is defined as "A condition in which the lining of the bladder becomes inflamed and starts to bleed. The blood can be seen in the urine. Symptoms include pain and a burning feeling while urinating, feeling a need to urinate often, and being unable to control the flow of urine. Haemorrhagic cystitis may be caused by anticancer drugs, radiation therapy, infection, or being exposed to chemicals, such as dyes or insecticides" (NCI Dictionary of Cancer Terms 2016 https://www.cancer.gov/publications/dictionaries/cancer-terms?cdrid=695987).

Haematuria can be symptomatic or asymptomatic. It can be described as microscopic (not visible to the eye but detected on a dipstick and in the microscope) or macroscopic (red urine or visible blood or clots) (Table 9.3). Normally about 1 million erythrocytes are excreted daily in the urine. This is equal to one to three erythrocytes per high-power field (magnification ×400) under the microscope. Haematuria is defined as abnormal presence of blood in the urine, i.e. more than three erythrocytes per high-power field in the micro-

Table 9.3 Haematuria is graded as follows

Grade	Haematuria findings
I	Microscopic
II	Macroscopic
III	Macroscopic with clots
IV	Requiring instrumentation for clot evacuation Leading to urinary retention Requiring surgical intervention May also include elevated creatinine levels and renal impairment

Droller et al. (1982).

scope. To be confirmed as microscopic haematuria, two positive samples on consecutive days are needed. The haematuria can be visually detected (macroscopic) as red urine at levels as low as 1 mL blood per litre urine. The visible blood does however not necessarily correspond to the degree of blood loss through the urine. Red urine may also have other causes which will not be described here.

Cystitis is the term used to describe inflammation of the bladder. The inflammation can be caused by an infection or as a reaction to certain drugs or radiation therapy.

The following symptoms may be seen in all types of cystitis:

- Urinary urgency and frequency
- Burning or stinging with urination or right after
- Pain, dysuria (painful urination), lower abdominal or supra-pubic pain
- Nocturia, when sleep is disturbed twice or more at night due to a need to urinate
- Urinary incontinence
- General feeling of illness

9.3.3 Incidence

Reported incidences of HC after HSCT range between 5% and 70% depending on risk factors and use of preventive measures or not, but most materials describe an incidence between 5% and 30%.

9.3.4 Pathogenesis

The pathogenesis leading to HC is not completely known but is likely to be multifactorial. The onset is seen either early, within the two first weeks after start of conditioning treatment, or late, more than 2 weeks after HSCT. Conditioning treatment with chemotherapy, irradiation, cytopenia, viral infections due to immunosuppression and alloimmune reactions (immunisation by development of antibodies in response to an antigen, i.e. a protein from a donor, e.g. by receiving HSCT or transfusion) may all contribute to HC in the posttransplant period. Higher incidence of late-onset HC in HSCT with unrelated donors, older patients, and in patients with graft versus host disease (GvHD) and thrombocytopenia does support the conclusion that the pathogenesis is multifactorial (de Padua Silva 2010).

9.3.4.1 Drug-Related HC

Early-onset HC is usually a direct and immediate effect of the conditioning treatment. Conditioning therapy for HSCT often contains one or more alkylating agent. Cyclophosphamide, ifosfamide, busulfan, melphalan and thiotepa are among the most commonly used drugs in conditioning regimens and the major drug-related cause of HC. Use of other alkylating agents and etoposide may also increase the risk of HC. When cyclophosphamide or ifosfamide is metabolised in the body, it produces a metabolite called acrolein. Acrolein will cause direct toxicity to the inner lining of the urinary tract, the urothelium. The degree of damage is dose dependent, and the toxicity may increase with previous or concomitant radiation therapy and if busulfan is included in the conditioning regimen together with cyclophosphamide. The time of duration that acrolein is exposed to the bladder also contributes to the degree of damage. For cyclophosphamide, the maximal concentration of active metabolites is reached after 2–4 h of oral or intravenous administration. Most of the cyclophosphamide, 35–80% of the dose, is excreted in the urine as metabolites, and up to 20% is excreted as intact drug (Hassan and Ljungman 2003). In patients with decreased renal function, particularly in severe cases, decreased renal excretion may result in increased plasma levels of cyclophosphamide and its metabolites. This can cause increased toxicity. The following substances may also increase the concentration of toxic metabolites, possibly through inhibited breakdown or decreased renal excretion: allopurinol, cimetidine, hydrochlorothiazide and HIV protease inhibitors.

9.3.4.2 Nondrug-Related HC

When HC occurs more than 2 weeks after HSCT, a common cause in the immunocompromised host can be viral infection. Viral particles are frequently identified from the urine of HSCT recipients. Of these, reactivation of the polyoma BK virus (BKV) is the commonest and most consistent risk factor for HC following HSCT, as the virus is almost invariably present in the urine of patients with HC (Leung et al. 2005). The damaged urothelial cells provide a milieu for viral replication. Immunosuppression leads to viral reactivation and causes viruria. However, the exact pathogenetic link between BKV and HC remains enigmatic. Other viral agents such as adenovirus, cytomegalovirus (CMV) and other polyomaviruses similar to BKV may also but less often cause HC.

Alloimmunity after engraftment by attack from donor lymphoid cells against infected urothelial cells has not been confirmed as causing HC but may be an additional potential factor for development of this complication.

9.3.5 Diagnosis

The diagnosis of HC is confirmed by the presence of haematuria and symptoms of cystitis taking into account risk factors such as:

- Age (older patients)
- Chemotherapy (particularly cyclophosphamide- or ifosfamide-containing regimens)
- Irradiation
- Immunosuppressive drugs (anti-thymocyte globulin (ATG), cyclosporine (CyA), corticosteroids)
- Cytopenia
- Thrombocytopenia
- Infection
- Myeloablative conditioning
- Unrelated donor
- Mismatched donor
- GvHD
- Viruria (presence of virus in the urine) in particular with BKV, adenovirus and CMV

In order to confirm microscopic haematuria, two positive urine samples on consecutive days are needed. Urinary tract infection (UTI) should be confirmed by urine culture for bacteria and PCR-testing for virus. Yet, a diagnosis is occasionally derived from the exclusion of alternative causes.

9.3.6 Prognosis

In most cases of chemotherapy-induced HC with pre-engraftment onset and in polyomaviruria, the condition is self-limiting and the prognosis is good. If the viruria is caused by adenovirus, the prognosis is worse with the risk of progression to systemic adenovirus infection. In these cases early pharmacological intervention with antiviral drugs, e.g. cidofovir, is recommended.

9.3.7 Prevention of Chemotherapy (Cyclophosphamide/ Ifosfamide)-Induced HC

Hyperhydration with forced diuresis, i.e. 3 L/ m²/24 h with the goal of a diuresis of >250 mL/h, during and until the day after administration of an alkylating agent is the most important preventive action. If the diuresis is insufficient, diuretics should be administered. The forced diuresis will not just dilute the urine but shorten the time of duration for acrolein exposure to the bladder and thus prevent the toxic effects. During the days of hyperhydration, the patient shall be closely monitored for fluid balance, including weight, at regular intervals. An electrocardiogram (ECG) should be taken, and approved, prior to start of treatment, and vital signs (blood pressure, pulse, oxygen saturation and respiratory rate) should be checked throughout the day in order to ascertain circulatory stability. Electrolytes and renal function should be monitored by blood samples and electrolyte substitution given where required. A need for potassium substitution is not uncommon. The patient should also be assessed for any urinary or low abdominal pain or discomfort. All assessments mentioned above should be performed at least every 6 h. Informing the patient about the treatment and treatment goals as well as the importance of reporting any symptoms of HC will help ensure that appropriate actions and early intervention can be applied without delay.

For patients receiving cyclophosphamide- or ifosfamide-based regimens, the drug mesna (sodium 2-mercaptoethanesulfonate) can be used as pharmacological prophylaxis, although the additional benefit in the HSCT setting has not been scientifically proven in comparison with hyperhydration and forced diuresis. Mesna binds to the toxic metabolite acrolein and forms a non-toxic compound. By additional actions mesna also reduces the forming of acrolein in the urine. The drug itself has low toxicity (Mesna Summary of Product Characteristics 2017 (SPC) [in Swedish]).

In HSCT conditioning with cyclophosphamide, the recommended dose of mesna according to the Summary of Product Characteristics (SPC) is 20% of the cyclophosphamide dose and the first mesna dose should be administered immediately prior to the cyclophosphamide. Subsequent doses will then be given at 3, 6, 9 and 12 h after administration of cyclophosphamide (totalling 120% of the cyclophosphamide dose). It is important to adhere to the timing of mesna doses in order to ensure efficacy of the treatment. Mesna treatment should be continued during the cyclophosphamide treatment period plus the time predicted for the metabolites to reach non-toxic levels. This will usually occur between 8 and 12 h after completed cyclophosphamide administration. This treatment schedule for mesna may however vary according to conditioning regimen and doses as well as to patient individual factors.

An example of a checklist to be used during high-dose cyclophosphamide treatment is enclosed.

BK virus-induced HC may be prevented by the administration of quinolones (e.g. ciprofloxacin) (Dropulic and Jones 2008). Although quinolones are not strictly antiviral, fluoroqui nolones are capable of inhibiting the helicase activity of BKV large T antigen (TAg) protein, which seems to be crucial for separation of the double-stranded DNA genome during replication of the virus (Umbro et al. 2013). There is currently no consensus regarding this prophylaxis because many patients with BKV do not develop HC. The fact that there is a general increase of multidrug-resistant microorganisms makes the use of this prophylaxis a matter for careful consideration.

9.3.8 Treatment

The first intervention will be hyperhydration with forced diuresis to prevent clot formation. HC is usually painful and analgesia should be administered. If the patient is thrombocytopenic, a higher threshold level for platelet transfusion and intensive platelet support should be applied, in particular in haematuria grades III–IV. Catheterisation and bladder irrigation with 0.9% sodium chloride (normal saline) may be necessary to prevent clot obstruction. Catheter insertion should be performed so that the risk of additional injury to the urothelium is minimised. Treatment with bladder instillation of various compounds such as formalin, alum, silver nitrate, sodium hyalonurate, prostaglandins, GM-CSF, fibrin glue, cidofovir, ciprofloxacin or ribavirin has been reported as effective, but experiences are still limited (Carreras 2012). If obstruction occurs, cystoscopy can be performed. Selective embolisation of bladder arteries and catheterisation of both ureters to rest the bladder are actions that can be taken in severe cases. Cystectomy remains the last resort if all other treatment attempts fail.

In addition to actions mentioned above, treatment with systemic administration of palifermin, oral oestrogens and recombinant FVIIa may be used (Carreras 2012). Systemic antimicrobial drugs, e.g. cidofovir, ciprofloxacin and ribavirin, can be started, if the HC is confirmed or likely attributable to adeno- or BK virus. Decreased immunosuppression could be considered in particular in cases of relapsing viral cystitis. Note that anticoagulants such as tranexamic acid and aminocaproic acid are contraindicated in HC due to risk of clot formation and retention!

Another type of treatment that has proven effective is hyperbaric oxygen (Savva-Bordalo et al. 2012). The patient then receives 100% oxygen in a hyperbaric chamber but limited access to hyperbaric chambers, and the likely need and inability for the patient to move to another treatment unit often makes this intervention less of an option.

9.3.9 Nursing Aspects

During treatment with hyperhydration, the same need for close monitoring and assessments as in the prophylactic setting applies (see above). Assess the need for platelet transfusion prior to catheterisation as well as after. Blood transfusions may also be necessary with significant blood loss. Standard monitoring for signs of infection, injury, pain, clot formation and other potential complications from the urinary catheter is important. In cases of bladder irrigation keeping the fluids for irrigation at ambient temperature may alleviate discomfort. Complications of the irrigation can be prevented or minimised by close monitoring and recording of fluid balance. It is also important to maintain patient comfort by adequate pain management and general nursing interventions such as comfortable positioning and assistance with personal hygiene. The need for information and psychological support should be observed for both patient and family.

Since in particular viral HC may occur after discharge from the hospital, careful assessment of any signs and symptoms related to the urinary tract and that may indicate viral infection is just as important in the outpatient setting.

NB!
Administer mesna
at ordered intervals

Patient ID:

Assessments for treatment with high dose 2 g/m^2 or 4 g/m^2 cyclophosphamide (Cy)

Date: ___________		**Date:** ___________	
time:		**time:**	
12.00	ECG	**00.00**	Blood Pressure
	Blood Pressure		Pulse
	Pulse		Saturation
	Saturation		(Weight)
	Weight		Urine output *Administer diuretics if urine output <1500 mL*
	Urine output (after 1st day) *After 1st day: Administer diuretics if urine output <1500 mL*		
	Serum Sodium		
	Serum potassium		
	Serum creatinine		

time:		**time:**	
18.00	Blood Pressure	**06.00**	Blood Pressure
	Pulse		Pulse
	Saturation		Saturation
	Weight		Weight
	Urine output *Administer diuretics if urine output <1500 mL*		Urine output *Administer diuretics if urine output <1500 mL*
	Serum Sodium		Serum Sodium
	Serum potassium		Serum potassium
	Serum creatinine		Serum creatinine

9.4   Sinusoidal Obstruction Syndrome/Veno-Occlusive Disease

9.4.1   Introduction

Sinusoidal obstruction syndrome (SOS) is also known as veno-occlusive disease (VOD) and is referred to as SOS/VOD hereafter. Of the early complications that are considered to be of vascular endothelial origin, this is the most described. There are diagnosis and severity criteria (McDonald et al. 1984, 1993; Jones et al. 1987; deLeve et al. 2009; Mohty et al. 2016), although the EBMT criteria proposed in 2016 (Mohty et al. 2016) is expected to be further validated, and there is approved treatment available. Careful monitoring of HSCT patients allows early detection of SOS/VOD. Treatment can then be started without delay, ultimately improving patient outcomes. From pre-transplant assessment to medical management and overall care of the patient, nurses thus have an essential role to play as part of a multidisciplinary team (Wallhult et al. 2017).

There are specific differences between the clinical presentation of SOS/VOD in adults versus in children which has not been reflected in the older diagnosis and severity criteria. For this reason, EBMT has also developed a classification for diagnosis and severity criteria for SOS/VOD in paediatric patients (Corbacioglu et al. 2017). The information presented below is related to adults. For the paediatric population, please see original article and/or the VOD learning programme on the EBMT website. (Veno Occlusive Disease (VOD) Learning Programme 2017 http://www.ebmt.org/Contents/Nursing/Materials/LearningProgrammes/Pages/default.aspx.)

### 9.4.2	Definition and Pathogenesis

When drugs used in haematopoietic stem cell transplant (HSCT) conditioning regimens are metabolised in the liver, it results in toxic metabolites being produced by the hepatocytes. The metabolites trigger the activation, damage and inflammation of the endothelial cells lining the sinusoids (sinusoids being small capillary-like blood vessels in the liver). This trigger mechanism can start as soon as the conditioning treatment is administered. The activated sinusoidal endothelial cells release inflammatory cytokines, chemokines and the enzyme heparanase which break down the extracellular matrix that supports the structure of the sinusoids. The endothelial cells are then forced to round up, and gaps form between the cells. The gaps allow for red blood cells, white blood cells and other cellular debris to exit through these gaps in the sinusoid walls into the space of Disse. (The space of Disse is the perisinusoidal space that is located between the endothelium and the hepatocytes.)

When cells and debris accumulate in this space, the sinusoids become narrower. Due to the sinusoidal damage, endothelial cells can dissect off and embolise further downstream thus contribute to the narrowing. The damage also leads to an increase in the expression of tissue factor (TF) and plasminogen activator inhibitor-1 (PAI-1). This coagulopathy causes an increase in clot formation and a decrease in the breakdown of clots. The deposition of fibrin and the clot formation will contribute to the narrowing of the sinusoids and may ultimately lead to hepatic sinusoidal obstruction. The result is SOS/VOD which is characterised by obstruction of the sinusoids, portal vein hypotension and reduced hepatic venous outflow. Severe cases can progress to multi-organ dysfunction (MOD)/multi-organ failure (MOF) and death.

SOS/VOD usually develops before day +21 after HSCT with a peak incidence around day 12, but about 15–20% of the SOS/VOD cases have a late onset, after day +21.

### 9.4.3	Incidence and Prognosis

Although relatively rare, SOS/VOD is one of the main causes of non-relapse, transplant-related mortality. A mean incidence of 14% (Coppell et al. 2010) has been reported, but it varies with the diagnostic criteria, depending whether the Seattle (McDonald et al. 1984, 1993) or the slightly stricter Baltimore criteria (Jones et al. 1987) have been used. It will also depend on risk factors including intensity of conditioning regimen and type of transplant. After allo-HSCT with myeloablative conditioning (MAC), the incidence is approximately 10–15%, but if reduced intensity conditioning (RIC) is used, the incidence is <5%. This is the same incidence as for auto-HSCT.

Early-stage SOS/VOD, mild SOS/VOD, may not be particularly well-recognised since the symptoms are subtle, may not require treatment and spontaneously resolve within a few weeks. Unrecognised SOS/VOD may however progress, sometimes very rapidly, into moderate or severe. Severe SOS/VOD is associated with MOD/MOF and a mortality rate of 84%.

9.4.4 Risk Factors

The risk factors for SOS/VOD can be divided into patient- and disease-related and transplant-related risk factors (Mohty et al. 2015). As mentioned above, the risk factors, as well as the clinical presentation of SOS/VOD, differ between the adult and the paediatric population, and the risk factors presented here are related to adults.

The *patient- and disease-related risk factors* are:

- Older age
- Decreased performance status (Karnofsky score <90%)
- Metabolic syndrome
- Female receiving norethisterone (gestagen) to postpone menstruation period
- Genetic factors (GSTM1 polymorphism, C282Y allele, MTHFR 677CC/1298CC haplotype)
- Thalassemia
- Disease status beyond CR2
- Refractory disease or relapse
- Hepatic-related risk factors (Cirrhosis, hepatic fibrosis, active viral hepatitis, transaminases (AST and ALT) >2.5 of the upper limit of normal (ULN), serum bilirubin >1.5 ULN, coagulopathy (deficit of anti-thrombin (AT) III, tissue plasminogen activator (t-PA) and resistance to activated protein C), elevated ferritin level, iron overload, previous abdominal or hepatic irradiation, use of hepatotoxic drugs and previous use of gemtuzumab ozogamicin and inotuzumab ozogamicin. It can be noted that SOS/VOD has been reported after inotuzumab ozogamicin treatment also in non-transplant patients.)

The transplant-related risk factors are:

- Unrelated donor
- HLA-mismatched donor
- Non-T-cell-depleted graft
- MAC
- Conditioning regimen with busulfan and/or TBI
- Second HSCT

9.4.5 Diagnosis

Despite the fact that diagnostic criteria were developed in the 1980s and have been used in clinical practice and research studies, it is often hard to identify early or mild cases of SOS/VOD before it progresses to a more severe form. Some reasons are lack of sensitivity and specificity of the criteria, the dynamic manifestations that makes definition of the condition hard and that early signs and symptoms often are subtle and makes differentiation from other transplant complications difficult. Given the poor prognosis of severe SOS/VOD, it is however vital to identify mild cases before they progress to moderate, with signs of hepatic injury and requiring more aggressive intervention, or further progress to severe SOS/VOD with MOD/MOF. The most recent diagnostic criteria proposed by EBMT (Mohty et al. 2016) are the same as the Baltimore criteria (Jones et al. 1987) for classical SOS/VOD with onset within the first 3 weeks after HSCT, but if SOS/VOD develops after day +21, elevated serum bilirubin level is not always seen, why a modified version of the criteria can be used for diagnosis of late SOS/VOD (Mohty et al. 2016) (Table 9.4). The EBMT criteria will also better capture the dynamic manifestations of the disease and thus facilitate an early diagnosis as well as a more accurate assessment of severity. Treatment can then be started at a stage with greater chance for treatment response.

Differential diagnoses will need to be excluded by assessing risk factors, symptoms and lab tests since liver dysfunction can also be seen in sepsis, viral infection, graft versus host disease (GvHD) and iron overload and as a side effect from many of the drugs used in the HSCT setting. In addition to the signs and symptoms required for diagnosis haemorrhagic complications, thrombocytopenia with platelet refractoriness, pulmonary dysfunction, renal dysfunction and encephalopathy are "late" signs that can be seen in more severe cases of SOS/VOD. Further it is worth noting that all symptoms are also observed in other conditions and that many other complications may coexist with SOS/VOD. Examples of differential diagnosis for classical symptoms of SOS/VOD are listed in Table 9.5.

Table 9.4 SOS/VOD diagnosis criteria

Original Seattle Criteria (1984)	Modified Seattle criteria (1993)[2]	Baltimore Criteria (1987)[3]	EBMT Criteria for adults (2016)[4]	
Presentation before Day 30 post-HSCT	Presentation before Day 20 post-HSCT	Bilirubin ≥2 mg/dL (~34 µmol/L) before Day 21 post-HSCT	Classical SOS/VOD in the first 21 days post HSCT **with** Bilirubin ≥2 mg/dL (~34 µmol/L)	Late onset SOS/VOD >21 days post HSCT
				Classical SOS/VOD
and at least two of the following:	**of** two of the following:	**and** at least two of the following:	**and** two of the following:	**OR**
Jaundice	Bilirubin >2 mg/dL (~34 µmol/L)	Hepatomegaly	Painful hepatomegaly	SOS/VOD confirmed by liver biopsy **OR** two or more of the following:
Hepatomegaly *and* right upper quadrant pain	Hepatomegaly *or* right upper quadrant pain of liver origin	Ascites	Ascites	Bilirubin ≥2 mg/dL (~34 µmol/L)
Ascites ± unexplained weight gain	Unexplained weight gain of >2% baseline due to fluid accumulation	Weight gain ≥5% from baseline	Weight gain >5%	Painful hepatomegaly
				Ascites
				Weight gain >5%
				AND
				Hemodynamical or/and ultrasound evidence of SOS/VOD

[1]McDonald et al. (1984)
[2]McDonald et al. (1993)
[3]Jones et al. (1987)
[4]Mohty et al. (2016)

When SOS/VOD is diagnosed, it is important to classify the severity grade in order to intensify the monitoring and identify patients that will need therapeutic intervention. The EBMT severity grading criteria (Mohty et al. 2016) stress the importance of taking the time since the appearance of the symptoms into account. A rapid progression of symptoms, and in particular bilirubin kinetics (the rate of increase) with a doubling time of 48 h, should be classified as a more severe grade than if symptoms develop more slowly over several days (Table 9.6).

9.4.6 Prevention

The first strategy for prevention is to be aware of pre-existing risk factors and try and eliminate them as far as possible and potentially establish supportive or treatment measures prior to transplant. The patient- and disease-related risk factors, including hepatic, are often difficult or impossible to change, but the transplant-related risk factors should be carefully considered in the pre-transplant setting.

No proven medical prophylaxis exists but sodium heparin, prostaglandin E1, ursodeoxycholic acid and low molecular weight heparin have been tried, although data about effectiveness remains inconclusive (Carreras 2012, 2015). Defibrotide, approved for treatment of severe SOS/VOD, has also been used as prophylaxis (Dignan et al. 2013), and one randomised study in children has shown a reduction in SOS/VOD incidence (Corbacioglu et al. 2012).

Table 9.5 SOS/VOD symptoms

Symptom	Also observed in
Jaundice	Biliary infection
	Cholestasis
	Acute GvHD
	Cyclosporine
	Drug or TPN injury
	Haemolysis
Hepatomegaly and ascites	Congestive heart failure
	Fungal infection
	EBV lymphoproliferative disease
	Pancreatitis
	Portal vein thrombosis
Rapid weight gain	Congestive heart failure
	Renal failure
	Sepsis syndrome
	Capillary leak syndrome

Eisenberg (2008)

9.4.7 Treatment

As soon as SOS/VOD is suspected, supportive therapy should be initiated. In mild cases of SOS/VOD, close monitoring to detect progression and supportive management is often sufficient.

The monitoring should include:

- Daily weight
- Fluid intake and output
- Abdominal girth
- Blood tests including urea and electrolytes
- Assessment of all sites for bleeding
- Assessment of pain source and level

The supportive management consists of:

- Restricting fluid intake
- Avoidance of hepatotoxic drugs if possible
- Diuretics
- Analgesia
- Blood products
- Electrolytes
- Comfortable positioning
- Psychological support

Table 9.6 New EBMT criteria for severity grading of a suspected SOS/VOD in adults

	Mild[a]	Moderate[a]	Severe	Very severe – MOD/MOF[b]
Time since first clinical symptoms of SOS/VOD[c]	>7 Days	5–7 Days	≤4 Days	Any time
Bilirubin (mg/dL)	≥2 and <3	≥3 and < 5	≥5 and < 8	≥8
Bilirubin (μmol/L)	≥34 and <51	≥51 and < 85	≥85 and <136	≥136
Bilirubin kinetics			Doubling within 48 h	
Transaminases	≤2 × normal	> 2 and ≤5 × normal	>5 and ≤8 × normal	>8 × Normal
Weight increase	< 5%	≥5% and <10%	≥5% and <10%	≥10%
Renal function	<1.2 × baseline at transplant	≥1.2 and < 1.5 × baseline at transplant	≥1.5 and <2 × baseline at transplant	≥2 × baseline at transplant or others signs of MOD/MOF

Patients belong to the category that fulfils two or more criteria. If patients fulfil two or more criteria in two different categories, they must be classified in the most severe category. Patients weight increase ≥5% and <10% is considered by default as a criterion for severe SOS/VOD; however, if patients do not fulfil other criteria for severe SOS/VOD, weight increase ≥5% and <10% is therefore considered as a criterion for moderate SOS/VOD

Abbreviations: *EBMT* European Society for Blood and Marrow Transplantation, *MOD* multi-organ dysfunction, *MOF* multi-organ failure, *SOS* sinusoidal obstruction syndrome, *VOD* veno-occlusive disease

[a]In the case of presence of two or more risk factors for SOS/VOD, patients should be in the upper grade

[b]Patients with multi-organ dysfunction must be classified as very severe

[c]Time from the date when the first signs/symptoms of SOS/VOD began to appear (retrospectively determined) and the date when the symptoms fulfilled SOS/VOD diagnostic criteria

For more details about nursing interventions see below.

The only curative treatment for SOS/VOD is the drug defibrotide. Defibrotide protects the endothelial cells, reduces inflammation and restores thrombo-fibrinolytic balance (Richardson et al. 2013). The recommended dose is 6.25 mg/kg body weight administered as a 2-h, i.v. infusion every 6 h (to a total dose of 25 mg/kg/day). Recommendation for treatment duration is at least 21 days but should continue until the symptoms and signs of severe VOD resolve. Defibrotide is generally well tolerated (Keating 2014) but should not be used with products that affect platelet aggregation, e.g. non-steroid anti-inflammatory drugs (NSAIDs), anticoagulant therapy or other products that increase the risk of bleeding.

9.4.8 Nursing Aspects

It is important to perform a risk assessment considering the risk factors mentioned above and to take baseline measurements including defining a threshold of >5% for weight gain or what level and pattern of weight gain that represents a clinical concern. Most baseline measurements will be standard for HSCT patients, but in patients at high risk for SOS/VOD, assessments of abdominal girth, right upper quadrant (RUQ) pain and inspection of sclera should be added.

Standard daily monitoring should include temperature, pulse, blood pressure, respiration rate and saturation. One of the most important daily monitoring aspects is an accurate fluid balance including intake, output and weight since fluid imbalance is one of the earliest signs of SOS/VOD. A fluid retention which does not respond to diuretics represents an early sign of endothelial damage.

When performing abdominal girth measurement, it is advised to use a marked line for placement of the measuring tape and to choose one position (i.e. sitting/standing/lying) for the patient, to be used consequently. Abdominal discomfort, tenderness, pain (in particular RUQ pain) and inspection for collateral circulation and/or spiders should always be included in abdominal assessment. For nurses trained in palpation and percussion for ascites, bulkiness, liver margins and size these assessments should also be performed.

Sclera and skin should be assessed for bleeding/bruising and discoloration (jaundice).

Knowledge of the relevant reference ranges of daily laboratory values, particularly liver enzymes, serum bilirubin, blood count, electrolytes, urea and serum creatinine will enable early detection of significant change or trend in values since nurses are likely to take blood samples and see the results first and can alert medical colleagues.

All findings should be precisely documented and any changes promptly reported. This is especially important in patients identified as high risk as early detection of SOS/VOD may affect the overall outcome.

If SOS/VOD is suspected, the monitoring should be intensified and adequate vascular access established. In addition to standard lab tests, coagulation parameters should be performed daily. If possible, hepatotoxic drugs should be avoided and diuretics and pain medication administered as needed. Electrolyte replacement may be necessary, and in case of thrombocytopenia or bleeding, blood products will be administered. If fluid restriction is enforced, it is important to know the smallest volumes that can be safely delivered.

The patient may also need assistance to be comfortably positioned.

When SOS/VOD has been diagnosed, the supportive care and monitoring will be further intensified including assessing for failure in respiratory, cardiac and renal function. Defibrotide treatment will most likely be started, and patients in need for ventilatory support should be prepared for transfer to the intensive care unit (ICU).

Patients should be informed and educated to notify the staff of any signs and symptoms that may need closer monitoring or intervention. In case SOS/VOD is diagnosed, both patient and family will need reassurance and support.

9.5 Other Early Complications of Endothelial Origin

9.5.1 Introduction

A number of early complications to haematopoietic stem cell transplantation (HSCT) seem to be initiated by damage to the vascular endothelium. The most well defined and well described of these complications is sinusoidal obstruction syndrome (SOS)/veno-occlusive disease (VOD) described in a separate section of this chapter. Other syndromes in this group have been named engraftment syndrome (ES), diffuse alveolar haemorrhage (DAH), idiopathic pneumonia syndrome (IPS) and transplant-associated microangiopathy (TMA). The similarities in their clinical manifestations and the lack of established diagnostic criteria often make determination of incidence and differential diagnosis difficult (Soubani and Pandya 2010; Afessa et al. 2012). Although many times mild and with spontaneous recovery, these complications also share the risk for progression to multi-organ failure (MOF)/multi-organ damage (MOD) resulting in a poor outcome.

Ongoing research and efforts for better characterisation and treatment indicate that there will be future changes in terminology and diagnostic criteria, as well as interventions, for the early HSCT complications mentioned here.

9.5.2 Pathogenesis

Several factors in the HSCT setting activate the endothelial cells that line the blood vessels. Contributing factors are the conditioning treatment and use of other drugs such as granulocyte colony-stimulating factor (G-CSF) and calcineurin inhibitors (CNI), e.g. cyclosporine-A, and microbial products translocated through mucosal barriers. The result is that fluid and proteins leak out of tiny blood vessels and flow into surrounding tissues. If unrecognised, this may lead to dangerously low blood pressure and subsequently MOF and shock. The symptoms often appear around the time of neutrophil recovery, i.e. when the absolute neutrophil count (ANC) increases to $\geq 0.5 \times 10^9$/L, which is why the complex process of engraftment may also play a role in activation of endothelial cell damage. The activation of the endothelial cells leads to further damage and inflammation by the release of pro-inflammatory cytokines. Since the incidence of vascular endothelial syndromes is higher after allogeneic transplantation, alloreactivity (the immune response to non-self cells) is considered to play a role in activation and damage of endothelial cells.

9.6 Engraftment Syndrome (ES)

9.6.1 Definition

ES usually occurs after auto-HSCT although described in allo-HSCT as well, in particular when reduced intensity conditioning (RIC) and cord blood (CB) have been used.

Due to lack of diagnostic criteria, the term ES has been used as synonymous with capillary leak syndrome (CLS), auto-aggression syndrome, peri-engraftment respiratory distress syndrome (PERDS), aseptic shock syndrome and autologous graft versus host disease (AGVHD). Although there are differences, their common denominator is that they share some or all symptoms that have been attributed to ES.

Engraftment is defined as when the number of neutrophils in the patient's blood rises to an absolute neutrophil count (ANC) of $\geq 0.5 \times 10^9$/L.

Peri-engraftment can be defined as the period within 5 days of neutrophil engraftment.

9.6.2 Incidence and Prognosis

Due to the diagnosis difficulties, there is no reliable incidence figure and numbers between 10% and 70% have been reported. There is also a lack of survival data. Most cases are mild and respond well to corticosteroid therapy, but ES may progress and lead to transplant-related mortality and decrease in overall survival. Patients who require mechanical ventilation has a poor prognosis.

9.6.3 Risk Factors

A number of potential risk factors related to patient characteristics, disease, previous treatment, conditioning treatment, stem cell source and supportive drug treatment have been reported, but there is a lack of consensus which can in part be contributed to the lack of diagnostic criteria. Changes in HSCT practices with new drugs and alternate stem cell sources may impact the risk factors in the future.

Among the risk factors described are:

- Female gender
- Advanced age
- No or little prior chemotherapy
- Previous use of bortezomib and lenalidomide in multiple myeloma patients
- Cord blood transplantation
- CD34+ cell number and engraftment rate
- G-CSF treatment
- Amphotericin treatment
- Cyclosporine (CyA) treatment
- Auto-HSCT for amyloidosis, multiple myeloma, POEMS (polyneuropathy organomegaly endocrinopathy monoclonal protein and skin abnormalities) syndrome and auto-immune diseases

9.6.4 Diagnosis

There are two tools to aid diagnosis of ES; the Spitzer (2001) and the Maiolino et al. (2003) diagnostic criteria. The clinical manifestations are divided into major or minor clinical criteria (Table 9.7), but Maiolino only has one major criteria, non-infectious fever. The timing of symptoms relative engraftment also differs between the two, where Maiolino has a stricter timeframe from 24 h before to any time after neutrophil recovery compared to Spitzer's 96 h after (Table 9.8). However, in some patients others have described onset of symptoms from 7 days

Table 9.7 Engraftment syndrome criteria

Major criteria	Non-infectious fever	New fever (> 38°C) without documented infection or without response to anti-infectious treatment
	Skin rash	Maculopapular exanthema in >25% of body surface area
	Pulmonary oedema	Confirmed by X-ray or CT, Without signs of infection, cardiac failure or pulmonary embolism
Minor criteria	Weight gain	>2.5% from baseline
	Hepatic dysfunction	Bilirubin ≥2 mg/dL (34μmol/L) or transaminases (ASAT/ALAT) ≥2 times increase from baseline
	Renal dysfunction	Creatinine ≥2 times increase from baseline
	Transient encephalopathy	Without other cause
	Diarrhoea	≥2 liquid stools per day without documented infection

Table 9.8 Spitzer and Maiolino criteria

	Spitzer criteria	Maiolino criteria
Symptoms	3 major or 2 major and 1 minor	Non-infectious fever and 1 minor
Timing relative engraftment	Within 96 h after	24 h before or at any time after

before (for patients with POEMS) to 7 days after engraftment, and in cases with more severe symptoms, the early symptoms may have been overlooked, why the clinical criteria sometimes could be used regardless of appearance of symptoms in relation to time for engraftment (Chang et al. 2014). C-reactive protein (CRP) is not used for diagnosis in either criteria, but a sudden and significant increase in the CRP level has been found to support the diagnosis.

9.6.5 Prevention

Early recognition of signs and symptoms is the most important aspect since there is no standard prophylaxis for ES, although there is evidence that corticosteroids may prevent this complication.

9.6.6 Treatment

Before treatment is initiated, other diagnoses such as infection, drug rash, diarrhoea associated with infection or medication and intravenous (i.v.)-related fluid overload should be excluded. Broad-spectrum antibiotics should be used until infection is ruled out (Cornell et al. 2015). If cultures are negative, symptoms remain after 48–72 h of antibiotic treatment and other etiologies can be excluded, corticosteroid treatment can be initiated.

Methylprednisolone in doses of 1–3 mg/kg/day i.v. are recommended until symptoms begin to subside. Response to treatment is usually seen within 2–3 days. Corticosteroids could then be switched to oral administration and should be slowly tapered. Early intervention with steroids prevents progression to more severe manifestations, and in the vast majority (80%) of patients, there is then complete resolution in less than 6 days. In cases with no response to steroid treatment after 72 h, biopsies of affected organs may be necessary. If biopsies are performed for evaluation of diarrhoea, the findings may not be able to distinguish from GvHD. This does however not exclude ES since overlap and coexistence with GvHD is possible. If a biopsy supports the ES diagnosis treatment with additional immune suppressants should be started and continued until response. If the result of the biopsy is an alternative diagnosis, the patient should be treated accordingly.

In addition to pharmacological treatment supportive care with i.v. fluids, with electrolyte supplement as needed, and oxygen therapy may be necessary depending on the symptoms.

In cases of encephalopathy or severe ES with MOF, plasma exchange may be considered (Yeoung-Hau and Syed 2014).

9.6.7 Nursing Aspects

Daily nursing assessments are critical in early detection and diagnosis of all complications to HSCT. The patient's general well-being should be assessed, and listed below are the nursing assessments that should be carried out frequently, the findings that could indicate ES and actions that can be taken in order to detect or rule out the ES diagnosis (Table 9.9). All findings should be

Table 9.9 Nursing assessments and actions

Assessment	Action
Temperature	Monitor frequently, and in cases of fever ≥38 °C, obtain cultures from blood, urine, stools or other suspected sites of infection and keep the patient comfortable
Pulse and blood pressure	Monitor frequently in order to detect, e.g. circulatory symptoms of fluid overload, infection and pulmonary dysfunction
Respirations and saturation	Monitor frequently, and if symptoms of pulmonary dysfunction, e.g. dyspnoea, tachypnoea, change in breathing pattern, chest pain or cough, are present, a chest X-ray or pulmonary CT scan may be performed. In order to ensure adequate oxygenation, administration of oxygen therapy may be necessary
Weight and fluid balance	Assess the patient's weight daily and perform calculation of fluid balance at least once daily to note any trends. If oedema, ascites or other symptoms of fluid retention occurs diuretics should be administered as ordered
Skin	Perform assessment at least daily and note any rashes. If a rash is detected, review the patient's medication chart for medication that may cause drug rash Jaundice and yellow sclera are signs of liver dysfunction and bilirubin levels should be checked
Stools	Monitor frequency and consistency and obtain cultures and test for *Clostridium difficile* in cases of diarrhoea in order to rule out infection. Pale stools are a sign of liver dysfunction and bilirubin levels should be checked

(continued)

Table 9.9 (continued)

Assessment	Action
Lab tests	Be alert to any trends or changes in ANC, bilirubin, transaminases and creatinine and to result of cultures
Mental status	Assess regularly for confusion, lethargy, headache, visual disturbances, aphasia and note any changes
Patient information and education	Educate the patient about signs and symptoms of ES and explain why it is important to report any symptoms without delay. Explain actions taken in diagnosis and management of ES and provide emotional support to both patient and family

Thoele (2014)

documented and any abnormalities promptly reported to the treating physician.

If steroid treatment is started, the patient should be assessed for possible side effects such as hyperglycaemia and insomnia. Blood glucose should be monitored daily.

9.7 Idiopathic Pneumonia Syndrome

9.7.1 Definition

Pulmonary complications (PCs) are the leading cause of patients' admission to intensive care unit (ICU) after HSCT. PC can be divided into infectious or non-infectious. One of the non-infectious PCs is idiopathic pneumonia syndrome (IPS).

For the purpose of this chapter, IPS will be defined and described according to the definition by the American Thoracic Society (Panotskaltsis-Mortari et al. 2011) as "an idiopathic syndrome of pneumopathy after HSCT, with evidence of widespread alveolar injury and in which an infectious etiology and cardiac dysfunction, acute renal failure or iatrogenic fluid overload have been excluded". The alveolar injury is a result from the release of proinflammatory cytokines during engraftment increasing alveolar permeability and causing diffuse alveolar or interstitial infiltrates.

IPS also includes a subset of diagnoses of primary lung injuries classified according to the anatomical sites of inflammation. They can either be related to the pulmonary parenchyma (e.g. acute interstitial pneumonitis and acute respiratory distress syndrome (ARDS)), the airway endothelium (e.g. bronchiolitis obliterans syndrome (BO)), the vascular endothelium (e.g. different forms of ES (PERDS, CLS)) or be unclassifiable. Other less frequent non-infectious PCs have also been identified. None of these entities will be described here.

9.7.2 Incidence and Prognosis

PCs are common in HSCT recipients and a major cause of morbidity and mortality. IPS is more often seen in patients undergoing allogeneic HSCT with a mean estimated incidence of 1–10% (6% in auto-HSCT) (Chi et al. 2013). The overall outcome is different between auto- and allo-HSCT recipients, and where IPS in patients that have undergone auto-HSCT usually has a favourable prognosis, the mortality is 60–80% in the allo-setting (Carreras 2012). IPS has a progressive nature, and patients with progression to respiratory failure and need for mechanical ventilation have a very poor prognosis with 95% mortality.

9.7.3 Risk Factors

For IPS the following risk factors have been identified (Diab et al. 2016):

- Older age
- Low performance status (Karnofsky score)
- High-intensity conditioning regimen
- Total body irradiation (TBI)
- Allo-HSCT
- Acute graft versus host disease (aGvHD)
- Malignant disease

Pre-transplant pulmonary function abnormalities have also been associated with early respiratory failure and mortality (Chien et al. 2005).

9.7.4 Diagnosis

The most common signs and symptoms are fever, non-productive cough, rales, dyspnoea, tachypnoea and low saturation with an increasing need for oxygen support.

The diagnosis will be based on alveolar injury confirmed clinically, radiologically and/or functionally. X-ray will reveal diffuse pulmonary infiltrates. Infection must have been ruled out by negative cultures and tests in bronchoalveolar lavage (BAL) or lung biopsies (Zhu et al. 2008), and there should be no evidence of cardiac dysfunction, acute renal failure or treatment-related fluid overload. It is however considered possible that some cases of IPS may be caused by an unidentified underlying infection since infections may lack typical signs and symptoms in the neutropenic patient. The IPS diagnosis can thus be supported by lack of improvement despite broad-spectrum antibiotics and other antimicrobial drugs.

The typical onset will be around day +20, but IPS may also present later after HSCT, why it is important to be alert for this complication also after discharge from the hospital, in the outpatient setting.

There are no standard guidelines for diagnosis and evaluation of PC after HSCT, but the course of illness should be considered when differential diagnoses are to be excluded. When symptoms occur, IPS may rapidly progress to pulmonary dysfunction requiring mechanical ventilation.

9.7.5 Prevention

For patients at risk for IPS, careful consideration of treatment options pre- and posttransplant such as avoiding conditioning with TBI or high-intensity regimens and choice of GvHD prophylaxis may be beneficial. Monitoring of pulmonary function and symptoms after transplantation will enable prompt intervention.

In patients with decreased lung function prior to HSCT and suspected lung injury in the post-transplant setting, close collaboration with pulmonary specialist or the intensive care team may

prevent progression of pulmonary dysfunction (Elbahlawan et al. 2016).

9.7.6 Treatment

Beyond supportive care, there is no proven treatment for IPS. In auto-HSCT patients, corticosteroids can be effective, but this is usually not the case for allo-transplanted patients, irrespective of steroid dose. Studies with etanercept, a TNF-α-binding protein, given in combination with corticosteroids have reported improved pulmonary function in patients with IPS following allogeneic HSCT and may be considered (Carreras 2012) although a small but later study (Yanik et al. 2014) could not confirm the benefit of this treatment.

9.7.7 Nursing Aspects

The close monitoring and daily nursing assessments that apply for all HSCT patients should be employed. Depending on risk factors, extra attention may be needed to early and subtle symptoms of pulmonary dysfunction, such as decrease in saturation, shortness of breath and cough. Monitoring of daily weight and fluid balance, with administration of diuretics if necessary, will prevent and rule out fluid overload. Several different tests and examinations may be performed to establish or rule out the diagnosis of IPS. Sputum cultures and laboratory tests, such as polymerase chain reaction (PCR) for mycoplasma, and serum galactomannan for *Aspergillus* may need to be obtained, and chest X-ray or computed tomography (CT) scan performed to rule out infection. In case a BAL, with or without transbronchial biopsy, will be performed, information to the patient and preparation prior to the procedure as well as support both before and after and post procedure monitoring is important. The BAL may add substantial discomfort, in particular to an already seriously ill patient. Other lung function tests may also be repeated, for comparison with pre-transplant results.

When corticosteroids are administered, the blood glucose levels should be followed daily and the patient should be informed of and assessed for other side effects, e.g. insomnia. Oxygen therapy may need to be administered and noninvasive positive pressure ventilation necessary. Respiratory difficulties generate anxiety, and the patient should be offered psychological support as well as assistance with positioning and breathing techniques and exercises. Medication for anxiety may be necessary. Referral to a physiotherapist, respiratory therapist or other staff with expertise in pulmonary diseases should be made for advice on tools and exercises that may help the patient to maintain pulmonary function and prevent worsening of the condition.

If the condition shows no signs of improving, the patient should be prepared for transfer to the ICU.

Identification of patients at risk, prompt intervention to signs and symptoms of pulmonary dysfunction and close collaboration within the team will increase the chances of a positive outcome.

9.8　Diffuse Alveolar Haemorrhage

9.8.1　Definition

Diffuse Alveolar Haemorrhage (DAH) is a non-infectious pulmonary complication associated with haematopoietic stem cell transplant (HSCT) and other causes (Park 2013). It is differentiated from idiopathic pneumonia syndrome (IPS) through confirmation of pulmonary haemorrhage by bronchoscopy and bronchoalveolar lavage (BAL). The bleeding can be either insidious, causing a gradual pulmonary dysfunction, or a more acute bleeding into the alveolar space. Damage to the alveolar-capillary barrier from conditioning treatment and the engraftment process with recovery of neutrophils leads to entry of blood into the alveolar space.

9.8.2　Incidence and Prognosis

An approximate incidence of around 5% up to 20%, with a mortality rate ranging between 50% and 100%, has been reported for DAH in HSCT recipients (Afessa et al. 2002; Majhail et al. 2006; Carreras 2012). The incidence is similar between auto- and allo-HSCT.

The implication of prognostic factors has not been well studied, but early-onset DAH (within the first 30 days after transplant) in patients undergoing auto-HSCT has a favourable prognosis.

9.8.3　Risk Factors

Risk factors for the development of DAH in HSCT recipients include:

- Older age
- Total body irradiation (TBI)
- Myeloablative conditioning (MAC) regimens
- Acute graft versus host (aGvHD) disease

9.8.4　Diagnosis

Dyspnoea, dry cough and fever are the most common complaints. Haemoptysis is rarely observed in HSCT recipients. Hypoxemia may be present and diffuse or focal interstitial or alveolar infiltrates can be found on chest X-ray or computed tomography (CT) scan. With such findings, bronchoscopy with BAL and transbronchial biopsy is indicated although performing these invasive tests in patients with severe illness, and unstable respiratory status is a challenge.

The diagnosis is based on BAL findings which become progressively more blood stained, indicating blood in the alveoli. Other causes, such as heart failure and fluid overload, should be excluded. Infection needs to be ruled out by obtaining relevant cultures. Presence of hemosiderin-laden macrophages in BAL fluid is not diagnostic for DAH but may support the diagnosis.

It is often very difficult to differentiate DAH from IPS and the ES form of respiratory distress (PERDS). IPS is more common in allo-HSCT, after engraftment, and does not respond to corticosteroids and has a more progressive nature. In PERDS the majority of patients do not have BAL findings becoming progressively bloodier.

The mean onset of DAH has been reported on day 24 after transplant and 6 days after absolute neutrophil count (ANC) recovery.

9.8.5 Prevention

Reversal of some risk factors, e.g. choice of conditioning treatment, may be possible, but otherwise no prophylaxis exists.

9.8.6 Treatment

High-dose corticosteroids, using methyl prednisolone in doses of 250–500 mg every 6 h for 4–5-days followed by slow tapering, is considered first-line treatment even if efficacy can be questioned. With early diagnosis and treatment with steroid therapy, respiratory failure can often be prevented. Noninvasive ventilation may decrease mortality although the majority of patients with DAH require mechanical ventilation, and sepsis and MOF/MOD will cause death in a large proportion of patients (Rabe et al. 2010).

Other pharmacological therapies, as well as plasma exchange, have been tried for treatment of DAH. Recombinant factor VIIa (rFVIIa) has been administered and achieved temporary control of bleeding. Tranexamic acid or the TNFα-inhibitor etanercept have been used in addition to corticosteroids but have not proved to be effective.

Transfusion of platelets and red blood cells (RBC) may be necessary.

9.8.7 Nursing Aspects

Patients need frequent monitoring for early detection of any pulmonary symptoms. Respiration rate and saturation should be assessed together with temperature and other standard assessments. If cough is noted, this should be reported to the team and the treating physician. Cultures and blood tests may be necessary to rule out infection. Cultures should be performed according to signs and symptoms, but screening cultures can be collected to possibly enable detection of occult infection. The patient's circulatory status and fluid balance should be controlled by monitoring pulse, blood pressure, weight and input and output.

The patient should be instructed to report all symptoms, and if BAL and lung biopsy will be performed, patient information and support throughout the whole procedure is vital. Administration of transfusions, oxygen therapy and non-invasive ventilation should be performed as ordered and since dyspnoea and other breathing difficulties are associated with a great deal of anxiety patient support, sometimes with pharmacological treatment, is crucial. Proper positioning together with breathing exercises using appropriate breathing technique may alleviate some discomfort.

During high-dose corticosteroid treatment, blood glucose should be monitored, and it is important to be alert to steroid-related changes in the patient's mental status.

9.9 Transplant-Associated Microangiopathy (TAM)

9.9.1 Definition

Transplant-associated microangiopathy (TAM) is also known as haematopoietic stem cell transplantation (HSCT)-associated thrombotic microangiopathy (TA-TMA). In this text, the term TAM is being used. TAM is characterised by microangiopathic haemolytic anaemia with schistocytes (fragmented red blood cells) and thrombocytopenia from platelet consumption. These symptoms are due to endothelial dysfunction causing small vessels thrombosis in the microcirculation. TAM is a multi-visceral disease most often affecting the kidneys, but pulmonary, gastrointestinal and central nervous system (CNS) involvement can also be seen. Complement system dysregulation plays an important role in the severity of TAM. Defects in the complement system lead to formation of the lytic complex C5b-9. This complex can be detected in blood, and an increased level will support the TAM diagnosis.

9.9.2 Incidence

The incidence will vary with the criteria used to diagnose TAM. In retrospective data, the incidence is approximately 4% in auto-HSCT, 7% has been reported in allo-HSCT (Carreras 2012), whereas one prospective study has shown an incidence close to 40% (Jodele et al. 2015). Conditioning intensity, myeloablative (MAC) versus reduced (RIC), has not shown any difference in incidence in allo-HSCT.

9.9.3 Prognosis

As with many early complications in HSCT prompt recognition of early signs and symptoms with early diagnosis and intervention will increase the chances of a positive outcome. Cases of mild TAM where calcineurin inhibitor (CNI), e.g. cyclosporine, tacrolimus and sirolimus, is the cause generally have a good prognosis if CNI can be discontinued. If TAM is not related to CNI treatment, the prognosis is worse due to lack of effective treatment options. Exact figures for mortality rate are difficult to establish, but in patients with TAM and multi-organ involvement, the mortality is as high as >90%. Patients surviving TAM are as a consequence at greater risk for chronic kidney disease (CKD) and hypertension later on.

9.9.4 Risk Factors

Use of total body irradiation (TBI) in conditioning treatment, CNI, graft versus host disease (GvHD), infections (e.g. cytomegalovirus (CMV) and fungal infections) and unrelated donor transplant (in particular if mismatched) are all considered risk factors or triggers for TAM, although reported data is conflicting (Nadir and Brenner 2012; Rosenthal 2016).

9.9.5 Diagnosis

TAM usually has an onset between 1 and 2 months after HSCT but can be seen both earlier and later.

Several slightly different criteria for diagnosis of TAM are being used (Sahin et al. 2016). See adapted Table 9.10. The diagnosis is difficult but can be confirmed with a biopsy tissue sample although this invasive test may not always be an option for the seriously ill HSCT recipient. TAM has clinical similarities with idiopathic thrombotic thrombocytopenic purpura (TTP), and laboratory testing for the von Willebrand factor regulator ADAMTS13 can be performed to support the diagnosis. In classical TTP, there is a severe deficiency, while no significant decrease of ADAMTS13 is seen in TAM (Graf and Stern 2012).

Renal TAM should be suspected if the patient requires higher doses of antihypertensives than would be expected considering the situation and concomitant and/or nephrotoxic medication. Example of a differential diagnosis is virus-related nephropathy.

Symptoms such as tachycardia, chest pain and hypoxemia should lead to suspicion of lung involvement and pulmonary hypertension. The diagnosis can be supported by findings of cardiomegaly on chest X-ray, pericardial effusion on transthoracic echocardiography and blood tests.

Intestinal TAM presents with the same symptoms as acute GvHD (aGvHD), abdominal pain, diarrhoea, vomiting and gastrointestinal bleeding. The symptoms can also be mistaken for infectious colitis, but in TAM the cause of the bleeding is ischemia in the bowels due to the microangiopathy. In addition to the general diagnostic criteria, specific criteria for gastrointestinal TAM have been proposed. Besides the clinical symptoms, X-ray findings with signs of ileus and thick

Table 9.10 TAM diagnostic criteria

	Blood and Marrow Transplant Clinical Trials Network toxicity committee consensus definition for TMA (BBMT 2005[1])	International Working Group Definition for TMA (Haematologica 2007[2])	Probable TMA (Transplantation 2010[3])	Diagnostic Criteria for TA-TMA (Blood Rev. 2015[4])
				Tissue biopsy confirming microangiopathy *or* criteria below
1	Peripheral Blood Smear with RBC fragmentation and ≥ 2 shistocytes per high power field	>4% shistocytes in peripheral blood	>4% shistocytes in peripheral blood	LDH above Upper Limit of Normal (ULN)
2	Concurrent increase in LD	Thrombocytopenia <50 x10^9 /L or decrease of 50% from baseline	Concurrent increase in LD	Proteinuria on random analysis with ≥ 30 mg/dL
3	Concurrent renal dysfunction (doubling of serum creatinine from baseline) an/or neurologic dysfunction without other explanations	Sudden and persistant increase in LD	Thrombocytopenia <50 x10^9 /L or decrease of 50% from baseline	Hypertension
4	Negative DAT and IAT	Decrease in Hgb concentration or increase in RBC transfusion requirement	Negative DAT and IAT	Thrombocytopenia <50 x10^9 /L or decrease of 50% from baseline
5		Decrease in serum haptoglobin	Decrease in serum haptoglobin	Hgb below Lower Limit of Normal (LLN) or anaemia with transfusion requirement
6			Absence of coagulopathy	Shistocytes in peripheral blood or microangiopathy on tissue specimen
7				sC5b-9 above ULN
				1+2+3: Consider diagnosis of TAM and monitor very closely
				2+7: If present at diagnosis poor outcome is apprehended. Consider active treatment.

[1]Ho et al. (2005)
[2]Ruutu et al. (2007)
[3]Cho et al. (2010)
[4]Jodele et al. (2015)

mucosal wall and endoscopy with mucosal erosions and haemorrhages are included in the gastrointestinal TAM diagnostic criteria, but the only definite diagnostic test is a biopsy tissue sample.

As a result of generalised vascular injury in TAM, polyserositis with pericardial and pleural effusion and ascites can occur. It can easily be mistaken for GvHD, but where GvHD more seldom is associated with microangiopathic anaemia, proteinuria and hypertension, these symptoms are common in TAM.

9.9.6   Prevention

No specific prophylaxis exists, so vigilant monitoring of clinical signs and symptoms is neces-sary. CNI concentration in blood, lactate dehydrogenase (LD or LDH) and serum creatinine should be closely followed, i.e. two to three times/week, with laboratory testing. Additional blood tests with peripheral blood smear, haptoglobin and direct and indirect antiglobulin tests (DAT and IAT) should be performed if an increase is seen in CNI, LD and creatinine levels.

9.9.7   Treatment

There is currently no established treatment for TMA but supportive measures should always be taken. Traditionally the first step is to discontinue CNI, despite paucity of evidence for this action. It is also important to treat infections, GvHD and hypertension. Changing to other GvHD prophylaxis and use of antimicrobial drugs should be based on a risk-benefit assessment where, for example, nephrotoxicity is considered. Administration of diuretics may be necessary to treat fluid and sodium retention due to steroid treatment. Vasodilators and renin-angiotensin antagonists may also be used to treat hypertension.

It is recommended to restrict platelet transfusion in microangiopathic disease, but this is often impossible due to the need to prevent bleeding complications.

A potential treatment for TMA is eculizumab. Eculizumab stops the complement-activating cascade preventing formation of C5b-9. This leads to hampering of the intravascular haemolysis. Eculizumab has shown effect when started early after diagnosis (Jodele et al. 2015). Monitoring for effect by following serum concentration levels is important, and dose adjustments may be necessary to reach and maintain the desired therapeutic levels and effect.

In a small number of cases, successful treatment with rituximab and other monoclonal antibodies has been reported.

Treatment attempts have also been made with defibrotide at the same dosing as approved for treatment of severe sinusoidal obstruction syndrome/veno-occlusive disease (SOS/VOD) but with variable results.

Total plasma exchange (TPE) has been tried due to the clinical similarities between TAM and TTP, but where TTP can be successfully treated with TPE, it is not recommended for TAM due to poor response rates.

9.9.8 Nursing Aspects

Careful assessments will facilitate early diagnosis of, or ruling out, TMA and thus improves the outcome. Close monitoring of vital signs and being alert to any changes or trends is standard. Keeping track of fluid balance and weight is equally important. Blood pressure should be kept below 140/90 in adult patients (Jodele et al. 2015). The patient's urine should be monitored

for proteinuria and the patient instructed about what abnormal findings and symptoms to look for and to notify staff of any discomfort including signs of gastrointestinal bleeding. If invasive tests such as biopsies are to be performed, proper preparation and support is vital.

If pharmacological treatment with eculizumab is started, serum level concentration needs to be followed. Treatment with rituximab and defibrotide should be administered as ordered, and the patient should be monitored accordingly for effect and side effects.

Since the onset of TAM can occur after discharge from the transplant unit, it is important to be observant to symptoms and consider this diagnosis even in the outpatient setting.

References

Afessa B, Tefferi A, Litzow MR, et al. Outcome of Diffuse Alveolar Hemorrhage in Hematopoietic Stem Cell Transplant Recipients. Am J Respir Critical Care Med. 2002;166:1364–8. Originally Published in Press as https://doi.org/10.1164/rccm.200208-792OC on September 25, 2002.

Afessa B, Abdulai RM, Kremers WK, et al. Risk factors and outcome of pulmonary complications after autologous hematopoietic stem cell transplant. Chest. 2012;141(2):442–50. https://doi.org/10.1378/chest.10-2889.

Al-Dasoogi N, et al. Emerging evidence of the pathobiology of mucositis. Support Care Cancer. 2013;21:3233–41.

Bhatt V, Ventrell N, et al. Implementation of a standardised protocol for prevention and management on oral mucositis in patients undergoing haematopoitiec stem cell transplant. J Oncol Pharm Pract. 2010;16(3):195–204.

Carreras E. Chapter 11: Early complications after HSCT. In: Carreras E, Gluckman E, Masszi T, editors. EBMT-ESH handbook on haematopoietic stem cell transplantation. 6th ed. Genova: Forum Service Editore; 2012. p. 176–94.

Carreras E. How I manage sinusoidal obstruction syndrome after haematopoietic cell transplantation. Br J Haematol. 2015;168:481–91. https://doi.org/10.1111/bjh.13215. First published online 17 November 2014.

Chang L, Frame D, Braun T, et al ngraftment syndrome after allogeneic hematopoietic cell transplantation predicts poor outcomes. Biol Blood Marrow Transplant. 2014;20:1407–17. https://doi.org/10.1016/j.bbmt.2014.05.022.

Chi AK, Soubani AO, White AC, et al. An update on pulmonary complications of hematopoietic stem cell transplantation. Chest. 2013;144(6):1913–22. https://doi.org/10.1378/chest.12-1708.

Chien JW, et al. Pulmonary function testing prior to hematopoietic stem cell transplantation. Bone Marrow Transplant. 2005;35(5):429–35.

Cho BS, et al. Validation of recently proposed consensus criteria for thrombotic Microangiopathy after allogeneic hematopoietic stem-cell transplantation. Transplantation. 2010;90(8):918–26.

Clarkson JE, Worthington, HV et al. Interventions for treating oral mucositis for patients with cancer receiving treatment (review) Cochrane Library. 2011. Cochrane Database System Review (4)

Coppell JA, et al. Hepatic veno-occlusive disease following stem cell transplantation: incidence, clinical course and outcome. BBMT. 2010;16:157–68.

Corbacioglu S, et al. Defibrotide for prophylaxis of hepatic veno-occlusive disease in paediatric haemopoietic stem-cell transplantation: an open-label, phase 3, randomised controlled trial. Lancet. 2012;379:1301–9.

Corbacioglu S, et al. Diagnosis and severity criteria for sinusoidal obstruction syndrome/veno-occlusive disease in pediatric patients: a new classification from the European society for blood and marrow transplantation Bone Marrow Transpl. Advance online publication, 31 July 2017; 1–8.

Cornell RF, et al. Engraftment syndrome after autologous stem cell transplantation: an update unifying the definition and management approach. Biol Blood Marrow Transplant. 2015;21:2061–8.

Daniels R, et al. The sepsis six and the severe sepsis resuscitation bundle: a prospective observational cohort study. Emerg Med J. 2011;28:507–12. E-pub 2011, October 29.

deLeve LD, et al. Vascular disorders of the liver. Hepatology. 2009;49:1729–64.

de Padua Silva L. Hemorrhagic cystitis after allogeneic hematopoietic stem cell transplants is the complex result of BK virus infection, preparative regimen intensity and donor type. Haematologica. 2010;95:1183–90.

Diab M, et al. Major pulmonary complications after hematopoietic stem cell transplant. Exp Clin Transplant. 2016;14(3):259–70.

Dignan FL, et al. BCSH/BSBMT guideline: diagnosis and management of veno-occlusive disease (sinusoidal obstruction syndrome) following haematopoietic stem cell transplantation. Br J Haematol. 2013;163:444–57.

Droller MJ, Saral R, Santos G. Prevention of cyclophosphamide- induced hemorrhagic cystitis. Urology. 1982;20:256–8.

Dropulic LK, Jones RJ. Polyomavirus BK infection in blood and marrow transplant recipients. Bone Marrow Transplant. 2008;41:11–8.

Duyck J, Vandamme K, Muller P, Teughels W. Overnight storage of removable dentures in alkaline peroxide-based tablets affects biofilm mass and composition. J Dent. 2013;41(12):1281–9.

Elad S, Quinn B, et al. Basic oral care for haematology-oncology patients and hematopoietic stem cell transplantation: A postion paper from the jont task force of

the multinational association of supportive care/international society for oral oncology and the European group for blood and marrow transplantation. Journal of Supportive Care in Cancer. 2015;(1):223–36.

Eilers J, et al. Development, testing, and application of the oral assessment guide. Oncology Nursing Forim. 1988;15(3):352–60.

Eisenberg S. Hepatic sinusoidal obstruction syndrome in patients undergoing hematopoietic stem cell transplant. Oncol Nurs Forum. 2008;3:385–97.

Elad S, Raber-Durlacher J, Brennan MT, et al. Basic oral care for hematology-oncology patients and hematopoietic stem cell transplantation recipients: a position paper from the joint task force of the Multinational Association of Supportive Care in Cancer/International Society of Oral Oncology (MASCC/ISOO) and the European Group for Blood and Marrow Transplantation (EBMT). J Support Care. 2014;(1)223–236.

Elbahlawan L, et al. A critical care and transplantation-based approach to acute respiratory failure after hematopoietic stem cell transplantation in children. Biol Blood Marrow Transplant. 2016;22:617–26.

E-learning package Sepsis and Sepsis Six. http://sonet.nottingham.ac.uk/ Accessed online 11 Sept 2017.

Filicko J, Lazarus HM, Flomenberg N. Mucosal injury in patients undergoing hematopoietic progenitor cell transplantation: new approaches to prophylaxis and treatment. Bone Marrow Transplant. 2003;31:1–10.

Graf L, Stern M. Acute phase after haematopoietic stem cell transplantation - bleeding and thrombotic complications 2012. Hamostaseologie. 2012;32(1):56–62.

Hassan M, Ljungman P. Cytostatika. Stockholm: Liber; 2003.

Ho VT, et al. Blood and marrow transplant clinical trials network toxicity committee consensus summary: thrombotic Microangiopathy after hematopoietic stem cell transplantation. Biol Blood Marrow Transplant. 2005;11:571–5.

Jodele S, et al. A new paradigm: Diagnosis and management of HSCT- associated thrombotic microangiopathy as multi-system endothelial injury. Blood Rev. 2015;29(3):191–204.

Jones RJ, Lee KS, Beschorner WE, Vogel VG, Grochow LB, Braine HG, et al. Venoocclusive disease of the liver following bone marrow transplantation. Transplantation. 1987;44:778–83.

Keating GM. Defibrotide: A review of its use in severe hepatic Veno-occlusive disease following haematopoietic stem cell transplantation. Clin Drug Investig. 2014;34:895–904.

Kee PPL, et al. Diagnostic yield of timing blood culture collection relative to fever. Pediatr Inf Dis J. 2016;35(8):846–50.

Kuten-Shorrer M, Woo S-B, Treister NS. Oral graft-versus-host disease. Dent Clin N Am. 2014;58(2):351–68.

Lalla RV, Bowen J, Barasch A, et al. Evidence-based clinical practice guidelines for the management of Mucositis Secondary to Cancer Therapy (MASCC/ISOO review). Cancer. 2014;120(10)1453–61.

Leung AYH, et al. Polyoma BK virus and haemorrhagic cystitis in haematopoietic stem cell transplantation: a changing paradigm. Bone Marrow Transplant. 2005;36:929–37.

Maiolino A, et al. Engraftment syndrome following autologous hematopoietic stem cell transplantation. Bone Marrow Transplant. 2003;31:393–7.

Majhail NS, et al. Diffuse alveolar Hemorrhage and infection-associated alveolar Hemorrhage following hematopoietic stem cell transplantation: related and high-risk clinical syndromes. Biol Blood Marrow Transplant. 2006;12:1038–46.

McDonald GB, et al. Venoocclusive disease of the liver after bone marrow transplantation: diagnosis, incidence and predisposing factors. Hepatology. 1984;4:116–22.

McDonald GB, et al. Veno-occlusive disease of the liver and multi organ failure after bone marrow transplantation: a cohort study of 355 patients. Ann Intern Med. 1993;118:255–67.

Mesna Summary of Product Characteristics (SPC) [in Swedish]. Accessed online 11 Sep. 2017. https://lakemedelsverket.se/LMF/Lakemedelsinformation/?nplid=19900208000063&type=product.

Mohty M, et al. Sinusoidal obstruction syndrome/veno-occlusive disease: current situation and perspectives—a position statement from the European Society for Blood and Marrow Transplantation (EBMT). Bone Marrow Transplant. 2015;50:781–9. https://doi.org/10.1038/bmt.2015.52. published online 23 March 2015.

Mohty M, et al. Revised diagnosis and severity criteria for sinusoidal obstruction syndrome/veno-occlusive disease in adult patients: a new classification from the European Society for Blood and Marrow Transplantation. BMT. 2016;51:906–12. Published online 2016, May 16.

Nadir Y, Brenner B. Thrombotic complications associated with stem cell transplantation. Blood Rev. 2012;26:183–7.

National Cancer Institute (US). Oral mucositis chemoradiotherapy and hematopoietic stem cell transplantation patients management of mucositis accessed on line 3/04/16. http://www.cancer.gov/cancertopics/pdq/supportivecare/oralcomplications/HealthProfessional/page5#Section_85; 2013.

NCI Dictionary of Cancer Terms. https://www.cancer.gov/publications/dictionaries/cancer-terms?cdrid=695987. Accessed online 11 Sep 2016.

Nesher L, et al. Utility of routine surveillance blood cultures in asymptomatic allogeneic hematopoietic stem cell transplant recipients with indwelling central venous catheters at a comprehensive cancer center. Am J Infect Control. 2014;42:1084–8.

Panoskaltsis-Mortari A, et al. American Thoracic Society Committee on idiopathic pneumonia syndrome. An official American Thoracic Society research statement: noninfectious lung injury after hematopoietic stem cell transplantation: idiopathic pneumonia syndrome. Am J Respir Crit Care Med. 2011;183(9):1262–79.

Park MS. Diffuse alveolar Hemorrhage. Tuberc Respir Dis. 2013;74:151–62.

Peterson DE, Boers-Doets CB, Bensadoun RJ, Herrstedt J, on behalf of the ESMO Guidelines Committee. Management of oral and gastrointestinal mucosal injury: ESMO clinical practice guidelines for diagnosis, treatment, and follow-up. Ann Oncol. 2015;26(Supplement 5):v139–51.

Quinn B, Thompson M, Treleaven J, et al. United Kingdom oral care in cancer guidance: second edition. www.ukomic.co.uk. Accessed 03/09/16; 2015.

Quinn B, Potting C, Stone R, et al. Guidelines for the assessment of oral mucositis in adult chemotherapy, radiotherapy and haematopoietic stem cell transplant patients. Eur J Cancer. 2008;44(1):61–72.

Rabe C, et al. Severe respiratory failure due to diffuse alveolar hemorrhage: clinical characteristics and outcome of intensive care. J Crit Care. 2010;25:230–5.

Richardson PG, et al. Drug safety evaluation of defibrotide. Expert Opin Drug Saf. 2013;12(1):123–36.

Rhodes A, et al. Surviving sepsis campaign: international guidelines for management of sepsis and septic shock: 2016. Intensive Care Med. 2017;43:304–77.

Rosenthal J. Hematopoietic cell transplantation-associated thrombotic microangiopathy: a review of pathophysiology, diagnosis, and treatment. J Blood Med. 2016;(7):181–6.

Rovira M, et al. Chapter 12: Infections after HSCT. In: EBMT-ESH handbook; 2012. p. 196–215.

Royal College of Physicians. National Early Warning Score (NEWS) standardising the assessment of acute-illness severity in the NHS. 2012.

Rubenstein EB, Peterson DE, Schubert M, et al. Clinical practice guidelines for the prevention and treatment of cancer therapy – induced oral and gastrointestinal Mucositis. American Cancer Society. Cancer. 2004;100(Suppl 9):2026–46.

Ruutu T, et al. Diagnostic criteria for hematopoietic stem cell transplant-associated microangiopathy: results of a consensus process by an international working group. Haematologica. 2007;92:95–100.

Sahin U, et al. An overview of hematopoietic stem cell transplantation related thrombotic complications. Crit Rev Oncol Hematol. 2016;107:149–55.

Sambunjak D, Nickerson JW, Poklepovic T, Johnson TM, Imai P, Tugwell P, Worthington HV. Flossing for the management of periodontal diseases and dental caries in adults. Cochrane Database Syst Rev. 2011;(12):CD008829.

Savva-Bordalo J, et al. Clinical effectiveness of hyperbaric oxygen therapy for BK-virus-associated hemorrhagic cystitis after allogeneic bone marrow transplantation. Bone Marrow Transplant. 2012;47(8):1095–8.

Schorr CA, et al. Severe sepsis and septic shock management and performance improvement. Virulence. 2014;5(1):226–35.

Singer M, et al. The third international consensus definitions for sepsis and septic shock (Sepsis-3). JAMA. 2016;315(8):801–10.

Soubani AO, Pandya CM. The spectrum of non-infectious pulmonary complications following hematopoietic stem cell transplantation. Hematol Oncol Stem Cel Ther. 2010;3(3):143–57.

Spitzer TR. Engraftment syndrome following autologous hematopoietic stem cell transplantation. Bone Marrow Transplant. 2001;27:893–8.

Swedish "Pro Sepsis" Programme Group Sepsis. Care Program Severe Sepsis and Septic Shock – Early identification and initial intervention [För Svenska Infektionsläkarföreningen "Pro Sepsis" Programgrupp Sepsis. Vårdprogram svår sepsis och septisk chock – tidig identifiering och initial handläggning. Reviderat oktober 2015] 2015 edition.

Thoele K. Engraftment syndrome in hematopoietic stem cell transplantations. Clin J Oncol Nurs. 2014;18(3):349–54.

Toubert A. Chapter 14. Immune reconstitution after allogeneic HSCT. In: EBMT-ESH handbook on haematopoietic stem cell transplantation; 6th ed. Genova: Forum Service Editore 2012. p. 235–47.

Umbro I, et al. Possible antiviral effect of ciprofloxacin treatment on polyomavirus BK replication and analysis of non-coding control region sequences. Virol J. 2013;10:274.

Veno Occlusive Disease (VOD) Learning Programme. http://www.ebmt.org/Contents/Nursing/Materials/LearningProgrammes/Pages/default.aspx. Accessed online 11 Sept 2017.

Wallhult E, et al. Management of veno-occlusive disease: the multidisciplinary approach to care. Eur J Haematol. 2017;98:322–9.

Watson M, et al. Palliative adult network guidelines. 3rd ed. Tricord, London: West Sussex; 2011.

Yanik GA, et al. Randomized, double-blind placebo-controlled trial of soluble tumor necrosis factor receptor: Enbrel (Etanercept) for the treatment of idiopathic pneumonia syndrome after allogeneic stem cell transplantation: blood and marrow transplant clinical trials network protocol. Biol Blood Marrow Transplant. 2014;20:858–64.

Yeoung-Hau HL, Syed AA. Brain teaser: encephalopathy after stem cell transplantation. Am J Med. 2014;127(4):281–3.

Zhu K-E, et al. Incidence, risks, and outcome of idiopathic pneumonia syndrome early after allogeneic hematopoietic stem cell transplantation. Eur J Haematol. 2008;81:461–6.

Supportive Care

10

S. J. van der Linden, M. E. G. Harinck,
H. T. Speksnijder, Teija Schröder, Ien Schlösser,
Vera Verkerk, Micheala van Bohemen,
A. M. Rusman-Vergunst, J. C. Veldhuijzen,
and W. J. A. Quak

Abstract

Hematopoietic stem cell transplantation (HSCT) care is highly complex. This chapter focuses on the aspects of supportive care required following HSCT.

Assessment tools are key component of nursing practice and are necessary for planning and providing patient-centered care. HSCT care must be planned, implemented, and evaluated and is underpinned by collaboration with the entire multidisciplinary healthcare team.

With supportive care following HSCT, we ultimately aim to improve the quality of life of our patients in the posttransplant period.

Supportive care extends beyond symptom management and includes social, psychological, and spiritual care. The needs of the patient are multifactorial and can be complex, considering multiple issues at the e time and involving multiple disciplines.

S. J. van der Linden (✉) • M. E. G. Harinck
I. Schlösser • V. Verkerk • M. van Bohemen
A. M. Rusman-Vergunst • J. C. Veldhuijzen • W. J. A. Quak
Erasmus MC, Rotterdam, The Netherlands
e-mail: s.vanderlinden@erasmusmc.nl;
W.quak@erasmusmc.nl

H. T. Speksnijder, MSc, RN
Hogeschool, Utrecht, The Netherlands

T. Schröder, MA, RN
Helsinki University Hospital for Children
and Adolescents, Helsinki, Finland

© EBMT and the Author(s) 2018
M. Kenyon, A. Babic (eds.), *The European Blood and Marrow Transplantation Textbook for Nurses*,
https://doi.org/10.1007/978-3-319-50026-3_10

Throughout supportive nursing care, our clinical competence is critical and is complemented by experience, knowledge, and awareness.

Keywords

Supportive care • Assessment • Early warning scores • Oral care • Nutrition
Allied health professionals • Transfusion • Physiotherapy • Spiritual care
Complementary therapies • Music • Touch • Massage • Pediatric

10.1 Nursing Assessment

Highly complex nursing care is essential for the disease- and treatment-related health problems of patients with hematological diagnoses (Kluin-Nelemans and Tanasale-Huisman 2013). The diagnoses within hematology are diverse but generally associated with a specific set of symptoms. Hematological diseases can be broadly divided into malignant and nonmalignant hematological diseases. The underlying hematological disease and cumulative effects of previous therapy can influence the degree and range of side effects and symptoms experienced following HSCT conditioning therapy. These effects can manifest as physical complaints such as fatigue, fever, infection, and bleeding and can result in complex illness necessitating specialist care and treatment. Psychological concerns are common and can frequently manifest as low-level anxiety and depression and less often as features of significant trauma. As a key element of the multidisciplinary team, nurses are ideally placed to identify and assess symptoms due to illness or treatment at an early stage. HSCT nurses have extensive knowledge that contributes to treatment optimization. Assessment is undertaken frequently to reflect the dynamic nature and rapidly changing clinical picture and will take into account the patient's vital signs, blood results, and symptoms as well as knowledge of their baseline physical function. By taking the medical and social history of the patient into consideration, we can increase our awareness of the potential care problems that may arise. The understanding and assimilation of information derived from these sources in conjunction with standardized assessment tools and instruments enable measurable and objective care delivery.

10.2 Pain Assessment

In certain hematological diseases such as lymphoma or multiple myeloma, patients experience pain as a result of the compression of the lymph nodes or bone destruction. In some cases, patients are reluctant to report symptoms of pain to their attending physicians in case this is interpreted as a poor treatment response. It is imperative to consider both verbal and nonverbal signs and symptoms of pain to complete a comprehensive assessment.

The bedside nurse is well placed to assess their patient and explain the importance of adequate pain management using pharmacological and supportive measures. Improving the patient's comfort will enable them to better tolerate treatment and improve their experience.

In the HSCT setting, pain is most commonly experienced as a result of mucositis, but patients will also report other pain such as bone pain associated with GCSF, abdominal pain due to diarrhea, or general discomfort with fluid accumulation.

Not all reported pain symptoms or discomfort is treated in the same way. By explaining to our patients the possible cause of the pain and the treatment for it, we can also help to manage their expectations of the analgesia and other supportive interventions. We should inform our patients of the common side effects of analgesia like drowsiness and constipation and ways of reducing these effects.

When assessing pain, a standardized tool should be applied to ensure consistency across patients and between assessments. A comprehensive evaluation of the pain, location, characteristics, onset, duration, frequency, severity of pain, and exacerbating and relieving factors should be included. This assessment should be supported by the patient's nonverbal reactions such as facial expression, pallor, tempo of speech, body position, etc. as well as their vital signs.

According to Kluin-Nelemans and Tanasale-Huisman (2013), a nurse can give the patient information and tips and tricks in the field of pain relief to the patient:

- Check to what extent the pain is present on performing her/his daily routine (getting up, going to the shower, or getting dressed). The use of a pain scale can give insight to the extent of pain the patient endures. Ask the patient how she/he scores the pain from 0 (no pain) to 10 (maximum pain). If analgesia is administered, you can monitor the effect by reassessing the pain score.
- Consideration of pretreatment with analgesia before starting the daily routine may permit the patient to move independently or with more comfort.
- Nonsteroidal anti-inflammatory drugs (NSAIDs) *should not* be prescribed for the HSCT patient. These can cause diminished function of the thrombocytes and kidney damage and complicate the monitoring of infections.

- If the patient is immobile for long periods, pain can increase. The nurse should assess pressure area risk and consider offering a pressure area mattress and/or gel cushion to increase comfort and reduce pressure area deterioration.
- In addition to pharmaceutical pain relief, complementary care can also be offered to reduce pain: heat-cold packs, relaxation by music therapy, distraction, or gentle massages (if possible with low thrombocytes).

10.3 The Role of Early Warning Scores

Adult

Observing vital signs is a crucial task in the care of the HSCT patient. The patient's condition can change dramatically in a short period of time due to treatment and illness. Various measuring instruments allow us to monitor vital functions. The modified early warning score (MEWS) shows when values of vital functions deviate and indicates when intervention is required.

The MEWS (Subbe et al. 2001) scores various items (Table 10.1):

- Heart rate
- Blood pressure (systole)
- Breath rate
- Temperature
- Awareness (AVPU score)

Table 10.1 Modified early warning score

Score	3	2	1	0	1	2	3
Systolic blood pressure (mmHg)	<70	71–80	81–100	101–199		≥200	
Heart rate (bpm)		<40	41–50	51–100	101–110	111–129	≥130
Respiratory rate (bpm)		<9		9–14	15–20	21–29	≥30
Temperature (°C)		<35		35–38.4		≥38.5	
AVPU score				Alert	Reacting to voice	Reacting to pain	Unresponsive

Subbe (2001)

In addition, decreased urine production, SaO2 < 90% with adequate O2 therapy, and the nurse's awareness or "gut feeling" give increased value to existing scores (Ludikhuizen et al. 2012). If the score is moderately elevated, it is advisable to monitor the vitals more often and to inform the attending physician. When the score increases, continuous monitoring is necessary, and evaluation from an emergency intervention team or a medical emergency team should be requested. These teams are available in most HSCT centers and usually consist of a doctor and an intensive care unit (ICU) nurse/emergency nurse.

HSCT and Intensive Care The outcomes of HSCT patients have been greatly improved over recent decades due to new therapies and improvements in supportive care. An ICU admission is sometimes necessary to treat life-threatening situations that can arise following HSCT.

Reasons for admission might include:

- Respiratory failure secondary to infection
- Sepsis requiring intensive support
- Multi-organ failure
- Renal dysfunction
- Complications such as graft-versus-host disease after allogeneic stem cell transplant

Treatment in the ICU consists of:

- Mechanical ventilation
- Support of vital functions
- Treatment of sepsis/septic shock
- Continuation of chemotherapy

Over the past 20 years, the survival of the hematology patient on the ICU has been greatly improved, with reductions in mortality by 40–60% (Netters et al. 2010; Ven van der et al. 2009). When a hematological patient is admitted to ICU early in their course, the chance of survival is greater (Peigne et al. 2009). Early admission reduces further organ dysfunction and increases the probability of reversing existing organ failure by delivering timely and appropriate organ support. The modified early warning score (MEWS) may contribute to this early recognition and prompt referral to ICU.

When the patient is well enough to return to the HSCT unit, fear of relocation may occur. This can happen because the continuous monitoring of vital functions ceases and the ward environment is very different from that of the intensive care. The patient may experience stress and anxiety and should be prepared at ICU for the transfer to the HSCT unit taking into account the psychological effect of relocation to both patient and family (Coyle 2001).

Pediatric

As noted by Agulnik et al. 2016, hospitalized oncology and HSCT patients are a high-risk population with frequent clinical decline requiring unplanned PICU transfer and high mortality rates. Complications developed by these patients, such as sepsis and respiratory failure, are known to have better outcomes with earlier identification and management.

It is important to know the normal vital signs in children in different ages. That is the basis which helps to recognize the early warning signs in children. The use of the pediatric early warning system (PEWS) scores in clinical practice is a new concept (Murray et al. 2015). In reference to Agulnik et al. (2016), PEWS has been implemented in many pediatric institutions. Their study demonstrates that the PEWS tool is valid in identifying pediatric oncology and HSCT patients requiring unplanned PICU transfer.

The use of PEWS scores as an assessment tool has the potential to quantify the severity of illness in children. It is hoped that this results in facilitating early identification of patients at risk for clinical deterioration and prompt intervention to avoid the need to transfer to a higher level of care (Murray et al. 2015).

10.4 Nutritional Assessment

The malnutrition universal screening tool (MUST) is a validated screening tool for recognition and treatment of malnutrition. The MUST form must be filled in accurately upon admission, asking for length/height, weight, and weight loss and whether the patient has no food intake for several days.

The HSCT patient often has a reduced dietary intake during and following conditioning therapy, but this is often not considered at the time of admission.

Sometimes weight loss is difficult to assess due to fluid gain. It is not possible using conventional methods to determine what proportion of muscle or fat components account for the weight loss.

The measuring instruments deployed to obtain information about muscle function and muscle mass are the hand clamp and the bioelectrical impedance analysis (BIA).

The hand clamping force gauge (see Fig. 10.1) can be used to measure the maximum crushing force. The maximal squeezing force of the hand gives a good estimate of the peripheral muscle function and is related to the total amount of muscle mass in the body. Hand force depends on age and gender. It can also be influenced by other factors, such as disease. By obtaining dif-

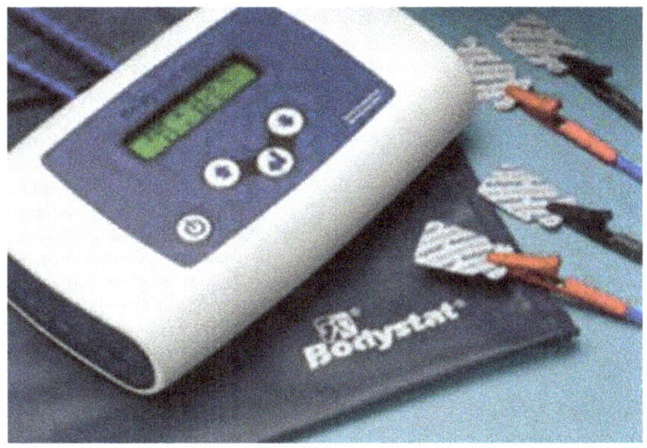

Fig. 10.2 Bioelectrical impedance analysis (BIA) (Photo credit https://www.habdirect.co.uk/bodystat)

ferent hand tightness measurements during the course of treatment, it can be determined whether the patient's muscle function increases or decreases.

A bioelectrical impedance analysis (BIA) (see Figs. 10.2 and 10.3) is a tool measuring the resistance that the body provides for an alternating current of 50 kHz. The fat-free mass is calculated using a formula incorporating the resistance, length, weight, gender, and age. With this measurement we can assess whether a patient with weight loss has lost muscle mass and/or fat mass. Determining the fat-free mass with the BIA is not reliable if there is an abnormal hydration status.

10.5 The Role of Allied Health Professionals

In the care of the HSCT patient, collaboration between different supporting disciplines is of great importance. Not only is medical and nursing care essential, but body, mind, and psychosocial care is necessary to facilitate the patient's recovery. Allied healthcare professionals (AHP) are essential members of the multidisciplinary team (MDT) and include:

- *Dietician*
- *Physiotherapist*
- *Occupational therapist*

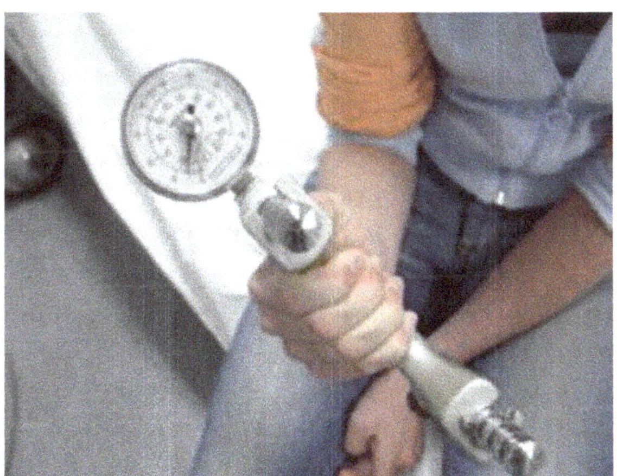

Fig. 10.1 Hand dynamometer (Photo credits www.nutritionalassessment.azm.nl)

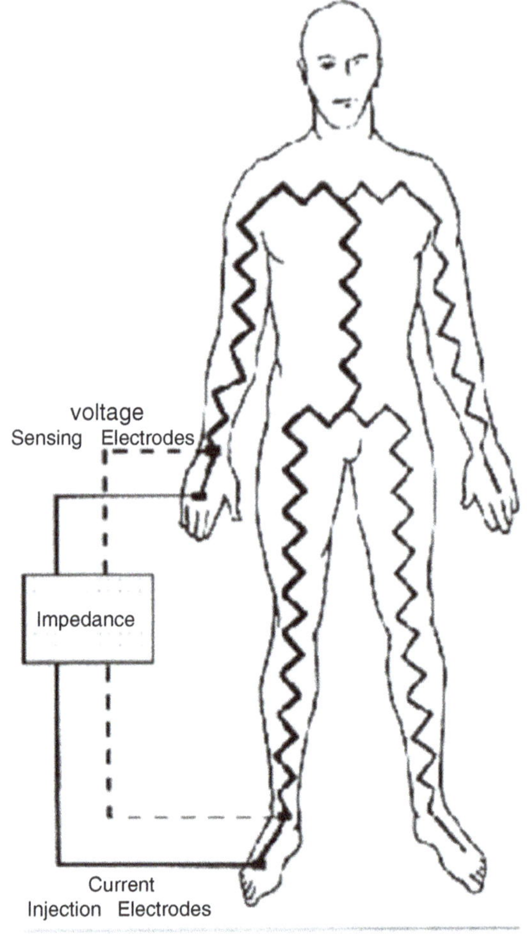

Fig. 10.3 BIA resistance (Photo credit http://www.nutritionalassessment.azm.nl/algoritme+na/onderzoek/lichaamssamenstelling/bia.htm)

- *Wound or tissue viability nurse*
- *Pain nurse* or specialist
- *Spiritual worker*
- *Social worker*
- *Counselor/psychologist*
- *Consultative psychiatric nurse (CPN)*
- *Psychiatrist*

10.6 Principles of Nutritional Support

Patients undergoing HSCT experience intensive treatment with chemotherapy, sometimes in combination with total body irradiation (TBI).

10.6.1 Through the Treatment with Intensive Chemotherapy, There May Be the Following Nutritional Problems

10.6.1.1 Reduced Resistance to Infection

Following intensive chemotherapy, the patient has reduced tolerance due to neutropenia and/or increased intestinal permeability. In neutropenia, the number of white blood cells decreases significantly, resulting in the so-called aplasia with an increased risk of infection. The patient is neutropenic if the neutrophil granulocytes (subdivision of the leukocytes) are less than 0.5×10^9/l. An increased permeability of the intestinal wall is caused by intensive chemotherapy damaging the gastrointestinal mucosa. As a result, pathogenic bacteria (bodily bacteria or bacteria from the diet) can enter the bloodstream (sepsis or blood poisoning). The patient has an increased risk of infection due to the reduced resistance. If the patient is expected to be neutropenic for longer than 7–10 days after chemotherapy, antimicrobial prophylaxis may be given because of the high risk of infection. In some centers, the patient may commence this prophylaxis (selective intestinal contamination, SDD) at the time of conditioning therapy. These specific antibiotics select out the patient's own aerobic, potentially pathogenic intestinal flora and remove them.

To prevent food-mediated infections, the Hygiene Nutrition Directive or "neutropenic diet" or "clean diet" guidelines are implemented. This directive is usually followed from the start of conditioning therapy until discontinuation of the SDD or neutrophil recovery. The National Consultation Dietitian Hematology and Stem Cell Transplantation in the Netherlands has written the Hygiene Nutrition Directive, which is the basis for all hospitals in the Netherlands. There are small differences between several hospitals.

10.6.1.2 Food Aversion, Taste and Smell Changes, and Bad Taste in the Mouth

Intensive chemotherapy, as well as other medications such as antibiotics and antifungal agents, adversely affects the senses of taste and smell.

The influence of the disease itself can also affect taste, and taste may be reduced and/or there may be increased sensitivity to all flavors and smells. Aversions to specific foods, enhanced flavor or taste sensation, or a bad taste (metal, cardboard, or sand flavor) are frequently reported. Sometimes, the taste perception does not match the taste memory. Patients may also be more sensitive to odors and can find that many foods or products like perfume or cleaning agents smell unpleasant.

10.6.1.3 Nausea and Vomiting

Cytotoxic treatment is often associated with complaints of nausea and vomiting. Highly emetogenic cytotoxic agents used in HSCT regimes include carmustine and cyclophosphamide; moderately emetogenic are busulfan (iv Busilvex), cytarabine, and (high-dose) melphalan. Nausea and vomiting can occur independently. Medication to reduce nausea and vomiting (antiemetics) and hydration infusions are given and often adjusted. Nausea and vomiting after chemotherapy can occur acutely (4–24 h) and is often severe. The symptoms may also occur later (2 or several days to sometimes a few weeks after the chemotherapy). There is usually no association between vomiting and the type of diet used. As the patient undergoes multiple chemotherapy cycles, anticipatory vomiting may occur. In this case, vomiting occurs prior to the treatment in response to previous chemotherapies and is triggered by memory, experience, smell, taste, and sometimes visual cues.

10.6.1.4 Reduced Appetite and Early Satiety (Full Feeling)

Intensive chemotherapy, as well as other medications, infections, and fever, can cause a reduced appetite and feeling of early satiety or fullness. As a result, a reduced dietary intake may occur, which may adversely affect the nutritional state.

10.6.1.5 Mucositis (See Oral Complications Section for Further Information)

Mucositis (oral and gastrointestinal) frequently occurs after conditioning therapy. The grade depends on the type of chemotherapy. Chemotherapies that are associated with mucosi-

tis are busulfan, etoposide, melphalan, and methotrexate. Mucositis can occur in the mouth and throat (orally) and in the rest of the gastrointestinal tract (gastrointestinal).

Oral mucositis can vary widely from sensitive gums (mucositis grade 1), the patient is often able to eat everything, until blisters and ulcerations in the mouth, and then the patient has even difficulty drinking sips of water (mucositis grade 4, according to the WHO scale). Good oral hygiene is very important to limit complications associated with oral mucositis. Mucositis usually occurs 4–10 days after the conditioning and lasts about 2–3 weeks. As soon as the leukocytes start to rise to normal values, the mucositis heals rapidly.

In severe mucositis, oral nutritional intake is usually inadequate, and the patient is recommended for nutritional intervention. Gastric feeding with a tube through the nose (tube feeding) is preferred over parenteral nutrition, because it is physiologically more natural and reduces the risk for intestinal atrophy. The main contraindication of tube feeding is the risk of bleeding due to ulcerations in the gastrointestinal tract.

Insertion of a nasogastric feeding tube is safe when there is mucositis grade 1 or 2 and if there are sufficient platelets (at least 40×10^9/l). Otherwise the patient first needs platelet transfusion for placement of the tube. When the severity of the mucositis is too great to introduce a tube, parenteral nutrition is the remaining option.

Diarrhea, due to gastrointestinal mucositis, is a common complaint following conditioning therapy. It is important to pay attention to dietary fiber, electrolytes, and hydration. Patients with severe watery diarrhea have reduced nutritional absorption through the gut, and parenteral nutrition may be indicated.

When the patient is discharged from the hospital after HSCT, dietary intake is often still not optimal and particularly after allogeneic myeloablative conditioned (MAC) stem cell transplantation. The patient often reports a dry mouth, nausea, vomiting, and early satiety. These patients often need nutritional monitoring and support for some time in the outpatient setting. Additionally, these patients often have increased energy demands due to the treatment, and further interventions may need to be considered such as tube feeding at home to limit further weight loss and restore nutrition.

In general, following autologous HSCT there are less complications and infection-related problems. However, following allogeneic HSCT it takes several months for the immune system to being to recover, and these patients are susceptible to infections for quite some time. In addition, the immune system is suppressed with medication to prevent graft rejection and to prevent or treat GvHD.

10.7 Transfusion

Introduction

Blood transfusion is an essential element of supportive care for many hematological disorders, and HSCT recipients will almost always require transfusion support during aplasia. Importantly, HSCT recipients will usually require product irradiation to prevent transfusion-associated GvHD (tGvHD). This section covers general information on blood transfusion. Please refer to your local and national transfusion directive or policy for further details.

Blood Products and Indication

Different types of blood products can be transfused: erythrocyte concentrate, platelet concentrate, and plasma. The most commonly used blood product is erythrocyte concentrate (Sanquin 2016). Erythrocyte concentrate is administered in severe anemia, where insufficient hemoglobin reduces oxygen transport capacity. There may be acute anemia, for example, due to bleeding, or chronic anemia, for example, due to a chronic disease.

Platelet concentrate is administered to correct thrombocytopenia to prevent or treat bleeding. The indication for administration of prophylactic platelets depends on the patient's condition and whether the patient requires a higher circulating platelet count to treat, limit, or prevent bleeding.

Plasma is administered to help correct coagulation factors. The indication for plasma transfusion is usually based on PT/APTT and fibrinogen content in the blood.

In summary, the indication for transfusion is based on the clinical situation of the patient and laboratory diagnostics.

Blood Groups and Pre-transfusion Investigations

In order to select the correct blood product for a patient, the determination of the ABO and Rhesus blood group is necessary. For transfusion of platelet concentrates and plasma, this is sufficient. In addition to the ABO and Rhesus blood group systems, there are many more systems such as *Duffy, Kidd,* and *MNS*. For the administration of erythrocytes, it is important to screen the patient prior to every transfusion for irregular antibodies in addition to the ABO and Rhesus blood groups. These antibodies are usually not naturally present in the blood but can be acquired at each pregnancy and may increase with chronic transfusion need. Depending on the number and type of antibody, it may be difficult to find the appropriate erythrocyte concentrate. Following allogeneic stem cell or cord blood transplantation, the stem cell donor blood group(s) as well as recipient blood group should also be taken into account. For example, in case of double cord blood transplantation, up to three different AB0 blood groups may need to be taken into account. In case of emergency and if there is no time for determining a blood group, erythrocytes with blood group "O negative" must be administered. Blood group O negative is the universal donor for erythrocytes.

Platelet antibodies such as the HLA (human leukocyte antigen) antibodies may also need to be considered. These antibodies may develop after prior transfusions and/or pregnancy. Sometimes HLA antibodies result in no or low increment after platelet transfusion. For these patients, platelet donors are selected as the best possible match with the patient at HLA level. This is an intensive process, and sometimes only a very small number of platelet donors are identified for a particular patient. In these cases, it may

Table 10.3 Symptoms that may indicate possible transfusion reaction

Mild	Moderate	Serious
Temperature rise >1 or <2 °C	Moderate clinical decline during transfusion	Severe clinical impairment during transfusion
Urticaria	Cold shivering	Dyspnea
Itch	Temperature rise >2 °C	Respiratory insufficiency
Exanthem/erythema		Hypotension/shock
		Low back pain

Vademecum (2017)

take longer than usual to obtain platelets for the patient, and in an emergency, "random donor" platelets may be prescribed until the matched platelets become available. For plasma transfusion, only the ABO blood group is important. Note: Blood group AB is the universal donor. In plasma, the Rhesus blood group does not need to be considered since the Rhesus blood group is on the membrane of the erythrocyte.

It is known that some drugs can interfere with the accuracy of pre-transfusion investigations in the laboratory. An example of this is daratumumab (monoclonal Ab anti-CD38). It is therefore important, upon request of serological testing, to provide the laboratory with all relevant medical information and transfusion history, including transplantation, pregnancy, previous serious transfusion reactions, and the use of relevant medication such as fludarabine (purine analog).

Processed Blood Products

Sometimes blood products need to be processed. In addition, erythrocytes and platelet concentrates need to be irradiated and may be washed in some cases. Erythrocytes and platelets are washed in the case of previous severe anaphylactic transfusion reaction or in a patient with IgA deficiency. When washing blood products, the plasma proteins are removed as far as possible. In plasma this operation is not possible. Erythrocytes and platelets are irradiated to damage the T cells in the blood product, preventing these T cells from causing transfusion-associated graft-versus-host disease in patients with risk factors such as HSCT, anti-thymocyte globulin (ATG), alemtuzumab and fludarabine use, and Hodgkin's lymphoma. Only thrombocyte and erythrocyte blood products can be irradiated.

Transfusion Reactions

Although today's blood products are very safe, a patient sometimes experiences side effects from transfusion. The table below (Table 10.3) shows the symptoms of a possible transfusion reaction that may occur during and up to several hours after transfusion.

Acute transfusion reactions may be caused by administration of an incorrect blood product, volume overload, or bacterial or viral contamination of the transfused product. In addition, there may be an unexpected reaction from the patient. If transfusion symptoms are observed during a transfusion reaction, the transfusion should be discontinued immediately and the doctor should be alerted. Always leave intravenous access in situ and then follow the instructions of the physician. It is very important to inform the blood transfusion laboratory about the possible transfusion reaction so that the cause can be investigated. This may prevent a transfusion reaction at a subsequent transfusion.

In addition to acute reactions, blood transfusions can create long-term effects. For example, if a patient gets a lot of erythrocyte concentrates over a longer period of time, developing iron overload can lead to increased iron stores in organs such as the heart, liver, and kidneys causing severe damage. This process occurs because erythrocyte concentrate contains iron, and the body does not have a system to break this excess iron down and remove it. However, this can be treated by monthly venesection when the blood counts have normalized after HSCT and if the hemoglobin is not sufficient, by medication such as Exjade or Desferral.

Hemovigilance

Hemovigilance is the systematic monitoring of side effects and adverse incidents throughout the donor to patient transfusion chain, as well as anything that contributes to safer and more effective use of blood products. In this context, hospitals report transfusion reactions and incidents to their National Hemovigilance Organization. Annually, serious transfusion actions are reported to the EU by the National Hemovigilance Organization.

Conclusion

For a safe blood transfusion, it is important that the correct indication is stated. The laboratory must have all relevant medical information to select the correct blood product. The nurse must verify:

1. The transfusion prescription
2. The identification of blood product
3. The patient and must always be performed by two nurses

In addition, the patient must be observed closely during transfusion and the doctor notified immediately of symptoms of possible transfusion reaction. The blood is an organ, and blood transfusion is an organ transplant which requires maximum care.

10.8 Physiotherapy and Exercise

Over the last years, several clinical trials have contributed to the growing body of evidence showing the beneficial effects of exercise in cancer patients and also in the field of HSCT. Exercise interventions at different time points during and after HSCT can improve physical performance, quality of life, symptom control, and fatigue. However, it is still not possible to give a clear advice regarding the best type, intensity, start, and duration of an exercise program (Steinberg et al. 2015; Wiskemann et al. 2015; Wiskemann

and Huber 2008; Cramp and Byron-Daniel 2012; Knols et al. 2005; Spence et al. 2010; Speck et al. 2010).

In the time period before and after the HSCT, a specialized oncology physical therapist can be useful to advise, coach, and support exercise (under supervision). By remaining mobile, complications can be prevented and the effects of the treatment can be optimized. Depending on the phase in which the patient is, the physical therapist will set goals (by using the "shared decision model" with the patients). The goal can be to stay at the same level during the treatment or improve condition before, during, or after treatment.

Due to the long hospitalization in isolation and the side effects from treatment, exercise can be a challenge. Most patients are not permitted to leave their room, so providing apparatus such as light weights, exercise bands, or static bikes can be helpful. The patient's condition changes day to day, so the physical therapist will need to adjust the expectations to ensure they remain realistic. It is important not to force exercise to maintain safety and prevent strain or injury.

10.9 Psychological/Spiritual Care

Introduction

Psychosocial issues can lead to such a loss of energy that patients become dependent on their partner or caregivers. This is further compounded by fatigue. In addition, physical symptoms such as pain can enhance the sense of dependence. Reduced appetite, insomnia, and side effects of medication can cause depressive feelings, while anxiety and fear can contribute to restlessness, forgetfulness, nausea, and tension. It is important to regularly evaluate these patient's care needs and any additional care or aftercare requirements.

- Patients often experience fear and powerlessness feeling a loss of control over the disease and its consequences. It is important to explain factual information about the diagnosis and treatment procedures, possible side effects, and practical guidance to improve understanding.

- Patients often experience the stages of mourning (denial, anger, negotiation, and acceptance) and react in their own way to their diagnosis. They may also experience these emotions during their transplant. Anxiety, sadness, powerlessness, and/or a disturbed body image can cause dysfunction, and it is essential to support the patient to reduce fear and/or discuss their feelings. Enabling a social network around the patient will provide a vital source of support both during and after hospitalization. Prompt referral to a psychologist or possibly a consultative psychiatric nurse (CPN) or a psychiatrist may be necessary for those patients with a history of psychological issues, in those who appear unable to cope emotionally, or where there are any concerns for psychological well-being.
- Patients with younger children or grandchildren are advised to discuss their diagnosis and treatment with them. There are different information materials aimed at children of different ages.
- Within the family unit, there may be a change in the role of the patient or family members. Offering a social worker can be helpful in finding support to manage these changes.
- Through diagnosis and treatment, patients can develop low self-esteem. The treatment may affect their physical appearance in a way that makes them feel uncomfortable. Tips on personal care should be discussed. There are several organizations that can assist in counseling. Advise the patient and provide them with resources and signposting where possible.
- Finding a trusted person or talking with other patients can help the HSCT patient in discussing her/his feelings or fears. Patients should be directed to relevant patient associations prior to commencing HSCT treatment.

Basic Information of Psychological Care for the HSCT Recipient

Beside the physical impact of the HSCT treatment, there is great impact on the whole psychosocial well-being of the patient (and their relatives). Physical problems continuously interact with the psychological state. The enduring nature of many physical problems demands a huge amount of resilience. This section describes the emotional impact of HSCT therapy and the importance of integrated care, with a focus on the role of the psychologist or consultative psychiatric nurse (CPN) and on the role of the bedside HSCT nurse.

Emotional problems such as depression and fear of relapse may occur and impact adversely on the patients' quality of life (QOL) (Syrjala et al. 2012). Emotional concerns are frequently referred to as psychological distress, which has been defined in Distress Management Version I (Practice Guideline Oncology of National Comprehensive Cancer Network (NCCN) 2002) as "a multi-determined unpleasant emotional experience of a psychological (cognitive, behavioral, emotional), social, and/or spiritual nature that may interfere with the ability to cope effectively with cancer, its physical symptoms, and its treatment."

"Distress extends along a continuum, ranging from common feelings of vulnerability, sadness, and fears to problems that may become disabling such as depression, anxiety, panic, social isolation, and spiritual crisis" (NCCN 2002).

This description gives sufficient reason to organize an interdisciplinary team of caregivers around this special patient group. "Meeting the needs of a patient requires the multiple competences that many caregivers from different professions will have to share in order to offer the best quality of comfort and care. It is a common practice in which each team member will inculcate his own competencies. This is the essence of interdisciplinary" (Porchet 2006). Braamse, psychologist at Vrije Universiteit, Amsterdam (VUmc), wrote her doctoral thesis about psychological aspects of HSCT in patients with hematological malignancies (2015). Hematological malignancies as well as treatment procedures are associated with impairment in patients' QOL. According to the World Health Organization (WHO), QOL reflects a subjective concept, defined as an "individual's perception of their position in life in the context of the culture and value systems in which they live and in relation to their goals, expectations, standards and concerns" (WHO 2017). Impairments are caused by the original disease, prior treatment, and intensive conditioning therapy. Certain subgroups of patients have more difficulties adjusting to their disease and treatment and consequently experience a more impaired health-related QOL post-transplant compared with other patient subgroups. Suffering from (chronic) GvHD leads to problems with overall QOL and physical well-being. Braamse (2015): "Other subgroups that are at risk for worse psychological and social functioning are female patients, patients receiving low social support and patients experiencing pre-transplant psychological distress." This is consistent with other research (Hill et al. 2011; Nordin et al. 2001) on psychological and social functioning in cancer patients. Receiving low social support had been shown to increase the risk of depression and anxiety. Braamse (2015) indicates that most HSCT patients were not in need of active interventions to improve psychological distress: most patients chose watchful waiting instead of a special online intervention program or additional psychological care. Braamse (2015) concluded that a discrepancy appears to exist between symptoms patients report in the year after transplantation and their need for additional care: it seems that a substantial number of patients who report emotional problems after auto-SCT do not engage in help-seeking behavior." This highlights the great resilience of patients going through all different aspects related to undergoing a HSCT and their strength to cope with it without additional professional help.

Role of the Consultative Psychiatric Nurse for the HSCT Patient A consultative psychiatric nurse (CPN) visits the HSCT patients in the outpatient clinic, during the "waiting zone" before admission. The patients are screened by protocol which asks them to share their experiences about:

- Hearing the diagnosis
- Treatment
- Impact on different aspects of life

- Physical condition
- Sleeping pattern
- Influence on relationships and work
- Communication with caregivers

The CPN gives psychoeducation on various topics, for example, coping, loss of control, and loss of social roles. The screening includes some questions which indicate if there is a risk of psychiatric decompensation or other increasing problems. The CPN discusses the assessment outcome and possible needs with the patient as well as helpful resources. Extra support by the allied health professionals or other disciplines may also be suggested.

When there is preexistent psychopathology, a special care plan will be described in collaboration with the physician, the psychiatrist, and nurses from the ward. The CPN writes the conclusions and advice in the patient record.

During the hospitalization of these patients, the CPN visits them for a brief consultation and observes how the patient is coping. This is an informal way of counseling. CPNs take part of the weekly interdisciplinary meeting to discuss the complex cases with the nurses and other disciplines. The main goal of the meeting is to give practical advice about the communication and structuring the daily nursing care. The meeting also functions as a mechanism for supporting each other in our work with this patient group, which has great impact on all caregivers.

The experience of the CPN is that many HSCT patients after hearing the news about their diagnosis have a "rollercoaster experience." At this point, there is often less time to think about the impact of therapy options due to the pressure to commence therapy. In the weeks between chemotherapy with its (side) effects and waiting for HSCT, patients often begin to consider their dilemma and contemplate their situation. Meanwhile, their physical condition is improving, and they are afraid of losing this as they begin their HSCT journey. Most patients share their experience (while they visit the CPN in the out-clinic setting) about the two emotional pathways: realizing that it is a possibility that they can die and trying to stay strong and positive toward the treatment. They lose their innocence toward staying in isolation and dealing with lots of physical problems. Last but not least, they struggle with their social role and how to manage the loss of or changes to it.

Patients report many examples of when they felt understood by their doctors and nurses. But many patients also report experience of misunderstandings and difficult and complicated communication with caregivers.

Deweirdt and Vincke (2008) stated how patients report the importance of a family member being allowed to stay for rooming-in while the patient was anxious. For the patient it is important that their caregivers provide basic, personal attention, inserting in their experience, their concerns, and their irritations.

The phase of recovery varies between patients. Some of them have the feeling of being elderly or aged. Others use their first energy to spend time at work or with friends, which can affect home relationships and partner interaction.

HSCT patients are frequently readmitted because of infections, GvHD, or other complications. After a long stay in the hospital, each new readmission can add an enormous psychological burden. It is understandable that patients sometimes lose courage. In some cases, patients speak about their boundaries being further threatened by the treatment. They find it difficult to discuss because the doctor did so much good work and can mean that they don't want to refuse further treatment. It can be the role of the CPN to help patients communicate their wishes.

The Collaboration Between a CPN and Hematology Nurses on the HSCT Wards

Case Examples for This Population

Case One

Patient A, male, 21 years old, non-Hodgkin lymphoma (NHL).

Relapsed NHL (initially diagnosed aged 16). He is a student and living independent near the campus. He has a steady relationship for a year, but because of his treatment and functional decline, he has moved back home to live with his mother. His parents are divorced and don't communicate well. He enjoys online gaming until late at night and subsequently wakes up late in the morning.

During his hospitalization he had some difficulty with the ward routine such as waking up early in the morning and was unfriendly toward the nurses. His mother was very concerned, so she stopped working. She visited her son daily and remained by his bedside for the entire visit even when his girlfriend arrives.

He had fever for several days and mucositis requiring opioid administration, and he experienced nightmares due to analgesia. His thoughts and reactions were slower and at night, he became more anxious. He couldn't eat normally.

In this case the CPN can help the nurses with coordinating the communication and the daily routine and to observe for the signs of confusion or hallucinations that might occur despite his young age.

Case Two

Women B, 44 years old, acute myeloid leukemia (AML).

She has a known bipolar personality diagnosis for which she is prescribed lithium. Lithium has a specific therapeutic range and must be closely monitored through lithium blood levels. Nurses on general wards are often uncertain about the care of patients with a psychiatric diagnosis and about their own (communication) tools and skills. It is understandable that they are unsure about their observations because behavior change can occur as a result of the HSCT and existing psychopathology. The patient and the CPN can work together to process this and support the ward team in the care of these patients.

In these cases the patterns of reaction on the changed psychosocial situations are very understandable. Patients are not doing things wrong, but sometimes their reactions or behavior may not have a positive effect on recovery. For each case it is important that the HSCT nurses use their own observations to contribute to patient care.

In the nursing practice, it can be helpful to consider the following:

- Does the patient really understand the need to strictly follow a set medication regime after SCT?
- How is the hygiene at home in relation of infection risk?

- In normal life enjoying food impacts on quality of life. How can the nurse help their patient with the difficulties they experience around food?
- Diarrhea caused by GvHD has various effects on the psychological well-being of the patient. How can you help to support?
- The pattern of activities changes significantly in comparison with normal life, and the hospital room and environment can inhibit mobility.
- The sleep pattern and routine are disrupted because of intravenous therapies which can stimulate the need of going to the toilet. Other contributing factors are worrying about the diagnoses and social impact in their lives.
- Some patients do not understand their treatment regimen, either due to preexistent loss of cognitive functioning, dementia, low IQ, or the sheer complex nature of their therapy. This can cause increased anxiety and loss of control.
- Self-image is often a concern: roles and relationships change rapidly, and often there are feelings of being "on hold," at the sideline.
- How do we facilitate intimacy and address sexual functioning concerns?

Nurses understand that body and mind continually interact, and they need to develop skills to structure and interpret their observations. They should discuss this in multidisciplinary meetings and consider appropriate interventions. Nurses need to be taught how to use evidence-based tools that assess and address this aspect of care.

The patient is the best source of information about the impact of their concerns, coping in normal healthy life and what might help them at that moment. To promote self-management and shared decision-making, it is necessary that nurses are aware of the diverse resources and how to use them in their own work setting. Even when there are many professionals involved in a patient's care, it does not necessarily follow that they will work in a multidisciplinary manner. Interdisciplinary working is time demanding: time for meetings, dialogue, and questioning teamwork (Porchet 2006).

Coolbrandt (2005) wrote a thesis about keeping and losing courage, a qualitative research in HSCT patients at Gent University Hospital.

Coolbrandt (2005) noticed the active role of the nurses in the recovery story of HSCT patients. Like their medical counterparts, nurses contribute to the positive story and support patients in their therapy. Nurses protect the positive story by advising what the patient might expect. When things are going badly, they intervene by explaining the situation. Sometimes, it is appropriate to normalize a situation and the patients feel less panic. Nurses give positive feedback; patients told that it helped them when the nurses are optimistic. Nurses give comfort when they reassure that symptoms will resolve, and they identify solutions improve symptoms. Nurses are often searching for the balance between "realistic hope and hopeful realism." This study of Coolbrandt (2005) is followed by a study in the same ward about the way hematology nurses care for HSCT patients through the most difficult part of treatment (Deweirdt and Vincke 2008). We already know, but this study confirms the great importance of an empathic attitude and expertise. This empathic attitude is characterized by understanding what the patient is going through, willingness to adjust the schedule if necessary for the patient, and to pay attention to the person behind the patient. The shown expertise, that nurses can normalize concerns and complications, creates confidence in the collaboration between patient and caregivers.

Psychologist Braamse (2015) learns that for some patients, there's often no immediate solution for the problems. Patients have to go through the situation – and they know that very well. They don't expect their nurses and relatives to wear their burden. Patients know that the isolation is inherent of their illness and treatment. But they still need the presence from caregivers and close relatives or to feel them nearby. In this way, they can feel the autonomy to choose their own way of coping with the situation. That autonomy is often affected by the disease and treatment.

Nurses can always reflect on themselves with the following basic questions:

- What do I observe?
- What do I signal?
- Which interventions can I do?
- What do I report in the dossier?

- Who can I ask for extra support? And
- Which attitude is needed? Do I have it?
- Which knowledge is needed? Do I have it?
- Which skills do I need? Do I have them?
- What do I need from my colleagues?
- Who can I ask for counseling and coaching when I need it?

These questions can help you to go back to your nursing base when the complexity of the cases makes you problematize things too much. When you feel powerless because of the multiple problems, you don't have to forget that your presence is also an intervention.

10.10 Therapeutic Interventions, e.g., Complementary Therapies, Music, Touch, and Massage

In some countries there are well-being and relaxation departments for the oncologic patients. The goal is to provide the patients with a wide range of recreational activities and with that maximize their well-being during the treatment. Most of the time, such teams consist of a coordinator, an art therapist, a music therapist, and a group of volunteers. In the hospital they can make a "living room" where patients and their family can come to relax and optionally can partake in a creative activity or a workshop. It consists of four different subdivisions: activity therapies, art therapies, music therapies, and complementary therapies/care. Each division will be specified below.

10.10.1 Activity Therapies

Activity therapies consist of three different pillars: creative activities, social activities, and a rental service.

Creative Activities Patients can choose from a wide range of creative activities. They can do this on their own, with a volunteer, or with other patients (workshop). For this patient group, most activities take place in the patient room.

Some of the creative activities that we offer include mosaic, jewelry making, painting, drawing, mandala, knitting, and crochet. Special creative volunteers help and provide the patient with creative material. Also workshops can provide special creative activities like (dry)flower arranging and seasonal workshops.

A creative activity provides the patient with a welcome distraction to get through the day. It also helps to keep the mind of negative things, and it is a way to make something nice for their loved ones.

Social Activities Patients regularly stay for long periods of time during their treatment. Some of the patients don't have a big social network and are at risk of becoming lonely during their stay. An initiative "life well-being and relaxation" has special "social" volunteers that visit the patients on a regular basis. The volunteers work with a cart that is filled with all kinds of magazines. With that cart the volunteer visits every patient on the ward. They make contact with new patients, hand out magazines, and tell what can be offered to them during their stay. They make extra time to visit and talk to lonely patients. Most patients really look forward to the weekly meetings with the volunteers.

Rental Service (in Some Hospitals/Organizations) Patients have the possibility to rent items that will make their stay more pleasant. They can get laptops, game consoles, e-readers, tablets, and audio book players. Patients can rent Dvd's directy from a webpage. Offering board games, puzzles, and handy tools like a book seat (a handy device that makes it possible to put a book or a tablet on the bed without the need of holding it) is some of the special offers you can give to the patient.

10.10.2 Art Therapies

Art therapy focuses on the power of the image, where color and form play an important role. Art therapy can give support when the body, mind, and soul are out of balance because of the physical and mental pressure that comes with being ill. With art therapies a guiding question or a specific theme forms the basis for the therapy. Some possible themes are acceptance, come closer to your inner self, enlightenment, relaxation, and how to handle emotions. With art therapies the process is the most important aspect. It does not matter if the patient is creative or not; it only matters that the patient is willing and open for the therapy.

There are many different creative forms a patient can choose from: drawing, painting, felting, and molding. A combination of said techniques is also possible. Making a collage or writing poetry can also be offered. The materials that can be used are diverse: pastel chalk, aquarelle pencil, and aquarelle and acrylic paint. The art therapist decides together with the patient what material and technique to use.

Patients make regular use of art therapies. Because of their long stay in the hospital, the art therapist can offer lots of therapeutic sessions to the patients which make it easier to work on a certain set goal.

10.10.3 Music Therapies

Music therapy focuses on the power of melody, harmony, and rhythm. Music therapy can give support when the body, mind, and soul are out of balance because of the physical and mental pressure that comes with being ill. With music therapies a guiding question or a specific theme forms the basis for the therapy. Some possible themes are acceptance, come closer to your inner self, enlightenment, relaxation, and how to handle emotions. With music therapies the process is the most important aspect. It does not matter if the patient is creative or not; it only matters that the patient is willing and open for the therapy.

There are many different musical forms a patient can choose from, both in an active form and the recipient. The music therapist can play alongside the bed of the patient; the patient can choose to just listen, but he/she can also sing or play along with an instrument. It is possible for the patient to borrow an instrument, so that they can enjoy play-

ing their own music during the stay in the hospital. Listening to music alongside the music therapist is also a possibility (the therapist has a blue tooth speaker box for these occasions), and the patient can compose and then record his/her own song on CD. This is a great opportunity because the music is not only beneficial for the moment but also acts as a nice memory for a later time.

The musical instruments the patients can choose from are as follows: guitar, keyboard, sound bars, and a lyre (a kind of harp).

Patients make regular use of the music therapies. A lot of patients find the music that the art therapist plays very soothing, and they can let their emotions run free. Some patients even request that the music therapist plays music on their deathbed or at their funeral.

10.10.4 Complementary Therapies/Care

Because of the side effects of the disease or HSCT treatment, some complementary therapies like massage, manicure, and pedicure are limited or not possible for the patient group. The complementary therapies that can be used by the patients are:

Aromatherapy With the use of aromatherapy, the patient can experience a wide range of different aromas. Every aroma has its own use. Some will sooth or calm, while others will activate the patient. The use of electric scent streamers in the patient room distributes the aromas.

Therapeutic Touch Therapeutic touch is a technique to help people relax, relieve their pain, and help them heal faster. It is sometimes called a "laying on of hands" and is based on ancient healing practices. Therapeutic touch is thought to promote healing through balance in the body.

Philips Living Color Lamp The Philips living color lamp can change the color of the room to match the mood of the patient. Patients can change the colors with a remote, so that they can alternate between colors. Just like aromatherapy colors can also influence the well-being of the patients.

10.11 **Skin Care** (see also Chap. 11 GvHD about skin care)

Introduction

Our skin is important in many ways. Grégoire (1999) stated that the skin is the first line of defense against harmful influences of our environment. The skin prevents us from overheating, undercooling, or drying out. The skin has a sense of touch, so we can feel things and also perform complex actions, for example, with our hands and face. Our skin is unique to us and who we are as a person, recognizable to the people around us or through identification by fingerprints and scars.

The skin exists of three layers:

- The epidermis
- The dermis (leather skin)
- The subcutaneous connective tissue

Grégoire (1999) wrote in his book about pathology and physiology of the layers of the skin. The epidermis is the outer layer. This consists for the most part of horn cells. These cells are constantly newly formed in the lower layer of the epidermis. The cells multiply by division. The newly formed horn cells always move slightly to the surface of the skin because they are pushed upward by the continuous production of new cells. When the cells reach the top of the epidermis, they die. Our skin will form a very strong layer (like an armor), which is difficult to penetrate for pathogens and, in addition, counteracts dehydration of the skin. This dead horn layer is extra thick on some areas of the body, such as on the soles of the feet and on the palms of our hand.

There are also other cells in the lower layer of the epidermis between the horn cells: the melanocytes. The pigment cells make small pigment pellets that they pass on to the horn cells to place the pigment like an umbrella above their core nucleus. Vulnerable hereditary material in the nucleus is shielded against the damaging effect of ultraviolet radiation in the sunlight.

The Grégoire (1999) wrote about the leather skin (dermis) as a solid construction of connective tissue and is much different in content than the epidermis which consists of a few types of cells. The leather skin is also the most important part of the active defense system of the skin: through which special white blood cells play an important role, viruses and bacteria can be recognized and directed harmlessly. The leather skin also ensures the elasticity and tensile strength of the skin. When the skin ages or is damaged by sunlight, the elasticity and resilience decrease. The leather skin is not constantly renewed, as happens with the epidermis. Damage to the leather skin will therefore always be visible as a scar. However, if only the epidermis becomes damaged, it will heal completely.

The subcutaneous connective tissue is the layer that separates the skin of the muscles and tendons in our body. There are blood vessels (food and oxygen supply), lymph vessels (drainage of waste), and nerves (touch sensation, pipeline, temperature sensation). The blood supply is ingenious and precisely regulates the supply of nutrients and oxygen to the leather skin and the lower layers of the epidermis. The blood vessels in the skin also play an important role in the body's temperature control. By dilating the blood vessels, extra heat can be delivered to the outside, and with vasoconstriction, the release of heat can be reduced so that no energy is lost.

Skin and Chemotherapy

When a patient receives chemotherapy, problems of the skin are common. The skin contains many fast-growing cells which will be affected by the chemotherapy.

Possible complaints are:

- A dry, flaky skin
- Rash
- Faster discoloration or skin damage by the sun
- Brown spots and brown discoloration
- White spots without pigment
- Acne
- Redness
- Itching
- Hyper-/hypopigmentation

Usually, after the end of chemotherapy, the skin will recover quickly.

The basic advise for chemotherapy patients (Erasmus MC (Care guide) (2009):

- The use of perfume or roller deodorant, after-shave, and razor blade is not advised. As a result of treatment, the skin may become more sensitive to these products and may lead to irritation or damage. When this happens, it increases the risk of infection. The use of shower gel, shampoo, and body lotion is allowed.
- Makeup may be used, as long as the skin and nail bed can be well observed. For example, eye shadow and noncolored lip balm are allowed, as they cover a very small part of the skin and are not specific. Rouge, powder, and similar products may not be used, as they cover a larger surface of the skin and possible skin abnormalities may be masked.
- Recommend wearing bath slippers and plenty of clothes. Clothes need to be changed when they are visibly dirty. However, in the presence of fever (perspiration), dry skin (skin scales), or cream use, changing the outfit is desirable. Washing can be done in a normal washing machine, with other people's clothes. However, they must be washed at least 40 °C.

Skin Responding at the Treatment

The skin changes depend on the type of chemotherapy the patient receives. For example, the skin is drier, darker (= pigmentation problem), or look dusky or gray. Also, the nails can change in structure. This is due to the effects of the chemotherapy. It is good to advise the patient to adjust the daily care of the skin to the changes that have occurred.

You can advise the patient (Erasmus MC (Care guide) (2009):

- Not to use very hot or very cold water during shower or bathing.
- Avoid alcohol-based products. They will dry out the skin.
- Do not use any perfumed soap during shower or bathing. A little (almond) oil in the bath water can help to keep the skin smooth.
- Use mild, unperfumed, moisturizing body lotion or cream.

Skin and Rash

If the patient endures itching, scaling, splitting, and burning, you can advise:

- Use soothing and protective creams and ointments. They keep the skin smooth and prevent the skin from drying out. Examples of non-dry skin creams: lanette cream and cetomacrogol cream. Examples in very dry skin: Vaseline lanette cream.
- Do not treat skin rash with anti-acne agents.

Skin and Acne

Chemotherapy can cause acne. This is a side effect that creates uncertainty in our patients. You can advise:

- Leave the skin alone.
- Wash the skin with not too cold or too warm water and do not use any soap. Or use a pH-neutral shower gel.
- Carefully dry the skin with the towel.
- Do not scratch or squeeze.
- A dermatologist may be able to recommend specific topical therapy.

Advice on Itching

Because of the treatment, the skin can dry out it which can cause itching or a prickling sensation that can be uncomfortable. You can advise:

- Do not scratch. Tell the patient to cut the nails very short and keep them clean.
- Itching gets worse sometimes by heat or by contact with clothes or bedding.
- Use a cool ointment or menthol powder (on localized areas) to relieve the itching. This only applies if the skin is not broken.

Skin and Risks of Bleeding and Infections

Chemotherapy may (temporarily) increase the risk of infection and bleeding. Observe the patient for wounds, blisters, or discolorations. In case of sudden redness of the skin or the occurrence of blisters, contact the attending physician. A little extra care for the skin is recommended.

Skin and the Sun

Advise caution with sun exposure and encourage the application of high SPF sunscreen (30–50). The patient needs to be careful in direct sun and also if they are in the shade due to reflected light. During the periods the patients undergo chemotherapy, they can take a walk or work in the garden but advise them against sunbathing. They should avoid the sun between 12 and 15 o'clock. Chemotherapy can cause the loss of hair and thinning of the hair on the scalp. The scalp is more at the risk for sunburn. After chemotherapy, the sun can cause more discoloration of the skin. Our patients must always protect their skin. Wearing a (sun) hat or cap and covering the arms are recommended. Using a sunscreen with a protection factor of 30 or more is extremely important.

10.12 Discharge from Inpatient Care

When a patient is discharged following HSCT, this is often an anxious time. They are now leaving the "safe" environment of doctors and nurses. Some of the patients feel that they don't have any trust in their own body to let them know when they are not well.

It is advisable to inform the patient about the general aspects/living rules so that they can pick up their daily routine at home: housework or social events.

School, study, and work

- Patients who are no longer neutropenic and when their physical condition allows may slowly take up their studies or activities.

Domestic work

- Patients can pick up and expand household tasks. For most patients, a full-day job is too heavy. Ask them to start slowly. It can be very stimulating for patients to feel "useful" again.
- If the patient is neutropenic, cleaning the residences from pets (birdcages, dog basket, etc.) should be discouraged. Cat's litter boxes and bird cages can easily transmit germs (toxoplasmosis). If nobody can't take over this task, recommend the patient to clean the animal shelter with (household) gloves.
- The patient can do some gardening but advise to avoid contact with sand and/or soil with their bare hands (toxoplasmosis) and avoid moving leaves and debris which may release fungal spores. Ask them to use garden tools and wear (household) gloves.
- Fresh flowers and plants can stay in the home, but give the patients advice to regularly refresh the water of the flowers.

Social

- Patient should be advised if they want to take some outdoor trips, such as holidays or camping visits, to discuss this with their treating physician. This is especially important if the patient wants to go abroad following HSCT. The patient must consider the hygienic conditions or vaccinations that may be needed in the visiting country.
- The patient needs to avoid visits of family and/or friends from sick (contagious) people until they are out of their leukopathic phase and while they remain immunocompromised.

Driving

- The patient should consult with their attending physician when to resume driving. Some medications or having anemia can affect the ability to concentrate so that driving is not safe.

Sports activities

- Give the patient information about building up their physical strength and condition. Some rehabilitation sports programs can be given in the living area of the patient. The patient can also seek information from a physiotherapist in the area to improve their physical condition.

10.13 Readmissions to Hospital

Patients are often unsure about the rules of life and their physical condition during and after HSCT. It is important that patients from the outpatient clinic receive clear information when they can resume certain activities in their social and general life. It is important to inform the patient fully about the rules of life so that they can pick become independent more quickly after this intensive treatment period.

In the home situation, side effects or problems may occur after HSCT. The patient should contact the hospital or attending physician. In many HSCT centers, emergency call procedures are well established. The patient should be aware of these. According to the Erasmus MC (2009) Zorggids (care guide), the contact moments should be as follows:

10.13.1 Urgent Complaints

Following HSCT, they should contact immediately (inside and outside office hours) with the following complaints:

- Fever (temperature above 38.5 °C)
- Cold shivers
- Blood in stool or urine
- Nosebleed
- Hematomas or bruising without bumping
- Difficulty moving the arms and/or legs
- Sudden shortness of breath
- Persistent and constant vomiting
- Persistent diarrhea
- Sudden/new skin rash

10.13.2 Complaints

Following HSCT the patient should contact (within office hours) at:

- No stool for longer than 3 days
- Symptoms of anemia, such as severe tiredness or dizziness

- Pain in the mouth
- Difficulty and pain with swallowing
- Painful and burning sensation during urination
- Burning and/or painful eyes
- Insufficient drinking or passing urine

10.14 Pediatric Considerations

Advances in treatment and improved prognosis increase the number of children and families living through the experience of childhood cancer. Increased survival rates come at the cost of aggressive combinations of chemotherapy, radiotherapy, and surgery, each of which may be associated with adverse effects and psychosocial difficulties for families (Kieman et al. 2010).

Hematopoietic stem cell transplantation (HSCT) may affect children and their families inducing depression, anxiety, burnout symptoms, and post-traumatic stress symptoms, as well as post-traumatic growth (PTG) which includes feelings of inner strength, closer relationships with family members and friends, and a greater appreciation for life, factors that might lead to a general feeling of growth (Riva et al. 2014). Furthermore, these treatments can lead to physical late effects, which may also have psychosocial consequences to the patient and the family long after treatment has ended (Kieman et al. 2010).

It is important to understand the general impact of childhood cancer on families, like the emotional impact, the specific impacts for individual family members and extended family, and the disruption to family life. How the illness impacts on the social lives and networks of the family and the social implications for families needs to be taken into consideration (Kieman et al. 2010).

There are many specific psychological interventions to help children deal with cancer treatment. As quoted by Weinstein and Henrich (2013) in their research, the interventions that are mostly used to help children before they undergo a painful or anxiety-inducing procedure are educating children by explaining the procedure, providing emotional support to children by listening and answering children's fears and worries or holding their hands, and distracting children through passive forms such as music, television, and books or through active forms such as playing, telling stories, singing, and using bubbles. Weinstein and Henrich (2013) explains the least commonly reported strategies that nurses used were breathing exercises to relax the child using books, tapes, and videos to educate children on their treatment and hypnosis. All these psychological interventions are effective in reducing pain and anxiety, along with enhancing acceptance of medical treatments (Weinstein and Henrich 2013).

Also Weinstein and Henrich (2013) stated that one of the primary benefits of these psychological interventions is that children shift from a passive and helpless state of pain and anxiety to a state of control and empowerment with an active adaptive attitude toward life. Through these interventions, children are considered an active participant within their own care. By preparing children psychologically for medical procedures and teaching them coping strategies, nurses may help reduce the risk of developing maladaptive behaviors and psychopathologies. Kieman et al. (2010) indicate that physicians and nurses working in pediatric oncology are in a unique position to identify and manage psychosocial issues in childhood.

In order to prevent feelings of isolation and helplessness, the children's rights in hospital (EACH 2016) stresses that steps should be taken to mitigate physical and emotional stress. The staff should avoid or reduce situations or actions described by the child as stressful. The staff should learn to recognize and act upon the fears or concerns of the child and families whether or not explicitly expressed. To mitigate emotional stress, the child and family should be offered emotional support.

It is important to work together with a multidisciplinary team members like the child life therapists, psychologists, and social workers who all can help to provide psychological support to the child and their families (Weinstein and Henrich 2013). Contacts should be offered to social services, psychologists, and therapeutic healthcare professionals as well as religious support or counseling when requested, taking into account the family's cultural background and contact with self-help groups, relevant support groups, and patient or consumer organizations (EACH 2016).

For children it is important to try to make the life in hospitals as close to normal life as possible. School is an important part of it for school-aged children. School is also an important part of adolescents' and young adults' lives, and being diagnosed with cancer in childhood may affect perceptions of school. Cancer and its treatment have a negative impact on mental and physical health and often lead to an increased absence from school. Furthermore, treatments with radiation and chemotherapy, especially among patients diagnosed with a central nervous system (CNS) tumor, may significantly affect neurocognitive function and levels of education (Winterling et al. 2015).

Results from Winterling et al. (2015) studies show that survivors appear to achieve education levels comparable to those of control groups although some studies indicate that survivors more often repeat a school year and receive additional academic support.

Furthermore, worry over missing school is a great concern for adolescents starting chemotherapy.

References

Agulnik A, Forbes PW, Stenquist N, Rodriguez-Galindo C, Kleinman M. Validation of a pediatric early warning score in hospitalized pediatric oncology and hematopoietic stem cell transplant patients. Pediatr Crit Care Med. 2016;17(4):e146–53.

Al-Dasoogi N, Sonis ST, Bowen JM, Bateman E, Blijlevens N, Gibson RJ, Logan RM, Nair RG, Stringer AM, Yazbeck R, Elad S, Lalla RV. Emerging evidence of the pathology of mucositis. Support Care Cancer. 2013;21:3233–41.

Braamse AMJ. Psychological aspects of hematopoietic stem cell transplantation in patients with hematological malignancies. Amsterdam: Ipskamp Drukkers Enschede; 2015.

Coolbrandt A. Moed houden en moed verliezen: een kwalitatief onderzoek bij stamceltransplantatiepatiënten. Masterthese; 2005.

Coyle MA. Transfer anxiety: preparing to leave intensive care. Intensive Crit Care Nurs. 2001;17:138–43.

Clarkson JE, Worthington HV, Littlewood A, Clarkson JE, McCabe MG. Interventions for treating oral mucositis for patients with cancer receiving treatment (review). Cochrane Library; 2011.

Cramp F, Byron-Daniel J. Exercise for the management of cancer-related fatigue in adults. Cochrane Database Syst Rev. 2012;11:CD006145.

Deweirdt N, Vincke J. Patiënten door het ergste heen helpen. *Een onderzoek naar de ondersteuning van hematologische verpleegkundigen aan stamceltransplantatie-en acute myeloïde leukemiepatiënten.* Universiteit Gent; 2008.

EACH and The European Association for Children In Hospital. (2016-last update). EACH Charter & Annotations. Available: https://www.each-for-sick-children.org/each-charter/introduction-each-charter-annotations.html. [10/13, 2016].

Erasmus MC Zorggids (Care guide). Hematology intended for patients with hematologic disease, including acute and chronic leukemia, (non) Hodgkin lymphomas and multiple myeloma. 2nd ed. Team Patient Communication; 2009.

Grégoire L. Inleiding anatomie/fysiologie van de mens. Integraal. 1999;2:232–45.

Hill J, Holcombe C, Clark L, Boothby MRK, Hincks A, Fisher J, Salmon P. Predictors of onset of depression and anxiety in the year after diagnosis of breast cancer. Psychol Med. 2011;41(7):1429–36. Universiteit Gent.

Kluin-Nelemans JC, Tanasale-Huisman EA. Hematologie. Bohn Stafleu van Loghum. 2013;2:156, 158, 245, 248–9, 253–5.

Knols R, Aaronson NK, Uebelhart D, Fransen J, Aufdemkampe G. Physical exercise in cancer patients during and after medical treatment: a systematic review of randomized and controlled clinical trials. J Clin Oncol. 2005;23(16):3830–42.

National Cancer Institute (US). (2013). Oral mucositis chemoradiotherapy and hematopoietis stem cell transplantation patients management of mucositis. Accessed on line 3/04/16. http://www.cancer.gov/cancertopics/pdq/supportivecare/oralcomplications/HealthProfessional/page5#Section_85.

Ludikhuizen J, Smorenburg SM, de Rooij SE, de Jonge E. Identification of deteriorating patients on general wards; measurement of vital parameters and potential effectiveness of the modified early warning score. J Crit Care. 2012;4:424.e7-424.e13.

NCCN (2002) website https://www.nccn.org/patients/resources/life_with_cancer/pdf/nccn_distress_thermometer.pdf

Netters FJS, Huls G, Tichelaar YIGV, Reyners AKL, Kluin-Nelemans JC, Zijlstra JG. Evidente toename in overleving van hematologische patiënten opgenomen op de intensive care. Nederlands tijdschrift voor hematologie. 2010;8:339–44.

Nordin K, Berglund G, Glimelius B, Sjödén PO. Predicting anxiety and depression among cancer patients: a clinical model. Eur J Cancer. 2001;37(3):376–84.

Murray JS, Williams LA, Pignataro S, Volpe D. An integrative review of pediatric early warning system scores. Pediatr Nurs. 2015;41(4):165–74.

Peigne V, Rusinova K, Karlin L, Darmon M, Fermand JP, Schlemmer B, Azoulay E. Continued survival gains in recent years among critically ill myeloma patients. Intensive Care Med. 2009;35:512–8.

Porchet F. Interdisciplinary communication. Berlin/Heidelberg: Springer; 2006. The World Health Organization Quality of Life Assessment (WHOQOL): position paper from the World Health Organization. Soc Sci Med. 1995; 41:1403–9.

Riva, R. Forinder, U, Arvidson, J. Mellgren, K., Toporski, J. Winiarski, J. Norberg, A. Patterns of psychological responses oin paretns of childer that underwent stem cell transplantation. Psycho-Oncology. 2014;23(11):1307–13.

Rubenstein EB, Peterson DE, Schubert M. Clinical practice guidelines for the prevention and treatment of cancer therapy – induced oral and gastrointestinal mucositis. Cancer. 2004;100(Suppl 9):2026–46. American Cancer Society.

Sanquin. (2016). Website. https://www.sanquin.nl/repository/documenten/nl/over-sanquin/over-sanquin/37356/Sanquin_jaarverslag_2016.pdf.

Speck RM, Courneya KS, Masse LC, Duval S, Schmitz KH. An update of controlled physical activity trials in cancer survivors: a systematic review and meta-analysis. J Cancer Surviv. 2010;4(2):87–100.

Spence RR, Heesch KC, Brown WJ. Exercise and cancer rehabilitation: a systematic review. Cancer Treat Rev. 2010;36(2):185–94.

Steinberg A, Asher A, Bailey C, Fu JB. The role of physical rehabilitation in stem cell transplantation patients. Support Care Cancer. 2015;23(8):2447–60.

Subbe CP, Kruger M, Rutherford P, Gemmel L. Validation of a modified early warning score in medical admissions. QJM. 2001;94:521–6.

Syrjala KL, Martin PJ, Lee SJ. Delivering care to long-term adult survivors of hematopoietic cell transplantation. J Clin Oncol. 2012;30(30):3746–51.

Vademecum. (2017). Website. https://www.vademecumhematologie.nl/artikelen/transfusiebeleid/transfusiereacties/soorten-transfusiereacties/.

Ven van der, M, Silderhuis V.M., Brouwer, R.M. Patiënten met een hematologische maligniteit op de Intensive Care. Ned tijschrift Geneeskunde. 2009;153:A582.

Weinstein AG, Henrich CC. Psychological interventions helping pediatric oncology patients cope with medical procedures: a nurse-centered approach. Eur J Oncol Nurs. 2013;17(6):726–31.

Winterling J, Jervaeus A, Sandeberg af M, Johansson E, Wettergren L. Perceptions of school among childhood cancer survivors: a comparison with peers.

J Pediatr Oncol Nurs. 2015;32:201–8. https://doi.org/10.1177/1043454214563405.

World Health Organisation (WHO). (2017). http://www.who.int/mental_health/publications/whoqol/en/.

Wiskemann J, Kuehl R, Dreger P, Huber G, Kleindienst N, Ulrich CM, Bohus M. Physical exercise training versus relaxation in allogeneic stem cell transplantation (PETRA study)- rationale and design of a randomized trial to evaluate a yearlong exercise intervention on overall survival and side-effects after allogeneic stem cell transplantation. BMC Cancer. 2015;15:619.

Wiskemann J, Huber G. Physical exercise as adjuvant therapy for patients undergoing hematopoietic stem cell transplantation. Bone Marrow Transplant. 2008;41(4):321–9.

Graft-Versus-Host Disease (GvHD)

11

John Murray, Jacqui Stringer, and Daphna Hutt

Abstract

Acute and chronic graft-versus-host disease (GvHD) is a major cause of morbidity and mortality in patients who undergo allogeneic haematopoietic cell transplantation (HCT) and affects approximately 30–40% of recipients. Its diagnosis is complicated, and staging of the disease varies dependent upon the transplant centre involved. Standardisation through the use of National Institute of Health (NIH) guidelines helps clinicians diagnose and treat their patients more effectively. For the majority of patients who go on to develop GvHD, corticosteroids remain the first-line treatment for both acute and chronic GvHD. Recipients that are refractory to systemic steroids have a plethora of second- and third-line options available to them. A 'standard of care' approach has not yet become agreed globally due to poor evidence from small and limited randomised control trials. Supportive care is paramount, and the nurse is often at the centre of the patients care and in the best position to guide and advise the patient and family through this often long-term complication.

Keywords

Acute graft-versus-host disease • Chronic graft-versus-host disease

11.1 What Is GvHD?

11.1.1 Definitions

Acute GvHD is a reaction of donor immune cells against host tissues. The three main tissues that acute GvHD affects are the skin, liver and gastro-intestinal tract (Jacobsohn and Vogelsang 2007).

Chronic GvHD is a syndrome of variable clinical features resembling autoimmune and other

J. Murray (✉) • J. Stringer
The Christie NHS Foundation Trust, Manchester, UK
e-mail: John.murray@christie.nhs.uk;
Jacqui.stringer@christie.nhs.uk

D. Hutt
Department of Paediatric Haematology-Oncology
and BMT, Edmond and Lily Safra Children Hospital,
Sheba Medical Center, Tel-Hashomer, Israel
e-mail: dhutt@sheba.health.gov.il

© EBMT and the Author(s) 2018
M. Kenyon, A. Babic (eds.), *The European Blood and Marrow Transplantation Textbook for Nurses*,
https://doi.org/10.1007/978-3-319-50026-3_11

immunologic disorders. Manifestations of chronic GvHD may be restricted to a single organ or site or may be widespread, with profound impact on quality of life (Jagasia et al. 2015).

11.2 Background to GvHD

The *New England Journal of Medicine* reported the infusion of bone marrow into patients by E.D. Thomas and colleagues in 1957, following radio- or chemotherapy. Preclinical animal studies revealed that transplantation of splenocytes from non-oncogenic donor strains facilitated haematopoietic recovery but led to a severe illness characterised by anorexia, reduced weight, diarrhoea, ruffled fur and eventual death. It was labelled at the time 'secondary' or 'runt's disease' and later became known as graft-versus-host disease (GvHD). It was clear that the effect was not one of the conditioning therapies but was associated with an immune-mediated syndrome (Wolf et al. 2012).

GvHD remains a leading cause of non-relapse mortality and is associated with a high morbidity that increasingly affects quality of life (Lee et al. 2003; Dignan et al. 2012).

However, the success of allogeneic HSCT depends on simultaneous graft-versus-tumour (GvT) effects. Therefore, broad-based immunosuppressive strategies are less attractive as these may dampen the GvT benefit. Relapse accounts for a significant proportion of treatment failures after HSCT; thus strategies for GvHD prevention with minimal impact on GvT are the holy grail of transplantation (Magenau and Reddy 2014).

Historically, GvHD is termed 'acute' before day 100 and 'chronic' any time after day 100. However, it has since been recognised that there can sometimes be 'overlap' between the types, so signs and symptoms are used to aid and determine the diagnosis. The skin is the most common organ affected followed by the gastrointestinal (GI) tract and then the liver. Typically, the skin develops a rash which often but not always appears on the palms of hands and soles of the feet first and can rapidly spread to the rest of the

body. GI and liver GvHD symptoms such as nausea, vomiting, diarrhoea, abnormal liver enzymes and jaundice are similar in both acute and chronic forms of GvHD.

According to the 2014 NIH consensus, the broad category of acute GvHD includes classic acute GvHD (maculopapular erythematous rash, gastrointestinal symptoms or cholestatic hepatitis), occurring within 100 days after HCT or donor leukocyte infusion. The broad category of acute GvHD also includes persistent, recurrent or late-onset acute GvHD, occurring more than 100 days after transplantation or donor leukocyte infusion. The presence of GvHD without diagnostic or distinctive chronic GvHD manifestations defines the broad category of acute GvHD (Vigorito et al. 2009; Jagasia et al. 2015).

11.3 Acute GvHD

Overview: acute graft-versus-host disease (aGvHD) occurs following an allogeneic haematopoietic stem cell transplant and is a reaction of donor immune cells against host tissues and remains a major cause of morbidity and mortality (Greinix 2008). High-dose chemotherapy +/− radiotherapy inflicts cellular damage, and this leads to an inflammatory process; the activated donor T cells interact with the host epithelial cells. Approximately 35–50% of haematopoietic stem cell transplant (HSCT) recipients will develop aGvHD (Dignan et al. 2012). There are several factors that can influence the development of aGvHD: the stem cell source, age of the patient, conditioning regimen and GvHD prophylaxis used. All aGvHD can be associated with culture negative fever. Commonly the three most cited organs are skin (rash/dermatitis), liver (hepatitis/jaundice) and GI tract (abdominal pain/ diarrhoea), and these may occur in isolation or in combination. Biopsies of skin and GI tissue (more rarely liver) are often obtained, although the diagnosis of aGvHD is regularly made based upon clinical signs and symptoms. A biopsy is useful to help differentiate from other diagnoses which may mimic GvHD, such as viral infection (hepatitis, colitis) or drug reaction (causing skin rash). The modified Glucksberg-Seattle criteria (Przepiorka et al. 1995) are widely used and give a stage and grade (grade 0–IV) for each organ and its degree of involvement. Those with grade III/IV aGvHD tend to have a poor overall outcome. Upon development of signs and symptoms, immunosuppression should be optimised. Oral or intravenous corticosteroids are frequently initiated, and although steroids remain the gold standard of initial therapy, they are effective in only 40% of patients (Weisdorf et al. 1990). Many protocols suggest a steroid treatment failure, if there is no improvement in symptoms after 3–7 days of treatment. At this point salvage (second-line), immunosuppressive therapy for which there is currently no worldwide consensus is implemented. Additional management issues are to pay attention to wound infections in skin GvHD and fluid/nutrition management in gastrointestinal GvHD. About 50% of patients with aGvHD will eventually develop manifestations of chronic GvHD (Jacobsohn and Vogelsang 2007).

11.4 Pathophysiology of GvHD

GvHD happens because the donated cells are not identical to the cells of patient (the host). GvHD is the body's response, a manifestation of the fight between the T cells of the donor and host's immune system.

T cells are white blood cells that usually protect us against foreign bodies, like bacteria, fungi and viruses. The T cells in our bodies are able to recognise the proteins on the cells as either belonging to us or not belonging to us. Those that belong to us are allowed to live within us in harmony, and our immune systems do not usually (except autoimmune disorders) defend themselves against these cells.

The donated haematopoietic stem cells are closely matched (except in a haplo-identical transplant) to those of the recipient, and unless they are from an identical twin, the donor cells will express slightly different cell surface pro-

teins. These small differences are recognised by the body as 'non-self', and subsequently these cells get questioned and stopped repeatedly by the body's policing or immune system.

This is the basis behind all the components of our immune system and why and how we fight any external invader trying to enter our body. The greater the differences in the tissue types, the greater the chance of the recipient developing GvHD.

In the 1960s, Billingham (1966) proposed three central tenets for the development of GvHD. The essential components are:

(i) The presence of immunocompetent cells from the donor
(ii) The inability of the recipient to reject donor cells
(iii) The histocompatibility differences between the donor and recipient

Donor T cells are now recognised as occupying a central role in mediating GvHD following interactions with activated host and donor antigen-presenting cells (APC). A complex network of cytokines, chemokines, cellular receptors and immune cell subsets then modulate T-cell/APC interactions that result in the initiation and maintenance of GvHD (Magenau and Reddy 2014).

The three phase process for aGvHD comprises:

initial tissue damage from the conditioning therapy

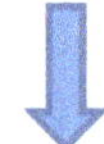

Activation of host APC

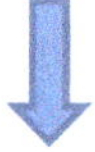

Activation and then proliferation of donor T cells

Finally, inflammatory cytokines are released such as interleukin-1 and tissue necrosis factor alpha that produce tissue necrosis.

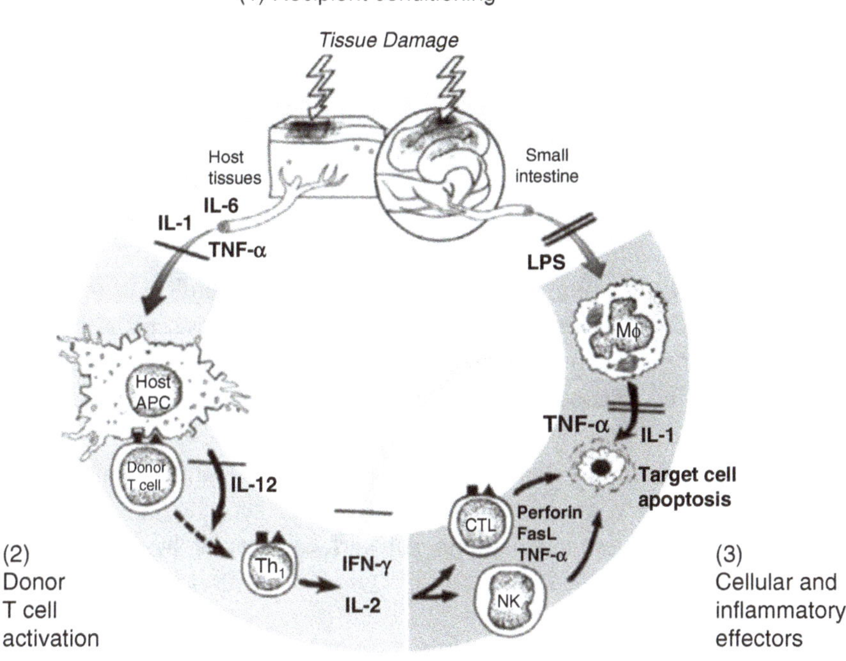

Fig. 11.1 The three phases of acute GVHD, as described by Ferrara and colleagues (From Hill and Ferrara 2000. Reproduced with permission)

Acute GvHD is modulated in part by the presence of cells capable of inhibiting immune responses, most notably regulatory T cells (Magenau and Reddy 2014) (Fig. 11.1).

Both prevention and treatment of aGvHD attempt to disrupt the three-step pathophysiological cycle. Most current treatment options of aGvHD affect more than one event in this cycle through relatively non-specific immunosuppressive and anti-inflammatory mechanisms (Greinix 2008).

Reduced intensity conditioning will usually contain drugs that deplete T cells, such as Campath-1H or ATG. This reduces the initial risk of aGvHD but increases the risk of infective complications such as CMV and also the risk of late-onset aGvHD and chronic GvHD.

Incidence: the incidence of serious (grade III/IV) aGvHD is about 30% with a fully matched (8/8) unrelated donor but 40% with one or two allelic mismatches at class I. This compares to about a 20% incidence for recipients of HLA-identical sibling transplants (Al-Kadhimi et al. 2014).

11.4.1 Risk Factors

Factors that can increase the likelihood of aGvHD include older recipient/donor, sex mismatch and specifically a multiparous female donor into a male patient. Furthermore, the intensity of the preparative regimen does appear to correlate with increased incidence of aGvHD. This effect may occur due to greater tissue damage from the preparative regimen, predisposing these tissues to more inflammation from the alloreactive cells. Higher doses of radiation also gives rise to more GvHD. Equally, more recent use of non-myeloablative preparative regimens has led to lower incidence of aGvHD in some studies (Jacobsohn and Vogelsang 2007).

11.4.2 Signs and Symptoms of aGvHD

Acute GvHD mainly affects the skin, gut and liver but can affect almost any part of the body.

11.4.2.1 Skin

Acute GvHD can cause a rash which is usually flat and red and often occurs on the hands, feet and around the ears and upper chest, at first. This can quickly spread to cover the whole body. It is often, but not always, itchy and sore and can feel like sunburn. A biopsy may be taken but is not always diagnostic. On examination the features may include apoptosis at the base of epidermal rete pegs, dyskeratosis, exocytosis of lymphocytes, satellite lymphocytes adjacent to dyskeratotic epidermal keratinocytes and perivascular lymphocytic infiltration in the dermis (Ferrara and Deeg 1991).

11.4.2.2 Gastrointestinal

Signs and symptoms include weight loss, stomach discomfort and pain, nausea, vomiting and diarrhoea. The diarrhoea can be profuse with secretions and may also result in bleeding from ulceration of the mucosa. The effects of high-dose therapies and infection need to be excluded. Biopsy in this group of patients is more informative and may show apoptotic bodies at crypt bases, crypt ulceration and flattening of surface epithelium (Dignan et al. 2012).

11.4.2.3 Liver

Jaundice from hyperbilirubinaemia is the hallmark of advanced liver GvHD with a cholestatic pattern of elevated conjugated bilirubin, alkaline phosphatase and gamma-glutamyl transpeptidase (GGT) and may be associated with pruritis. There is a wide range of differential diagnoses which should be considered and excluded such as veno-occlusive disease, drug toxicity and infection. It is often extremely difficult to perform biopsy due to the increased risk of bleeding, but, if taken, histology shows endothelialitis, lymphocytic infiltration of the portal areas, pericholangitis and bile duct destruction (Dignan et al. 2012).

11.4.3 The Benefits of aGvHD

There is a fine line with aGvHD. The symptoms and side effects can be unpleasant and sometimes harmful and, in severe cases, life-threatening. However, it is well documented that some level of aGvHD is beneficial. It has been found that relapse rates post allograft were lowest in patients with aGvHD versus those without. As mentioned earlier, a graft-versus-tumour effect exists that can be exploited. It is suspected that there are reactions to polymorphic minor histocompatibility antigens expressed either specifically on haematopoietic cells (and therefore not causing GvHD) or more widely on a number of tissue cells that have antitumour activity, thereby preventing disease relapse (Baron et al. 2012).

11.4.4 Classification of Acute GvHD: Grades I–IV

Regardless of the benefits, aGvHD carries a significant transplant-related mortality (TRM) with grades 0–I (mild) having a TRM of approx. 28% and grade II, III and IV (very severe) TRM of 43% 68% and 92%, respectively (Greinix 2008). Classification is performed using the revised Glucksberg-Seattle criteria (Przepiorka et al. 1995), which measures how severe signs and symptoms are in the skin, gut and liver (see Appendix 11.A.1). The treatment for aGvHD will depend on the grade, and the grade itself is predictive of overall survival.

11.4.5 Prevention of GvHD

Prophylaxis: prevention is always better than cure. Contemporary GvHD prophylaxis at most centres is based on calcineurin inhibitors (CNIs) along with short-course methotrexate (MTX). This works by interfering with calcium-dependent interleukin-2 (IL-2) gene activation and de novo purine metabolism, respectively; CNIs and MTX act synergistically to non-selectively inhibit lymphocyte activation and proliferation. The combination of ciclosporin and MTX or tacrolimus and MTX as prophylaxis for aGvHD compared to any single-agent treatment has been shown to be superior (Greinix 2008). With standard prophylaxis, approximately 40% of patients receiving HLA-matched HSCT will develop GvHD requiring high-dose corticosteroids.

11.4.6 Drugs Used as Part of Conditioning Therapy to Prevent GvHD

Ciclosporin (CsA): is given as an intravenous infusion commencing usually 1–2 days prior to HSCT infusion to load the blood stream and is eventually converted to an oral preparation when the patient is able to tolerate tablets again. Ciclosporin binds to cyclophilin and prevents generation of nuclear factor of activated T cells (NF-AT), which is a nuclear factor for initiating gene transcription for lymphokines including interleukin-2 and interferon gamma. This action leads to suppression of cytokine production and subsequent inhibition of T-cell activation (Greinix 2008).

Mycophenolate mofetil (MMF): used mainly in reduced intensity transplant conditioning regimens is an antimetabolite that results in noncompetitive reversible inhibition of inosine monophosphate dehydrogenase. This leads to selective inhibition of lymphocytes purine synthesis and proliferation. Patients have less mucositis and faster neutrophil recovery compared to methotrexate (Greinix 2008).

Tacrolimus: is an alternative to ciclosporin within the conditioning regimens at some centres. It binds to FK506 protein 12, a different protein to the one that CsA does but their final common pathway is identical. They both prevent the generation of NF-AT, a nuclear factor for initiating gene transcription for lymphokines like IL-2 and interferon gamma leading to suppression of cytokine production and thus inhibition of T-cell activation (Greinix 2008).

Sirolimus: is used within conditioning regimens and is a natural macrolide antibiotic that exerts its immunosuppressive effect by inhibiting cytokine-driven signalling pathways of the T and B cell via mTOR blockade and specifically inhibiting the progression of cells from the G1 phase to the S phase. The advantage is that sirolimus has a completely different toxicity profile to calcineurin inhibitors and can be used in combination with them (Dignan et al. 2012).

Methotrexate (MTX): is an anti-proliferative agent given intravenously on days 1, 3, 6 and 11 after HSCT for those patients receiving a full-intensity transplant. It prevents the division and clonal expansion of T cells. It is important to receive all four doses, but severe mucositis (grade IV) often prohibits administration of the 4th and final dose and is given at the clinician's discretion.

Campath 1-H or alemtuzumab: is given in a variety of doses from 30 to 90 mg within the conditioning regimen dependent upon the cell source and degree of mismatch between donor and recipient. It is an unconjugated humanised IgG1 kappa monoclonal antibody that targets the CD52 antigen on the T and B lymphocytes as well as on monocytes, macrophages, eosinophils and dendritic cells. The major disadvantage of this drug is the increase of infections due to the extended period of lymphopenia. CMV reactivations and infections are particularly troublesome in this patient cohort necessitating strict surveillance (Dignan et al. 2012).

Antithymocyte globulin (ATG): decreases T cells and also leads to viral infections. Epstein-Barr virus (EBV) reactivations can be problematic and can result in post-transplant lymphoproliferative disease (PTLD).

11.4.6.1 Initial Treatment of Acute GvHD

Despite all of the recent advances in the understanding and treatment of GvHD, steroids remain the best and first-line therapy. The mechanism of action of steroids for aGvHD is unclear but most likely relates to the suppression of cytokines such as prevention of synthesis of interleukin-1 by antigen-presenting cells and lymphocyte activities (Greinix 2008).

Grade I: should not require systemic treatment. If CsA levels are optimised, then topical steroids in conjunction with an emollient may be introduced along with antihistamine for itchy skin. It is important, however, to ensure the emollient is acceptable to the patient and to reinforce the necessity of using the creams or lotion regularly. For a topical treatment to be effective, it must be applied. If the preparation (cream or lotion) is not liked by the patient, then compliance is poor, and it will not be effective. Precautions such as avoiding scented soaps and perfumes can minimise the risk of additional skin irritation. Reminders to maintain a good fluid intake to avoid dehydration are important as are prompts to wear natural clothing next to the skin – silk, for example, is relatively non-irritant and thermoregulating.

Grade II: anything at or above grade II is likely to require systemic treatment. If the patient progresses from grade I to grade II following optimisation of CNI and topical therapy, then systemic corticosteroids are indicated. Patients presenting with grade II signs should commence systemic steroids for their anti-inflammatory properties. The starting dose is open to discussion, and local guidelines should be followed. Some patients with GI symptoms may benefit from budesonide as a steroid-sparing treatment as it is regarded as a non-absorbable therapy.

Grades III and IV: requires treatment with systemic steroids. If GI symptoms are the major feature, then the steroids should be given intravenously to prevent problems with absorption because of vomiting, diarrhoea and abnormal mucosal lining.

Steroids were first seen to be an effective treatment in the 1980s and remain effective globally in approximately 40% of people, with 30% having a long-lasting response and a probability of survival at 1 year of 53%. The skin being the most responsive at 40% with a response rate of 15–35% for those with liver involvement and 45% in GI. The lower the grade of aGvHD and the fewer organs affected result in a better response to steroids. There is currently no standard time for assessing the effectiveness of the steroids with a time gap of 3–7 days often given as indicative of treatment failure and requiring escalation to second-line therapies. The GvHD may at this point be labelled as 'steroid refractory disease' which carries a dismal long-term prognosis (Magenau and Reddy 2014) with infection being the leading cause of mortality followed by organ failure in nonresponders (Greinix 2008). Below is a list of second- and third-line treatment options for those who have had their CNI optimised and have failed to respond to corticosteroids for at least 7 days. The evidence for many of the second- and third-line treatments is sparse and comes from small patient series with heterogeneous populations. If patients fail a second-line therapy, then a further second-line therapy should be tried before moving on to third-line options (Dignan et al. 2012). Long-term survival has not been improved following addition of second-line treatments in comparison to steroids alone (Greinix 2008).

11.4.7 Second-Line Therapies for aGvHD

Extracorporeal photopheresis: 8-methoxypsoralen (8-MOP) is a photoactivated drug that covalently binds to DNA pyrimidine bases, cell surface molecules and cytoplasmic components in the exposed nucleated white cells causing a lethal defect. It is added to a patient's blood following withdrawal by a cell separator; this is then exposed to ultraviolet light A (UVA) and returned to the patient. The blood is separated into buffy coat as well as red cells and plasma, which are returned to the patient. The buffy coat is exposed to the UVA in the presence of the 8-MOP. Once reinfused, the cells undergo apoptosis over the next 24–48 h (Greinix 2008).

The mechanism of action is not currently fully understood but may relate to apoptosis of leucocytes. When the cells are reintroduced into the patient, they continue to phagocytose. The reinfusion of these cells and subsequent phagocytosis by antigen-presenting cells (APCs) may regulate immune homeostasis through modulation of cytokine production and tolerance induction of APCs (Bladon and Taylor 2006). This possible mechanism of ECP-induced immune tolerance includes inhibition of pro-inflammatory cytokine secretion, increased secretion of anti-inflammatory cytokines, reduced stimulation of effector T cells, induction of accelerated death of effector cells and stimulation of regulatory T-cell generation (Greinix 2008). ECP is a safe treatment as it has fairly minimal side effects, hypotension, fevers, drop in haemoglobin, photophobia and tiredness post procedure. The procedure is performed in most centres by highly trained apheresis nursing staff. The patient is assessed and accepted onto the ECP service following local policy. Venous access is assessed, and if this is inadequate via the antecubital fossa, a central venous catheter will be placed.

Further second- and third-line therapies include:

Second-line therapies				
Antitumour necrosis	Infliximab	Etanercept		
Mammalian target or rapamycin inhibitors mTOR	Sirolimus			
Mycophenolate mofetil (MMF)				
Interleukin-2 receptor antibodies	Daclizumab	Denileukin diftitox	Inolimomab	Basiliximab
Third-line therapies				
Mesenchymal stem cells MSC				
Alemtuzumab				
Pentostatin				
Methotrexate				
Tyrosine kinase inhibitor	Imatinib			

Often at least two second-line therapies will be used before moving on to a third-line treatment

11.4.8 Nursing Care Considerations for aGvHD

In addition to systemic treatments, there are often topical management techniques as well as general care that nurses can offer to patients that will lead to relief from frequently troublesome symptoms of aGvHD. Below are a few pointers for consideration when seeing patients with aGvHD affecting their skin, gastrointestinal system, eyes, mouth or genitals.

11.4.9 Cutaneous

Basic skin care:

The key issue with patients who have cutaneous aGvHD is to maintain the integrity of the skin, and the following suggestions are key factors in doing this: Regular application of preferred emollients (e.g. QV, Hydromol, Diprobase). Advise application of a thin layer (enough to make the skin appear 'shiny'), in the direction of hair growth. Try not to 'rub' as this will increase any pain or itch. As guidance for amounts, it would be suggested that an adult would use on average 500 g/week and a child, 250 g/week. Use of bath/shower preparations (e.g. Dermol, QV, Hydromol) rather than soap, use of high SPF sun-screen (e.g. SunSense SPF 50+) and localised use of topical antipruritic agents (e.g. Dermacool 0.5–1%) if required. If the skin is still flaky, the patient can be advised to apply lipids (e.g. coconut oil) in addition to the emollients. Topical immunomodulation (e.g. steroid/tacrolimus cream) should be prescribed as per local protocol; however, there are a few general rules about the use of topical steroids: think about the potency/duration of the product used in relation to the age of the patient and the area of the body it is being applied to. Always apply thinly – once daily is usually enough. Think about whether the skin is weepy, when a cream/lotion is appropriate or dry/scaly in which case an ointment may be preferable. Steroids should be applied at a different time to emollients (at least a 30 minute gap between) to ensure effective absorption and remember that broken skin is a contraindication to use.

Topical management of specific stages of cutaneous aGvHD:

1. Maculopapular rash (pruritic/painful). Most common areas: soles of feet, palms of hands, cheeks, ears, neck, trunk and upper back.

Emollients are key to management at this stage. With sensitive, irritated skin, an emollient which is too thick will just not be used, whereas one which is too 'thin' will be perceived as ineffective. It is worth offering sample packs with a variety of products to trial, either made up by the hospital or provided by a specific company (e.g. QV products by Crawfords). In situations where pruritis is a major issue, a product with high water content can be useful as they are more cooling but will need regular application.

Topical steroids, each hospital will have its own protocol for prescription of topical steroids and this should be adhered to.

Menthol cream (0.5–1%, e.g. Dermacool), these products can be useful for management of painful and pruritic skin but must be used with care as they can make the patient feel very cold with widespread use so are better used only on focal areas of extreme itch/pain.

Medical grade silk clothing (e.g. Dermasilk, Espere Healthcare), it is important to explore the holistic care of the patient. Many clothing materials can cause irritation – even natural materials such as cotton. If there are widespread areas of the torso affected, it is worth suggesting the use of medical grade silk as this is manufactured to cause minimal irritation and, in some countries, can be prescribed. If this is not available, clothing made from bamboo can be suggested as an alternative.

2. Erythroderma: intense generalised redness of the skin; inflammation that gives rise to erythema and scaling all over the body. Classically involves greater than 90% of the body surface.

The topical management of erythroderma is similar to the advice mentioned above, with emphasis on the regular application of easily applied emollients and increasing fluid intake. However, because erythroderma is so widespread, the use of menthol creams is limited – unless there are specific areas of the body which are causing particular distress.

In addition to the products above, in an attempt to maintain skin integrity, organic coconut oil or other natural lipids (e.g. olive oil) can be useful supplements to the emollients. Equally good quality creams containing aloe vera gel are often very soothing (note: do not use aloe vera gel alone as this will dry the skin).

3. Bullous/desquamation (stage IV): formation of large blisters and separation of the dermis/epidermis from the basal layer causing massive fluid loss.

These patients need treating as a person with severe burns. Your hospital may have a protocol specifically for this but an example would be to irrigate with sterile water, apply an antibacterial cream (e.g. Flamazine) and protect the area from the air to minimise pain and risk of infection. The cream can be applied directly to sterile theatre gauze and wrapped around the patient to prevent trauma.

11.4.10   Oral

Patients with oral aGvHD complain of a sore mouth that is not dissimilar to the pain suffered with oral mucositis post chemotherapy/radiotherapy. Tolerance of spicy food stuff is poor, toothpaste burns and hot drinks such as tea and coffee are almost impossible to take. It is important to rule out infection as this will cause pain to be worse. Frequent swabs for virus, bacterial and fungal infection should be taken and acted upon promptly. To aid with oral pain management, the use of caphosol, Gelclair, lidocaine, paracetamol mist and Difflam mouth wash can be used.

Advise patients to frequently swill the mouth after eating to remove any debris using plain water. This is refreshing and ph7 so comfortable to do. Encourage the use of products to aid production of saliva as the mucosa is usually very dry. Artificial saliva or sugar-free gum and in some centres pilocarpine may be used.

Many medications have side effects of dry mouth. Look to see if there are any alternatives that could be prescribed for your patient.

Early referral to the dentist is vital as the risk of dental caries and secondary oral cancers is higher in patients with oral GvHD. Advice to perform regular oral exercises to reduce the risk of contractures.

11.4.11 Gastrointestinal

Patients who develop diarrhoea will have stool samples sent to exclude infective components. Once ruled out and treatment started, nursing care may aid in a more rapid recovery and maintenance of weight. Ensuring an adequate oral input with high-calorie supplements, strict fluid balance is of primary importance. The options of enteral feeding or intravenous total parental nutrition in the short term to rest the bowel need to be kept in mind if the above actions are not sufficient, with procedures such as a radiologically inserted gastrostomy (RIG) used for long-term issues. Those with upper GI disturbance, nausea and vomiting need advice on small and frequent meals as well as supplements. Patients who develop grade IV GI aGvHD will benefit from use of flexi-seal faecal collection devices.

11.4.12 Eyes

Patients with dry and gritty eyes will benefit from regular and frequent use of lubricating eye drops. Infection should be excluded and treated if apparent. Wearing dark glasses will reduce irritants such as wind and block any debris that it may blow into the patient's eyes. There are a variety of graded dark glasses that may be obtained through an optician that can block up to 90% of light and reduce photophobia significantly. It is often useful to wear glasses inside the house to reduce discomfort. Cold compress with ice packs and chamomile tea bags are useful in some instances.

11.4.13 Genito-urinary System

This is an under-reported area of GvHD from patients; some basic nursing input can help with symptoms of pain and discomfort experienced. Asking patients if this is a problem for them is the first step as patients are often reticent about mentioning genital problems to the medical team. Once infection has again been ruled out or treated, there are a variety of treatments that may offer some symptomatic benefit. With female patients, application of an emollient to the vulval region and use of dilators with a lubricant such as olive oil or coconut oil will help to minimise the risk of contractures. Vaginal moisturisers may make women feel more comfortable. Referral through to endocrinology for discussions about hormone replacement therapy (HRT) with oestrogen can be initiated by nursing staff. Men may mention tightening of the foreskin and gentle frequent retraction, and application of emollient is suggested alongside good hygiene.

11.5 Chronic Graft-Versus-Host Disease

The understanding of the pathophysiology of chronic graft-versus-host disease (cGvHD) is in its infancy, and progress to prevent and treat cGvHD remains limited (Greinix 2008). Chronic GvHD remains the major cause of late morbidity and mortality after allogeneic haematopoietic cell transplantation and is a serious and common complication occurring in 20–80% of patients (Lee and Flowers 2008). Chronic GvHD prevalence and severity has increased over the past 20 years in line with the increasing use of haematopoietic stem cell transplantation for treatment of older age patients, the widespread use of mobilised blood cells instead of marrow for grafting and improvements in survival during the first several months after allograft. Typically occurring in the first 12 months, it can be seen as early as 2 months and as late at 7 years at onset, although onset at >1 year from transplant occurs in <10% of cases (Flowers and Martin 2015). The risk of infection due to the delay in immune reconstitution and use of immunosuppressive therapies to treat cGvHD remains, however, the leading cause for death in this group of patients (Couriel et al. 2006b). Supportive care advances have decreased the morbidity, but survival has not changed significantly since the 1980s. Patients with cGvHD have a 5-year survival of 40–70% with only 50% being able to stop immunosuppression at 5 years, with 10% needing treatment beyond this time point. The other 40% either die or develop a further malignancy before cGvHD resolves (Martin et al. 2006).

As cGvHD only occurs in allografted patients and can be prevented by T-cell depletion from the donor graft, donor T cells responding to allogeneic antigens in the patient are of critical importance in the development of cGvHD (Kuzmina et al. 2011). Chronic GvHD was initially thought to be as a consequence of persistent recognition of antigenic tissue differences between donor and host. However, the role of alloreactivity versus autoreactivity in the pathogenesis of cGvHD remains an area of debate (Greinix 2008).

Meier et al. (2011) explain that:

> Donor-derived immunocompetent T cells react directly or through exaggerated inflammatory processes against tissue after allograft. The persistence of alloreactive T cells, a Th1-Th2 shift of the cellular immune response (cGvHD seems to be mediated prominently by the Th2 cytokine response), defective peripheral and central tolerance mechanisms (i.e. failure of control by regulatory T cells and /or impaired negative selection of T cells in the thymus), replacement of antigen presenting cells (APC) of the host by APC's of the donor leading to indirect antigen presentation of allo-antigens, an increasing role of B cells producing auto and allo-antibodies against the host and non-specific mechanisms of chronic inflammation leading to fibrosis of involved organs.

The importance of autoreactivity is suggested by clinical manifestations of cGvHD that frequently mimic those of autoimmune diseases, as well as the finding of autoantibodies derived from B cells after Th2-mediated stimulation and cytokine release (Greinix 2008).

The advances in understanding of this process will have an impact on patients overall survival. Using a multidisciplinary team approach for best care, identifying those at risk, monitoring, early recognition with prompt diagnosis and high-quality follow-up with an agreed management plan to prevent complications of therapy that can often lead to disabilities are vital to continue to make headway in this immensely challenging area (Flowers and Martin 2015).

11.6 Acute Vs Chronic GvHD

Historically if patients developed signs and symptoms of GvHD after day 100, this was labelled as chronic even if clinically the patient appeared to have acute features. The criteria for the diagnosis of cGvHD are based on pathological changes occurring in the skin, lung, mucous membranes, gastrointestinal tract and musculoskeletal system (Greinix 2008). The National Institute of Health (NIH) developed a set of criteria following a consensus meeting in 2005 to help address the problem of diagnosis and wrote several guidelines on the diagnosis and classification of chronic GvHD. They stated that acute and chronic GvHD should be distinguished by clinical features rather than time from transplant. There should be the presence of at least one diagnostic clinical sign of cGvHD or presence of at least one distinctive manifestation confirmed by pertinent biopsy or other relevant test. All other diagnoses should be excluded (Filipovich et al. 2005).

The broad category of cGvHD includes classic cGvHD; presenting with manifestations that can be ascribed only to cGvHD, however, it also includes an overlap syndrome, which has diagnostic or distinctive cGvHD manifestations together with features typical of aGvHD (Vigorito et al. 2009).

It is no longer useful to simply describe cGvHD as limited or extensive based on the number of organs involved as this was a system devised in 1980 following the study of 20 patients in a retrospective review (Shulman et al. 1980). A more reliable and reproducible scoring scheme was described to evaluate the individual organ severity over four grading scores 0–3 by the NIH:

- None; score 0
- Mild involvement (no significant impairment of daily living); score 1
- Moderate involvement (significant impairment of daily living); score 2
- Severe impairment (major disability); score 3

The clinical score describes how affected the patient is by their inability to perform activities of daily living. This evaluation covers the involvement of individual organs and sites. For example, if they are unable to work due to ocular loss, they would be scored as 3 severe (Carpenter 2011). The scoring should be undertaken initially at 3 months post-transplant and at 3 monthly intervals and more frequently if new signs or symptoms are found or there is a change in treatment.

The NIH in 2014 provided a further update with the Diagnosis and Staging Working Group Report. Following new evidence, refinements were made to address the areas of controversy or confusion such as overlap and classic chronic GvHD. The subcategories of 'overlap' as it was transient and often depended on the degree of immunosuppression and is subject to changes during the disease course and 'classic' cGvHD as patients may develop acute features when immunosuppression is tapered were removed. A revision was made to the diagnostic criteria for involvement of the mouth, eyes, genitalia and lungs. Schirmer's test has been removed from the severity scoring form, and an ophthalmology review is recommended. Also if an unequivocal explanation can be made for a specific abnormality that is not GvHD, then that organ should be regarded as not affected by GvHD (Jagasia et al. 2015).

Chronic GvHD commonly occurs in patients who have previously had aGvHD although it is not simply a case of evolution from one to another. Chronic GvHD usually occurs within 3 years of allograft and is a disease of deregulated immunity with protean manifestations that mimic autoimmune disorders such as Sjogren syndrome, primary biliary cirrhosis, wasting syndrome, bronchiolitis obliterans, immune cytopenias and chronic immunodeficiency (Jagasia et al. 2015).

Due to the ambiguity of diagnosis, the limited understanding of pathophysiology and the additional clinical complexities that accompany this group of patients, a systematic approach to management has been somewhat lacking (Couriel et al. 2006a). There is still no unified consensus on the diagnostic features, although recent work from the NIH (2014) has in some ways addressed this with an attempt to bring a standardised assessment to clinical practice.

Presentation with signs and symptoms of cGvHD nearly always occurs within the first year post allograft but can occasionally happen several years later. Single organs alone may be affected and can progress to other organs; however, cGvHD nearly always affects multiple sites, having major impact upon a patient's quality of life. The eyes, mouth, skin, GI tract and liver are the most frequently affected organs. There is a wide range in severity and how this relates to compromise in patients' QoL, with some manifestations being more problematic to treat. Fasciitis or cutaneous sclerosis, severe ocular sicca and bronchiolitis obliterans syndrome (BOS) often require extensive periods of time with multiple immunosuppressive agents to treat (Flowers and Martin 2015).

11.6.1 Diagnosis of cGvHD

For a diagnosis of cGvHD to be made, the NIH 2014 working group suggest that at least one diagnostic manifestation of cGvHD or at least one distinctive manifestation, with the latter confirmed by pertinent biopsy, laboratory tests, evaluation by a specialist or radiology in the same or other organ, be present, unless stated otherwise. It is important with any organ considered for a diagnosis of cGvHD that other causes for the symptoms are excluded such as infection, recurrent or new malignancy (Jagasia et al. 2015). The features should also differ from the typical dermatitis, enteritis and cholestatic liver manifestations of aGvHD (see Appendix 11.A.2 for the full tables of assessment).

11.6.2 Chronic GvHD of the Skin

In cGvHD the skin is the most frequently affected organ if the patient has received HCT and has a wide variety of manifestations (Pavletic et al. 2006). For a clinical diagnosis of skin cGvHD features of poikiloderma, lichen planus-like eruption, deep sclerotic features, morphea-like superficial sclerotic features or as lichen sclerosus-like lesions are needed (Jagasia et al. 2015).

Assessments of skin are performed to look at the four anatomic levels of involvement, and the score is based on the percentage of area involved and the differentiation between non-sclerotic and sclerotic features:

1. Erythematous rash (epidermal involvement)
2. Movable sclerosis (dermal involvement)
3. Non-movable sclerosis, hidebound skin or involvement of subcutaneous tissue and facia (subcutaneous involvement)
4. Ulceration (full-thickness loss of epidermal tissue)

Points 1–3 are assessed using the 'rule of 9s' body surface area score. Local skin involvement below 20% body surface and the absence of sclerotic features is classified as 'mild'. Skin involvement between 20% and 50% is 'moderate' with more than 50% becoming 'severe' (Greinix 2008). This scoring system is effective in adults but less so in children; however, it is still used in children over the age of 1 year. Ulceration is recorded by measuring the diameter of the largest ulcer (Pavletic et al. 2006). The skin is often very fragile and becomes damaged easily with poor healing of any wound. Distinctive features of cGvHD that are not seen in aGvHD are depigmentation although this occurs gradually and may only be perceptible over long time periods and papulosquamous lesions, although this alone is not enough for a diagnosis. It must be made in combination with other signs or confirmed with biopsy. Common features of both acute and chronic GvHD are erythema, maculopapular rash and pruritis (Jagasia et al. 2015). Itching is common and, therefore, should be recorded using a scale of 1–10 for severity with the patient asked what was the highest score this week (Pavletic et al. 2006).

Distinctive signs of nail cGvHD are longitudinal ridging, splitting or brittleness, onycholysis and loss of nails that is usually symmetric and affects most nails (Jagasia et al. 2015).

Loss of hair can be a devastating effect of cGvHD for patients, and in this context it is considered a distinctive feature alone. Hair has often returned following chemotherapy or radiother-apy, and the loss is often patchy and happens across the whole body. Patients may suffer with premature greying, thinning or brittleness of their hair (Jagasia et al. 2015).

11.6.3 Chronic GvHD of the Oral Cavity

For patients who have received stem cells derived from the bone marrow (BM), oral cGvHD is the most common site of involvement, and the oral cavity is the second most common site with PBSC (Meier et al. 2011). There are three components to mouth and oral mucosa assessment:

1. Mucosal involvement
2. Salivary gland involvement
3. Sclerotic involvement of mouth and surrounding tissues (Couriel et al. 2006b)

Within the oral cavity clinical diagnostic features include lichen planus-like changes. These are described as white lines and lacy-appearing lesions or plaque like changes. This can occur on any oral surface including the tongue and lips. The mouth will be dry (xerostomia) and have mucoceles, mucosal atrophy, ulcers and pseudo-membranes. Common features of both acute and chronic GvHD are gingivitis, mucositis, erythema and pain (Jagasia et al. 2015). If new lesions occur >3 years post-transplant, secondary malignancy should be excluded with biopsy. The lesion often starts as leukoplakia and can be confused with cGvHD but may be a squamous cell carcinoma (SCC) (Couriel et al. 2006b).

Chronic GvHD of the mouth is scored on three areas using the standard 0–3 scale with a percentage of area involved:

1. Erythema
2. Lichenoid
3. Ulcers

Oral sensitivity is measured on a self-score system from 1 to 10, with worst it has been for the past week (Pavletic et al. 2006). The consequences of oral cGvHD in cases of hyposalivation and xerostomia are in relation to the function of saliva and lack thereof. Poor protection against oral infections and mechanical and chemical epithelial injuries can occur. Remineralisation is impaired that can lead to dental caries, speech may be altered and eating becomes problematic (Meier et al. 2011; Treister et al. 2013).

11.6.4 Chronic GvHD of the Eyes

New onset of dry, gritty or painful eye with cicatricial conjunctivitis, keratoconjunctivitis sicca and confluent areas of punctate keratopathy are distinctive features and may occur in isolation with no other active cGvHD (Couriel et al. 2006b). Lacrimal dysfunction or destruction is responsible for dry eye symptoms (Pavletic et al. 2006). Patients may describe photophobia, burning, irritation; pain, a foreign body sensation, blurred vision and paradoxically excessive tearing. Scoring of eyes is based on frequency of use of eye drops and the occurrence of keratoconjunctivitis sicca. Asymptomatic keratoconjunctivitis sicca or need for eye drops less than three times per day is classed as 'mild', whilst symptomatic and the need for more than three times daily eye drops +/− punctual plugs is 'moderate'. Those with 'severe' ocular cGvHD are unable to work because of ocular symptoms or require special eyewear to relieve pain or have loss of vision due to keratoconjunctivitis sicca (Greinix 2008).

11.6.5 Chronic GvHD of the Genitalia

Patients who suffer from oral cGvHD are also very likely to have some degree of genital cGvHD. This affects both men and women and is significantly under-reported. In women vaginal scarring and clitoral/labial agglutination occur, and in men phimosis and urethral/meatus scarring are features. In both sexes, lichen planus-like and lichen sclerosis features are diagnostic. It is essential due to the under-reporting of symptoms that patients are examined for early signs especially if oral features are present. Studies suggest

that 3–15% of women have vulvar or vaginal cGvHD (Couriel et al. 2006b). The diagnosis relies heavily on sign and symptom reporting. Symptoms in women may include dryness, burning, pruritis, pain to touch, dysuria and dyspareunia. Signs include patchy or generalised erythema, mucosal erosions or fissures, labial resorption, circumferential fibrous vaginal banding, vaginal shortening and complete vaginal stenosis. Female genital tract involvement is scored as 'mild' if any erythema on vulvar mucosal surfaces, vulvar lichen planus or vulvar lichen sclerosis exists. Those with any erosive inflammatory changes of the vulvar mucosa or fissures in the vulvar folds are scored as 'moderate'. Severe scores are when there is labial fusion, clitoral hood agglutination, fibrinous vaginal adhesions, circumferential fibrosis vaginal banding, vaginal shortening, synechia, dense sclerotic changes and complete vaginal stenosis (Couriel et al. 2006b).

In the absence of diagnostic manifestations of cGvHD in other organs, histological evidence is strongly recommended and ruling out of oestrogen deficiency or infection with yeast, HPV or bacteria (Couriel et al. 2006b). A referral pathway to the gynaecologist and if possible one with an interest in assessing these patients should be implemented.

Men may have painful intercourse and a burning sensation on micturition. Signs include noninfectious balanoposthitis, lichen sclerosis-like or lichen planus-like features, phimosis or urethra or meatus scarring or stenosis (Jagasia et al. 2015). Signs of lichen planus-like features are classed as 'mild', lichen sclerosis-like features or moderate erythema is 'moderate', and 'severe' signs are phimosis or urethral or meatal scarring.

11.6.6 Chronic GvHD of the Gastrointestinal (GI) Tract

Gastrointestinal tract symptoms occur frequently, and oesophageal web, stricture or concentric rings demonstrated on endoscopy or imaging are diagnostic features for GI cGvHD. Patients may have dysphagia, odynophagia, heartburn, anorexia, nausea, vomiting, abdominal pain, cramping, diarrhoea, weight loss and malnutrition, and these are all common features present in both acute and chronic GvHD as well as other aetiologies. It is important to make a firm diagnosis before commencing treatment. Diarrhoea should be investigated with stool culture and virology examination to exclude *C. diff* and CMV in particular (Couriel et al. 2006b). Patients may also suffer from pancreatic atrophy and exocrine insufficiency that causes malabsorption and can respond to pancreatic enzyme supplementation (Jagasia et al. 2015). For upper GI, early satiety, anorexia or nausea and vomiting are scored on occasional symptoms with little reduction in oral intake during the past week being 'mild'; a 'moderate' score of cGvHD as intermittent symptoms with some reduction in oral intake during the past week; and 'severe' if the patient has persistent symptoms throughout the day with a marked reduction in oral intake on almost every day of the past week. Lower GI disturbance with diarrhoea will score 'mild' if the patient has occasional loose or liquid stool on some days throughout the week. If the patient is having intermittent loose or liquid stool throughout the day, on almost every day of the last week without requiring intervention to prevent or correct volume depletion scores as 'moderate'. Those with 'severe' disease have voluminous diarrhoea on almost every day of the past week requiring intervention to prevent or correct volume depletion.

11.6.7 Chronic GvHD of the Liver

The liver has no firm diagnostic features of cGvHD, and all other causes need to be excluded, e.g. viral infections, biliary obstruction and drug toxicity. A biopsy if possible can help but carries a high risk of bleeding and is therefore not frequently performed; imaging may be useful to exclude liver abscess, infiltration or gall bladder disease (Couriel et al. 2006b). Patients may present in two ways, with a liver function test showing a steep rise in serum ALT, with or without jaundice or transaminitis, or as a progressive cholestatic picture with elevation of serum alkaline

phosphatase and GGT followed by jaundice (Jagasia et al. 2015). Any elevation of liver enzymes greater than twice normal may be regarded as 'mild', 2.5 times upper limit of normal as 'moderate' and 'severe' if five times.

11.6.8 Chronic GvHD Pulmonary System

Historically for a firm diagnosis of pulmonary cGvHD, a biopsy was essential to prove bronchiolitis obliterans (BO); however, as there was a high risk of bleeding, it is now accepted that a diagnosis of bronchiolitis obliterans syndrome (BOS) can be made following pulmonary function testing (PFT). Pre-transplant screening is essential to obtain a baseline PFT with post-transplant PFT at 3 months and 1 year or more frequently if the patient develops signs as patients remain asymptomatic with an insidious onset of symptoms (Flowers and Martin 2015). A new onset of an obstructive lung defect is indicative of BOS. Clinically the patient may be short of breath on exertion and have a cough or wheeze, but these may be later effects. There are strict criteria for BOS and all need to be met for a diagnosis:

1. FEV1/VC < 0.7 or the 5th percentile of predicted.
   (a) FEV1 = forced expiratory volume in 1 s.
   (b) VC = vital capacity (forced vital capacity (FVC) or slow vital capacity (SVC), whichever is greater).
   (c) The 5th percentile of predicted is equivalent to the lower value of predicted confidence interval.
   (d) For paediatric patients or elderly populations, use < predicted confidence interval using NHANESIII calculations.

2. %FEV1 <75% of predicted with >10% decline over less than 2 years. %FEV1 should not correct to >75% with salbutamol, and the rate of decline for the corrected values should still remain at >10% decline over 2 years.

3. Absence of infection in the respiratory tract, documented with investigations directed by clinical symptoms, such as radiologic studies (radiographs or computed tomographic scans) or microbiologic cultures (sinus aspiration, upper respiratory tract viral screen, sputum culture, bronchoalveolar lavage).
4. Either one distinctive manifestation of chronic GVHD or another supporting feature of BOS.

Air trapping by expiratory chest high-resolution CT or small airway thickening or bronchiectasis or trapping on PFT where there is a residual volume of >120% or residual volume/total lung capacity >120% predicted is supporting evidence for BOS (Jagasia et al. 2015).

11.6.9 Chronic GvHD of the Musculoskeletal System

Diagnostic features of the musculoskeletal system include fascial involvement usually of the forearms or legs, but frequently affecting the abdomen and chest wall with sclerosis of the overlying skin and subcutaneous tissue and joint stiffness or contractures that can develop and severely impact on quality of life (Jagasia et al. 2015). The degree of functional impairment is scored as 'mild' if there is mild tightness of arms or legs, normal or mild decreased range of movement (ROM) and does not affect activities of daily living (ADL). Where there is tightness of arms or legs or joint contractures, erythema thought due to fasciitis, a moderate decrease of ROM and mild to moderate limitation of ADL scores as 'moderate'. For 'severe' then the patient will have contractures with significant decrease of ROM and significant limitation of ADL, e.g. unable to tie shoe laces, button a shirt or dress self.

11.7 Scoring of Chronic GvHD

The global scoring system of NIH 2014 was developed to be suitable for clinical trial assessments and reflects the clinical impact of cGvHD on the

Table 11.1 NIH global severity of chronic GvHD

Mild chronic GvHD
   1 or 2 organs involved (not lung) *plus*
   Score in involved organs 1 *plus*
   Lung score 0
Moderate chronic GvHD
   3 or more organs involved *plus*
   Score of 1 in each organ
      OR
   Atleast 1 organ (not lung) with a score of 2
      OR
   Lung score 1
Severe chronic GvHD
   1 organ with a score of 3
      OR
   Lung score of 2 or 3
Key points
1. In skin: Higher of the two scores to be used for calculating global severity.
2. In lung: FEV1 is used instead of clinical score for calculating global severity.
3. If a non-GvHD documented cause unequivocally explains the entire organ abnormality, then the organ is not scored for global severity. If the abnormality is thought to be multifactorial, it is scored without attribution from non-GvHD causes.

Jagasia et al. (2015) with permission

patient's functional status and organ impairment and is defined by Jagasia et al. 2015 as (Table 11.1):

11.8 Assessment of Response

Pavletic et al. (2006) proposed a set of measures for assessing the response to treatment of cGvHD patients. These should be performed at 3 monthly intervals or whenever a major change occurs. Organ-specific measures should be recorded from clinical signs and symptoms, and a global rating of mild/moderate/severe made. Assessment with non-specific ancillary measures such as grip strength, 2-min walk test (or Activity Scale for Kids (ASK)) and Karnofsky score with a quality of life score (QoL) are recommended. Quality of life assessment tools such as SF-36 or FACT-BMT in adults or CHRIs (Child Health Ratings Inventories) in children can be used.

11.9 Treatment of Chronic GvHD

The long-term aim of cGvHD therapy is for the patient to develop immune tolerance and reduce the morbidity. This is recognised by the ability to withdraw immunosuppression without a flare of symptoms. Most therapeutic options focus on the development of immunosuppressive agents and the ex vivo removal of the unfractionated donor T-cell population from the stem cell graft (Greinix 2008). The mainstay of treatment has for more than 30 years been the use of systemic steroids, usually with a starting dose of 1 mg/kg per day with or without calcineurin inhibitor (CNI). Steroids have a multitude of side effects such as toxicities, diabetes, weight gain, bone loss, myopathy, hypertension, mood swings, cataracts, avascular necrosis and an increase in infections (Flowers and Martin 2015).

Treatment for cGvHD is far from satisfactory with only approximately 50% of patients responding to systemic steroids with or without calcineurin inhibitors and less than 20% of patients alive without disability at 4 years. Combinations of steroids with azathioprine, thalidomide, mycophenolate mofetil or hydroxychloroquine in randomised trials have not yielded any benefit over steroids alone for survival or duration of therapy (Flowers and Martin 2015). Despite this, steroids still offer the best first-line treatment choice for those with cGvHD and should be started as soon as a diagnosis is made.

There are a number of second-, third- and fourth-line therapies available, and approximately 50% of patients will require alternatives within 2 years of initial therapy due to progression of cGvHD (Flowers and Martin 2015).

11.9.1 Second-Line, Third-Line and Other Therapies for Chronic GvHD

Below is a brief list of second- and third-line therapies for cGvHD; it is not exhaustive by any means, and many treatments are used following limited evidence from small non-randomised trials. The choice for further therapies is in most part governed by the features of cGvHD and the toxicities that may be inflicted as well as the availability of the drug locally. The lack of consistently effective treatment in this setting underscores the need for high-quality clinical trials. Please refer to local policies and guidance with respect to second-line and subsequent therapies.

Extracorporeal photopheresis (ECP) is widely used in mucocutaneous cGvHD as a second-line therapy in steroid refractory patients and has been shown to be effective in up to 80% of patients (Couriel et al. 2006b). A UK consensus paper supported the findings and recommended ECP use in this group, with paired sessions every 2 weeks with reassessment at 3 months (Scarisbrick et al. 2008).

Imatinib, a tyrosine kinase inhibitor licenced for use in chronic myeloid leukaemia (CML), has gained in popularity over the past few years. Experiments have shown reduction in fibrosis possibly from a dual inhibition process of transforming growth factor beta and platelet-derived growth factor pathways (Dignan et al. 2012).

Sirolimus mTOR inhibitors such as sirolimus may be used in combination with other agents but with caution in CNI due to increased risk of thrombotic microangiopathy and hyperlipidaemia.

Rituximab is commonly used in haematology for B-cell malignancy and is a potent anti-CD20 monoclonal antibody, and there is some limited evidence of its use in cGvHD for musculoskeletal and cutaneous manifestations (Dignan et al. 2012).

Mesenchymal stem cells (MSC) (Ringden and Keating 2011) have generated considerable interest in treatment of aGvHD following initial studies from the group at the Karolinska Institute. There was some evidence from early experiments that MSC worked in autoimmune disorders, and given the fact that cGvHD may resemble this in some ways, MSC have been used for cGvHD treatment but remain mainly within clinical trials.

Infliximab, an antitumour necrosis factor (TNF) antibody, is a chimeric human anti-TNFa-IgG1(j) monoclonal antibody that inhibits the binding of

TNF to its cellular receptors and has been used in some cases of GI GvHD (Dignan et al. 2012).

Thalidomide inhibits angiogenesis, expression of adhesion molecules, TNFa, interleukin-6, interleukin-12 and nuclear factor kappa B activity. A randomised clinical trial of thalidomide, ciclosporin and prednisolone compared to ciclosporin and prednisolone did not show any additional benefit in the primary treatment of cGvHD. Thalidomide has significant side effects including constipation, neuropathy, neutropenia, thrombocytopenia, tiredness and thrombosis (Dignan et al. 2012).

11.9.2 Topical Treatments for cGvHD of the Eyes

The aim of treatment is to give symptomatic relief of dry eye and care should be co-ordinated with an experienced ophthalmologist. Focus is placed upon increasing ocular surface moisture via lubrication and decreasing tear evaporation and tear drainage from the eye and decreasing ocular surface inflammation. Preservative-free drops coat the eye surface minimising dry spots on the cornea, decreasing ocular symptoms and improving vision. It may take several different trials of drops to find one that works as patients may be more sensitive to one solution. Temporary (with punctual plugs) or permanent (with cauterisation) occlusion of the tear duct may offer a solution to those with severe dry eye. Where there is inflammation of the ocular surface, direct application of steroid eye drops may be beneficial especially if the patient is on a taper of systemic immunosuppression and the eye symptoms flare (Couriel et al. 2006b).

Ciclosporin eye drops appear to offer a solution, but they cause irritation in most patients, and thus compliance is poor. If available, autologous serum eye drops may decrease surface inflammation.

11.9.3 Topical Treatments for Oral cGvHD

Management of oral cGvHD aims to alleviate symptoms of dry mouth, sensitivity and pain whilst maintaining oral function and restoring mucosal integrity (Meier et al. 2011). It may appear obvious, but the single most important action for patients is to maintain good oral hygiene (daily care and regular dental visits). Children's toothpaste causes less irritation and should be used with a soft toothbrush, with the addition of lip salve if appropriate. Suggest also avoidance of potential triggers for flares of cGvHD such as spicy or hot food or sharp foodstuffs that can cause damage. Sip water and chew sugar-free gum to improve xerostomia.

Often patients require systemic therapy as multiple sites are involved. However, the oral cavity can be refractory to systemic therapy; thus complementary topical treatment is needed. There are a variety of topical steroid mouthwashes that are the first line of therapy, including prednisolone, budesonide or betamethasone. Tacrolimus 0.1% mouthwash is well tolerated and has shown to be an effective option and may be used alongside steroid mouthwashes as second-line therapy. It is important to describe adequately how to use these preparations as in many cases this is not their usual route of administration. Several centres in Europe have access to phototherapy with ultraviolet A and B light. This stems from work in cutaneous cGvHD. A glass fibre extension of an UVA source is used for manual intraoral application three to four times a week (Meier et al. 2011).

To relieve oral pain, topical application of local anaesthetics such as lidocaine can be applied, either as a gel, mouthwash or spray. These should be used with caution as the gag reflex may be compromised and lead to choking and aspiration.

11.9.4 Ancillary and Supportive Care for cGvHD of the Skin

Chronic GvHD of the skin remains the most affected organ and is often debilitating when in extremis. Topical treatments are a vital therapy in addressing the manifestations of itch, rash, pain and dyspigmentation, whilst the use of physical therapy helps patients with limited range of movement maintain some degree of functionality. Other healthcare providers such as tissue viability and infection control teams can offer help, guidance and support when skin becomes friable and breaks down leaving ulcers, erosions and superadded infections. The patient with cutaneous cGvHD is at an increased risk of skin cancer, and regular monitoring and assessment are advised. Any suspicion should be followed up with biopsy. Advice with respect to UV exposure should be given regularly: avoiding direct sun exposure and using sun blocks and sunscreens and loose fitting clothing with hat and glasses.

Emollients are the backbone of skin care to maintain the integrity of unbroken dry skin and can be applied frequently throughout the day. It is therefore important to work with the patient to ensure the prescribed product is one they are happy with and addresses their issues; otherwise they are unlikely to use it regularly enough for it to be effective (see section on aGvHD). It is worth noting they may need more than one product; areas of extreme scaling or with plaques, for example, will require an ointment (commonly on the lower limbs), whereas areas with delicate skin will require a lighter product (e.g. the face). Whilst emollients tend to be petroleum based, using a product which incorporates lipids (e.g. coconut oil in QV cream) will help 'nourish' the skin in addition to providing a barrier.

Topical steroids are initiated in a stepwise fashion, attempting to deliver the least potent steroid to achieve the result desired. Lower strength steroid hydrocortisone can be applied to the face as can Eumovate under strict supervision, whilst the more potent Dermovate and Betnovate should be applied to the body only.

Pruritis is common and can be a distressing symptom. Itch usually responds to systemic therapy, i.e. antihistamines; however, topical antipruritic with menthol such as Dermacool (0.5–1%) may be applied if still problematic (Couriel et al. 2006b). It is important to note however that such products must be used with care. Widespread use can lead to alteration in thermoregulation, and the patient will feel very cold. It is therefore important to use a maximum of twice daily and on targeted areas only. Night time is often the worst, and as such, one application at bedtime may be sufficient.

Once the skin barrier has become breached, bacterial, viral and fungal tests should be taken and, if infection confirmed, treated rapidly. If swabs do not support an infective cause, it is important to rule out other pathologies; the ulcer may be as a consequence of vasculitis, malignancy, drug reaction or dermatitis and will need appropriate management (Couriel et al. 2006b).

One of the major challenges for topical management of chronic skin GvHD is the often severe sclerotic features – characterised by thickened, tight and fragile skin. This is often associated with poor wound healing, inadequate lymphatic drainage and skin ulcers from minor trauma or idiopathic origin. There is basic advice which should be given and regularly reinforced to all patients:

- Take care to minimise risk of bumps/knocks.
- Pat skin dry – no rubbing.
- Wear loose clothing to minimise risk of friction/irritation.
- Avoid the sun as much as possible.
- Maintain a good oral intake (water).
- Minimise/avoid the use of perfumes directly onto the skin (advise to spray onto clothes instead); make-up, if used, suggest minimal skin applications, researching into good quality products and protect the skin by initial application of a moisturiser.
- Provide clear, consistent and repeated reinforcement regarding the importance of regular use of emollients.

11.9.5 Wound Care

As previously stated, patients with cutaneous cGvHD are at high risk of skin breakdown. Any breaks must be taken seriously as they will quickly turn into chronic wounds if not managed effectively.

If a lesion is superficial, it may be possible to contain it by the use of a hydrocolloid dressing (e.g. DuoDerm extra thin). These are dressings which form a waterproof, protective layer over the lesion, are typically self-adhering and maintain a moist environment to encourage healing. They generally only require changing every

3–4 days, so although they do absorb exudate, they would not be appropriate for a highly exuding wound. Equally, it is advisable to clean the wound with a topical antimicrobial solution (e.g. Octenilin) to minimise risk of high bacterial load in the wound bed. Because of the fragility of skin affected by cGvHD, to minimise risk of maceration and to facilitate adherence of the dressing, it is advisable to apply a barrier film (e.g. Cavilon or Sorbaderm) to the surrounding epithelium prior to application of the dressing.

In the case of cavity lesions, extra precautions are required. Wound healing in this patient cohort will commonly be slower (see below), and as such lesions are at risk of bacterial colonisation/infection thus further delaying the healing process.

Healing results from the interaction of platelets, with cells such as neutrophils, macrophages, fibroblasts and keratinocytes combined with extracellular matrix (ECM) components, such as fibronectin, tenascin and collagens. Interface with ECM components is regulated by mediators such as cytokines and growth factors (e.g. interleukins, interferons and TNF-α) (Olczyk et al. 2014). The inflammatory response is triggered, and components such as growth factors facilitate proliferation, differentiation and metabolism of cells involved in the healing process. Others help regulate inflammatory processes and play a chemotactic role (encouraging cell movement) for neutrophils, macrophages, fibroblasts and epithelial cells (keratinocytes) to stimulate angiogenesis and the formation of ECM (Olczyk et al. 2014).

Because this cohort of patients will commonly be experiencing disruption to levels of the components required to facilitate healing due to systemic management of GvHD, wound healing becomes ever more complex and challenging.

In addition to the issue summarised above, if a wound becomes infected, this can initiate a 'flare' of acute GvHD requiring more intensive management and potentially compounding the situation.

Bioburden can be compounded if there is a significant amount of slough on the wound surface or in cases where the patient presents with a thick layer of eschar over the wound surface.

Debridement can contribute to a significant decrease in the bacterial load on the wound surface; there are several methods which can be used:

- *Autolytic debridement* (breakdown of bacterial cells), the use of moist dressing such as hydrogels or hydrocolloids may facilitate this.
- *Surgical debridement*, with scissors or scalpel, however this should be undertaken with caution and by experienced tissue viability nurses/ trained medical personnel.
- *Mechanical debridement*, pulse lavage, gentle washing, there are pulse lavage systems available; they have the benefit that they stimulate blood flow to the area, which can speed up granulation. Standing under the shower (especially a 'power shower') prior to dressing can have a similar effect, if the lesion is in an appropriate place.
- *Biological debridement*, with larvae of *Lucilia sericata* (green bottle fly). Use of larvae can be considered; however, it should only be used with the supervision of an experienced tissue viability nurse. Larvae of the green bottle fly, introduced into a wound (usually in a sterile bag), can remove necrotic, sloughy and/or infected tissue; they can also be used to maintain a clean wound after debridement. Larvae should only be considered when other avenues have been exhausted. They do not digest healthy tissue; however in some cases of cGvHD, the tissue in the wound bed has such a poor blood supply that it will not be differentiated by the larvae as healthy and they may start to digest it if not carefully supervised.

To pre-empt the risk of infection, there should be a very low threshold for using antimicrobial wound irrigation solution to cleanse wounds and surrounding skin. An additional precaution is to pack the wound with a hydrofibre (e.g. Aquacel), which turns into a gel on contact with exudate and contains any bacteria within the gel. These dressings can be obtained with ionic silver (Aquacel Ag) to facilitate extra protection. If the wound is 'dry', dampen the hydrofibre prior to packing to prevent adherence to the wound bed. Although hydrofibres minimise the risk of maceration, it is still preferable to protect the surrounding skin with a barrier film; this will also facilitate adherence of the secondary dressing to the classically flaky skin of someone with cGvHD.

If the wound is not responding, collagen dressings can be used to try and facilitate effective healing (e.g. Promogran Prisma). Collagen is a key component of a healing wound. Due to issues such as bioburden, repeated trauma and ongoing immunosuppression, wounds in the patient with cGvHD can halt at the inflammatory phase, thus compounding the chronicity of the wound and impeding the formation of the 'scaffold' needed for cell migration. This will ultimately limit any formation of extracellular matrix (ECM) and granulation tissue (Brett 2008). Collagen-based wound dressings are uniquely suited to address this issue by acting as a substitute substrate, plus collagen breakdown products are chemotactic for cells required for the formation of granulation tissue (Brett 2008). In addition, collagen-based dressings have the ability to absorb wound exudate and maintain a moist wound environment and do not require removal at subsequent dressing changes. However, it is important to note that they remain inactive when dry, so where there is minimal exudate in the wound, it is important to dampen them before application.

11.10 Vulvovaginal GvHD

As with cGvHD in other parts of the body, symptoms associated with vulvovaginal GvHD (vv GvHD) may be attributable to other pathologies; *Candida* infection, for example, can cause discharge or itch, whilst hormone reduction/ menopause may be responsible for vaginal dryness/soreness. Such co-morbidities require diagnosis and appropriate treatment.

In women with chronic vvGvHD, mechanical and chemical irritants should be avoided. Washing with warm water, using products from such ranges as Oilatum or Dermol if required (rather than soap), cleaning in a front-to-back direction and then air-dried is to be advised. Bacteriostatic gels such as Replens may be used in the vagina for comfort as this adheres to the vaginal wall and has a long-lasting effect. Vulval and vaginal topical management can include steroid/immunosuppressant cream. In extreme cases, surgical interven-

tions may be required to release strictures and adhesion formation. In all cases, particularly if the woman is not sexually active, dilators lubricated with, for example, a lipid, such as coconut oil, should be thought about as a way of maintaining vaginal patency and capacity.

Crucially, it is important that these matters are addressed in a sensitive manner as there is often a psychological impact and it may be affecting any partnership the patient is in. For this reason, anyone working with these women needs to be skilled in offering them the opportunity to disclose any emotional concerns and, if necessary, refer them for expert counselling.

Body image and sexual dysfunction are significant problems for both men and women posttransplant and are especially problematic upon development of cGvHD. Counselling and early involvement with psych-oncology services are important to aid in maintaining normality in an abnormal situation.

11.11 Chronic Lung GvHD

Chronic lung GvHD may be treated with bronchodilators, inhaled corticosteroids, systemic steroids, montelukast and referral to a physical rehabilitation programme (Couriel et al. 2006b). Lung GvHD has a somewhat dismal outcome as it is not very responsive to any modality. Nurses and physiotherapists can help patients manage the distress and possible panic situations the patient may feel due to increasing breathlessness, by teaching complementary self-management skills such as breathing techniques, focused relaxation and stress management.

11.12 Connective Tissue Involvement in cGvHD

Patients with cGvHD affecting skin, joints and connective tissue will benefit from inclusion in an exercise rehabilitation programme along with occupational therapy. Functional losses associated with muscle loss, weakness, contractures and limb swelling lead to fatigue and a decreased ability to perform activities of daily living and often preclude patients from being able to return to work. Rehabilitation should aim to improve strength and mobility of joints and muscles and ideally should occur before permanent and lasting damage has set in (Couriel et al. 2006b). Such programmes should include family members where possible, as exercises need to be carried out on a regular basis to be effective, with the patient often needing support to do this. It can also be psychologically helpful to any family/carers involved as it allows them to feel confident to be part of the care of their loved one.

In addition to exercise, regular massage can help maintain flexibility and function of affected limbs. If there is fascial involvement, any massage provided will need to access these tissue layers to be effective. It is therefore important that the therapist providing this treatment has been trained in using such techniques. Again, it is possible to teach family members appropriate massage skills, which will improve the efficacy of therapy provided.

11.13 Quality of Life

QoL is severely compromised in cGvHD, with reports of fatigue, pain and GI upset. FACT-BMT QoL questionnaire studies have revealed that physical, sexual and social functioning is also lower with higher rates of depression and anxiety and adverse effects on social and family interactions. Depressive symptoms are more severe and last longer and often manifest when patients complain of loss of memory or poor concentration. Fatigue may be considered as a separate entity but is often mixed in with QoL, anxiety and depression. It may be described as a persistent and subjective state of tiredness that interferes with usual functioning and can continue for several years after transplant (Couriel et al. 2006b). Using questionnaires to assess these issues with individual patients is something which nurses can instigate to identify the impact of psychological morbidity in specific cases. These can be used as a framework to enable patients to express their concerns and structure a support programme to help manage specific issues – including onward referrals to appropriate professionals.

11.14 The Future

Considering the increased utilisation of HSCT, the morbidity and mortality associated with GvHD and the limitations inherent to contemporary therapies, novel approaches are urgently needed. Rationally designed treatments that inhibit deregulated pathways in malignant cells are typically the focus of 'targeted' therapy. In GvHD, the 'target' is elusive, as the goal is to carefully contain an overzealous but biologically normal immunologic response (Magenau and Reddy 2014). Success in prophylaxis and treatment of GvHD will depend on whether GvHD can be prevented without losing the antitumour effect. Improvements in the understanding of the pathophysiology will move clinicians towards this goal. Risk stratification and the emergence of a bedside GvHD test based on proteomics may be on the horizon and will ultimately then improve the outlook for this difficult-to-treat group of patients (Greinix 2008).

11.15 GvHD in Children

Data and research on GvHD in the paediatric population are limited with only a few studies specifically focused on children. Most studies are small, and children are often grouped into larger adult series (Baird et al. 2010). In this short review, we will emphasise on the specific aspects of paediatric GvHD primarily focusing on cGvHD.

Most of the literature on cGvHD has focused on adults. Although the clinical manifestation of cGvHD in children is similar to that in adults, the consequences of treatment and nonresponses are remarkably different in a growing organism (Lawitschka et al. 2012). Children with cGvHD are of particular interest, given their longer life expectancy and developmental issues following the complications of cGvHD and its therapy (Jacobsohn 2010; Jacobsohn et al. 2011). Compared with childhood cancer survivors who did not undergo transplantation, HSCT survivors have a substantially increased burden of serious chronic conditions and impairments involving every organ. A history of GvHD or presence of cGvHD contributes to increase rate of long-term complications in the paediatric transplant survivors (Chow et al. 2016). Chronic GvHD has negative effects on an individual's physical and mental health and can lead to the development of functional impairments and activity limitations over their lifetime (Baird et al. 2010) as well as reduced quality of life (Inagaki et al. 2015). However, paediatric cGvHD remains an understudied area of research (Jacobsohn et al. 2011); therefore, large paediatric multicentre studies are needed (Watkins et al. 2016).

11.15.1 Incidence and Risk Factors

Overall the rates of cGvHD are lower in children than adults (Champlin et al. 2000; Rocha et al. 2000). However, the incidence of cGvHD in the paediatric population is still substantial and has increased recently in association with the expanded use of peripheral blood stem cells and unrelated donors (Baird et al. 2010). Zecca et al. (2002) in a large paediatric study reported a cumulative probability of cGvHD of 27%; this probability is nearly half of the estimated probability of 40–50% described in adults. Flowers et al. (2011) published a large single-centre study of risk factors for aGvHD and cGvHD. The sample included both adult and paediatric patients; cGvHD was defined according to the NIH cGvHD criteria (Filipovich et al. 2005). The incidence of moderate to severe cGvHD in the paediatric patient was 28% (Watkins et al. 2016).

The risk factors for cGvHD in childhood are still poorly defined. Zecca et al. (2002) reported the risk factors associated with cGvHD in children: male patients transplanted from a female donor experience more cGvHD. Children with non-malignant disorders had a reduced risk of developing cGvHD. This might be due to the fact that children with these diseases do not benefit from GvHD since they do not need any graft-versus-malignancy effect, and therefore the most effective

pharmacologic strategies for both prevention and treatment of aGvHD were used in these patients. The condition of mixed donor chimerism is associated with reduced susceptibility to GvHD. Some of the children with non-malignant disorders (those with aplastic anaemia or with congenital immuno-deficiencies) are given less intensive preparative regimens, and it has been hypothesised that the cytokine storm, which is dependent on the intensity of the conditioning regimen, triggers development of GvHD. Malignant diseases and the use of mye-loablative protocol as well as TBI as part of the preparative regimen have an increased risk of classic aGvHD (Faraci et al. 2012). Older recipient and donor ages are another risk factor for cGvHD (Watkins et al. 2016).

11.15.2 Treatment

The major emphasis in GvHD has been on prevention, as results with treatment have been disappointing. Currently most centres use a combination of a calcineurin inhibitor (ciclosporin or tacrolimus) with short-course methotrexate (Jacobsohn 2008).

The treatment of cGvHD in paediatrics is highly variable and mostly extrapolated from the experience in adults. Although there is no proven standard therapy, prednisolone and ciclosporin are commonly used as frontline therapy. As steroids remain the basis of cGvHD therapy, the consequences of long-term steroid use in children are well described, and long-term harmful effects on growth and bone density persist even after discontinuation of therapy.

Other potential treatment strategies include extracorporeal photopheresis (as discussed earlier in this chapter) and the infusion of allogeneic human mesenchymal stem cells (MSC) for the treatment of aGvHD and cGvHD. Multiple MSC infusions are safe and effective for children with steroid-refractory aGvHD, especially when employed early in the disease course. Early treatment may be associated with reduced treatment-related mortality and better overall survival (Ball et al. 2013). MSC offer new potential modalities of treatments for paediatric cGvHD refractory to standard treatments (Lawitschka et al. 2012). The treatment in paediatric patients must take into consideration the potential effect on growth, nutrition, organ function, bone metabolism, hormonal balance, psychosocial aspects and immune reconstitution (Baird et al. 2010; Lawitschka et al. 2012).

The nursing management and care of children with GvHD are complex and require expert skills and knowledge as well as adjustment to the child/adolescent developmental need. Patients and families, who initially felt great relief to be cured from their primary disease, now face the challenge of a chronic devastating illness for which preventative and treatment strategies are suboptimal (Baird et al. 2010). The treatment and support of the children and their families require a multidisciplinary team care that will be able to provide a comprehensive response to all their needs.

Appendix
Appendix 1: Classification of Patients with Acute GVHD

Stage	Skin/maculopapular rash BSA	Liver bilirubin (mg/dl)	Gut (ml diarrhoea/day)
0	No rash	<34 umol/L	<500 ml/day
1	<25% of body surface area	34–50 umol/L	>500–999 ml/day or persistent nausea with histological evidence stomach/duodenum
2	25–50% of body surface area	51–102 umol/L	1000–1500 ml/day
3	>50% of body surface area	103–255 umol/L	>1500 ml/day
4	Generalised erythroderma with bullous formation and desquamation	>255 umol/L	Severe abdominal pain with or without ileus

Acute GvHD clinical grading modified Glucksberg/keystone criteria			
Grade	Skin	Liver	Gut
0	None	None	None
I	Stages 1–2	None	None
II	Stage 3	Stage 1	Stage 1
III	–	Stages 2–3	Stages 2–4
IV	Stage 4	Stage 4	–

Glucksberg et al. (1974) modified criteria taken from the EBMT 2008 revised edition of handbook with permission

Appendix 2: Scoring of Chronic GvHD

	SCORE 0	SCORE 1	SCORE 2	SCORE 3
PERFORMANCE SCORE: **KPS ECOG LPS**	Asymptomatic and fully active (ECOG 0; KPS or LPS 100%)	Symptomatic, fully ambulatory, restricted only in physically strenuous activity (ECOG 1, KPS or LPS 80-90%)	Symptomatic, ambulatory, capable of self-care, >50% of waking hours of bed (ECOG 2, KPS or LPS 60-70%)	Symptomatic, limited self-care, >50% of walking hours in bed (ECOG 3-4, KPS or LPS <60%)
SKIN † **SCORE % BSA** _GVHD features to be scored by BSA:_ **Check all that apply:** Maculopapular rash/erythema Lichen planus-like features Sclerotic features Papulosquamous lesions or ichthyosis Keratosis pilaris-like GVHD	No BSA involved	1-18% BSA	19-50% BSA	>50% BSA
SKIN FEATURES SCORE:	No sclerotic features		Superficial sclerotic features "not hidebound" (able to pinch)	**Check all that apply:** Deep sclerotic features "Hidebound" (unable to pinch) Impaired mobility Ulceration

Other skin GVHD features (NOT scored by BSA)
Check all that apply:
  Hyperpigmentation
  Hypopigmentation
  Poikiloderma
  Severe or generalized pruritus
  Hair involvement
  Nail involvement
  _Abnormality present but explained entirely by non-GVHD documented cause (specify):_________________

	No symptoms	Mild symptoms	Moderate	Severe symptoms with
MOUTH _Lichen planus-like features present:_ **Yes** **No**	No symptoms	Mild symptoms **with** disease signs but not limiting oral intake significantly	Moderate symptoms with disease signs **with** partial limitation of oral intake	Severe symptoms with disease signs on examination **with** major limitation of oral intake

_Abnormality present but explained entirely by non-GVHD documented cause (specify):_________________

	SCORE 0	SCORE 1	SCORE 2	SCORE 3
EYES *Keratoconjunctivitis sicca (KCS) confirmed by ophthalmologist:* **Yes** **No** **Not examined**	No symptoms	Mild dry eye symptoms not affecting ADL (requirement of lubricant eye drops $\leq$ 3 × per day)	Moderate dry eye symptoms partially affecting ADL (requirement lubricant eye drops > 3 × per day or punctal plugs), **WITHOUT** new vision impairment due to KCS	Severe dry eye symptoms significantly affecting ADL (special eyeware to relieve pain) **OR** unable to work because of ocular symptoms **OR** loss of vision due to KCS

*Abnormality present but explained entirely by non-GVHD documented cause (specify):*_________________

	SCORE 0	SCORE 1	SCORE 2	SCORE 3
GI Tract ***Check all that apply:*** Esophageal web/ proximal stricture or ring Dysphagia Anorexia Nausea Vomiting Diarrhea Weight loss $\geq$ 5%* Failure to thrive	No symptoms	Symptoms without significant weight loss*(<5%)	Symptoms associated with mild to moderate weight loss* (5-15%) **OR** moderate diarrhea without significant interference with daily living	Symptoms associated with significant weight loss* >15%, requires nutritional supplement for most calorie needs **OR** esophageal dilation **OR** severe diarrhea with significant interference with daily living

*Abnormality present but explained entirely by non-GVHD documented cause (specify):*_________________

	SCORE 0	SCORE 1	SCORE 2	SCORE 3
LIVER	Normal total bilirubin and ALT or AP <3 x ULN	Normal total bilirubin and ALT $\geq$3 to 5 x ULN or AP $\geq$ 3 x ULN	Elevated total bilirubin but $\leq$3 mg/dL or ALT > 5 ULN	Elevated total bilirubin > 3 mg/dL

*Abnormality present but explained entirely by non-GVHD documented cause (specify):*_________________

	SCORE 0	SCORE 1	SCORE 2	SCORE 3
LUNGS** **Symptom score:**	No symptoms	Mild symptoms (shortness of breath after climbing one flight of steps)	Moderate symptoms (shortness of breath after walking on flat ground)	Severe symptoms (shortness of breath at rest; requiring O_2)
Lung score: % FEV1	FEV1$\geq$80%	FEV1 60-79%	FEV1 40-59%	FEV1 $\leq$39%

Pulmonary function tests
    Not performed
*Abnormality present but explained entirely by non-GVHD documented cause (specify):*_________________

	SCORE 0	SCORE 1	SCORE 2	SCORE 3
JOINTS AND FASCIA P-ROM score *(see below)* Shoulder (1-7):___ Elbow (1-7):___ Wrist/finger (1-7):___ Ankle (1-4):___	No symptoms	Mild tightness of arms or legs, normal or mild decreased range of motion (ROM) **AND** not affecting ADL	Tightness of arms or legs **OR** joint contractures, erythema thought due to fasciitis, moderate decrease ROM **AND** mild to moderate limitation of ADL	Contractures **WITH** significant decrease of ROM **AND** significant limitation of ADL (unable to tie shoes, button shirts, dress self etc.)

Abnormality present but explained entirely by non-GVHD documented cause (specify):________________

	SCORE 0	SCORE 1	SCORE 2	SCORE 3

GENITAL TRACT
(see Supplemental figure‡)
    Not examined
Currently sexually active
    Yes
    No
	No signs	Mild signs‡ and females with or without discomfort on exam	Moderate signs‡ and may have symptoms with discomfort on exam	Severe signs‡ with or without symptoms

Abnormality present but explained entirely by non-GVHD documented cause (specify):________________

<u>**Other indicators, clinical features or complications related to chronic GVHD (Check all that apply and assign a score to severity (0-3) based on functional impact where applicable non–0, mild-1, moderate-2, severe–3)**</u>

Ascites (serositis)___   Myasthenia Gravis___

Pericardial Effusion___   Peripheral Neuropathy___   Eosinophilia > 500/µl___

Pleural Effusion(s)___   Polymyositis___   Platelets <100,000/µl___

Nephrotic syndrome___   Weight loss>5%* without GI symptoms___   Others (specify) :_________

Overall GVHD Severity *(Opinion of the evaluator)*	❏ **No GVHD**	❏ **Mild**	❏ **Moderate**	❏ **Severe**

Photographic Range of Motion (P-ROM)

† Skin scoring should use both percentage of BSA involved by disease signs and the cutaneous features scales. When a Discrepancy exists between the percentage of total body surface (BSA) score and the skin feature score, OR if superficial sclerotic features are present (Score 2), but there is impaired mobility or ulceration (Score 3), the higher level should be used for the final skin scoring.

* Weight loss within 3 months.

** Lung scoring should be performed using both the symptoms and FEV1 scores whenever possible. FEV1 should be used in the final lung scoring where there is discrepancy between symptoms and FEV1 scores.
Abbreviations: ECOG (Eastern Cooperative Oncology Group), KPS(Karnofsky Performance Status), LPS(Lansky Performance Status); BSA(body surface area); ADL(activities of daily living); LFTs(liver function tests); AP (alkaline phosphatase); ALT (alanine aminotransferase); ULN(normal upper limit).

‡ To be completed by specialist or trained medical providers (see Supplemental Figure).

Name:_______________________________ **Date of birth:**______________ **Assessment date:**________________

	SCORE 0	SCORE 1	SCORE 2	SCORE 3
GENITAL TRACT (male or female)	☐ No signs	☐ Mild signs and females may have symptoms* WITH discomfort on exam	☐ Moderate signs and may have symptoms* with discomfort on exam	☐ Severe signs with or without symptoms*

Currently sexually active:
☐ Yes ☐ No

Check all signs that applies:

☐ Lichen planus-like features

☐ Lichen sclerosis-like features

☐ Vaginal scarring (female)

☐ Clitoral/labial agglutination (female)

☐ Labial resorption (female)

☐ Erosions

☐ Fissures

☐ Ulcers

☐ Phimosis (male)

☐ Urethral meatus scarring/ stenosis (male)

☐ *Abnormality present but <u>NOT</u> thought to represent GVHD (specify cause):*_______________________________

☐ *Abnormality thought to represent GVHD <u>PLUS</u> other causes (specify cause):*_______________________________

**Genital symptoms are not specific to cGVHD and can represent premature gonadal failure or genital tract infection.*

If a gynecologist is unavailable, external examination may be performed to determine "discomfort on exam" as follows:

a) Spread the labia majora to inspect the vulva for the above signs. Touch the vestibular gland openings (Skene's and Bartholin's), labia minora and majora gently with a qtip. Vulvar pain elicited by the gentle touch of a qtip is classified as discomfort on examination. Palpate the vaginal walls with a single digit to detect bands, shortening, narrowing or other signs of vaginal scarring.

b) If the woman is sexually active, determine whether qtip palpation or gentle palpation of scarred ridges elicits pain similar to that which the woman experiences during intercourse.

Female genitalia: Severity of signs:
1) Mild (any of the following); erythema on vulvar mucosal surfaces, vulvar lichen-planus or vulvar lichen-sclerosis
2) Moderate (any of the following); erosive inflammatory changes of the vulvar mucosa, fissures in vulvar folds
3) Severe (any of the following); labial fusion, clitoral hood agglutination, fibrinous vaginal adhesions, circumferential fibrous vaginal banding, vaginal shortening, synechia, dense sclerotic changes, and complete vaginal stenosis

Male genitalia: Diagnostic features include lichen planus-like or lichen sclerosis-like features and phymosis or urethral scarring or stenosis. Severity of signs: **Mild** – lichen planus-like feature; **Moderate** – lichen sclerosis-like feature or moderate erythema; **Severe** – phimosis or urethral/meatal scarring

Biopsy obtained: ☐ Yes ☐ No	**Site biopsied:**__________ **GVHD confirmed by histology:** ☐ Yes	☐ No
Change from previous evaluation: ☐ No prior or current GVHD ☐ Improved	☐ Stable	☐ Worse ☐ N/A (baseline)

Jagasia et al. (2015) with permission

References

Al-Kadhimi ZG, Chen W, Smith D, Abid M, Deol A, Ayash L, Lum L, Waller EK, Ratanatharathorn V, Uberti J. High incidence of severe acute graft-versus-host disease with tacrolimus and mycophenolate mofetil in a large cohort of related and unrelated allo-geneic transplantation patients. Biol Blood Marrow Transplant. 2014;20:979–85.

Baird K, Cooke K, Schultz KR. Chronic graft-versus-host disease (GvHD) in children. Pediatr Clin N Am. 2010;57:297–322.

Ball LM, et al. Multiple infusions of mesenchymal stromal cells induce sustained remission in children with steroid-refractory, grade III–IV acute graft-versus-host disease. Br J Haematol. 2013;163:501–9.

Baron F, Labopin M, Niederwieser D, Vigouroux S, Cornelissen JJ, Malm C, Vindelov LL, Blaise D, Janssen JJWM, Petersen E, Socie´ G, Nagler A,

Rocha V, Mohty M. Impact of graft-versus-host disease after reduced-intensity conditioning allogeneic stem cell transplantation for acute myeloid leukemia: a report from the Acute Leukemia Working Party of the European group for blood and marrow transplantation. Leukemia. 2012;26:2462–8.

Bladon J, Taylor P. The down regulation of IL1 and IL6, in monocytes exposed to ECP treated lymphocytes, is not dependent on lymphocyte phosphatidylserine externalisation. Transpl Int. 2006;19(4):319–24.

Billingham RE. The biology of graft-versus-host reactions. Harvey Lect. 1966–7;62:71–8.

Brett D. Review of collagen and collagen-based wound dressings. Wounds. 2008;20(12):347–56

Carpenter P. How I conduct a comprehensive chronic graft-versus-host disease assessment. Blood. 2011;118(10):2679–87.

Chow EJ, Anderson L, Baker KS, et al. Late effects surveillance recommendations among survivors of childhood hematopoietic cell transplantation: a children's oncology group report. Biol Blood Marrow Transplant. 2016;22:782–95.

Champlin RE, Schmitz N, Horowitz MM, et al. Blood stem cells compared with bone marrow as a source of hematopoietic cells for allogeneic transplantation. IBMTR Histocompatibility and Stem Cell Sources Working Committee and the European Group for Blood and Marrow Transplantation (EBMT). Blood. 2000;95:3702–9.

Couriel D, Carpenter PA, Cutler C, Bolaños-Meade J, Treister NS, Gea-Banacloche J, Shaughnessy P, Hymes S, Kim S, Wayne AS, Chien JW, Neumann J, Mitchell S, Syrjala K, Moravec CK, Abramovitz L, Liebermann J, Berger A, Gerber L, Schubert M, Filipovich AH, Weisdorf D, Schubert MM, Shulman H, Schultz K, Mittelman B, Pavletic S, Vogelsang GB, Martin PJ, Lee SJ, Flowers MED. Ancillary therapy and supportive care of chronic graft-versus-host disease: National Institutes of Health consensus development project on criteria for clinical trials in chronic graft-versus-host disease: V. ancillary therapy and supportive care working group report. Biol Blood Marrow Transplant. 2006a;12: 375–96.

Couriel DR, Hosing C, Saliba R, Shpall EJ, Anderlini P, Rhodes B, Smith V, Khouri I, Giralt S, de Lima M, Hsu Y, Ghosh S, Neumann J, Andersson B, Qazilbash M, Hymes S, Kim S, Champlin R, Donato M. Extracorporeal photochemotherapy for the treatment of steroid-resistant chronic GVHD. Blood. 2006b;107:3074–80.

Dignan FL, Clark A, Amrolia P, Cornish J, Jackson G, Mahendra P, Scarisbrick JJ, Taylor PC, Hadzic N, Shaw BE, Potter MN, On behalf of the Haemato-oncology Task Force of the British Committee for Standards in Haematology and the British Society for Blood and Marrow Transplantation. Diagnosis and management of acute graft-versus-host disease. Br J Haematol. 2012;158(1):30–45.

Flowers MED, Inamoto Y, Carpenter PA, Lee SJ, et al. Comparative analysis of risk factors for acute graft-versus-host disease and for chronic graft-versus-host disease according to National Institutes of Health consensus criteria. Blood. 2011;117:3214–9.

Flowers MED, Martin PJ. How we treat chronic graft versus host disease. Blood. 2015;125(4):606–15.

Filipovich AH, Weisdorf D, Pavletic S, et al. National Institutes of Health consensus development project on criteria for clinical trials in chronic graft-versus-host disease: I. Diagnosis and staging working group report. Biol Blood Marrow Transplant. 2005;11(12): 945–56.

Faraci M, Caviglia I, Biral E, et al. Acute graft-versus-host disease in pediatric allogeneic hematopoietic stem cell transplantation. Single-center experience during 10 yr. Pediatr Transplant. 2012;16:887–93.

Ferrara JL, Deeg HJ. Graft-versus-host disease. N Engl J Med. 1991;324:667–74.

Glucksberg H, Storb R, Fefer A, Buckner CD, Neiman PE, Clift RA, Lerner KG, Thomas ED. Clinical manifestations of graft-versus-host disease in human recipients of marrow from HL-A-matched sibling donors. Transplantation. 1974;18:295–304.

Greinix HT. Graft-versus-host disease. Bremen: UNI-MED Verlag AG; 2008.

Hill GR, Ferrara JLM. The primacy of the gastrointestinal tract as a target organ of acute graft-versus-host disease: rationale for the use of cytokine shields in allogeneic bone marrow transplantation. Blood. 2000;95:2754–9.

Inagaki J, Moritake H, Nishikawa T, et al. Long-term morbidity and mortality in children with chronic graft-versus-host disease classified by National Institutes of Health consensus criteria after allogeneic hematopoietic stem cell transplantation. Biol Blood Marrow Transplant. 2015;21:1973–80.

Jacobsohn DA. Acute graft-versus-host disease in children. Bone Marrow Transplant. 2008;41:215–21.

Jacobsohn DA. Optimal management of chronic graft-versus-host disease in children. Br J Haematol. 2010;150:278–92.

Jacobsohn DA, Arora M, Klein JP, et al. Risk factors associated with increased nonrelapse mortality and with poor overall survival in children with chronic graft-versus-host disease. Blood. 2011;118(16):4472–9.

Jacobsohn DA, Vogelsang GB. Acute graft versus host disease. Orphanet J Rare Dis. 2007;2:35.

Jagasia MH, Greinix HT, Arora M, Williams KM, Wolff D, Cowen EW, Palmer J, Weisdorf D, Treister NS, Cheng S, Kerr H, Stratton P, Duarte RF, McDonald GB, Inamoto Y, Vigorito A, Arai S, Datiles MB, Jacobsohn D, Heller T, Kitko CL, Mitchell SA, Martin PJ, Shulman H, Wu RS, Cutler CS, Vogelsang GB, Lee SJ, Pavletic SZ, Flowers MED. National Institutes of Health chronic graft-versus-host disease consensus for clinical trials: I. The 2014 diagnosis and staging working group report. Biol Blood Marrow Transplant. 2015;21(3):389–401.

Kuzmina Z, Greinix HT, Weigl R, Körmöczi U, Rottal A, Frantal S, Eder S, Pickl WF. Significant differences in B-cell subpopulations characterize patients with chronic graft-versus-host disease–associated dysgammaglobulinemia. Blood. 2011;117(7):2265–74.

Lawitschka A, Ball LM, Peters C. Nonpharmacologic treatment of chronic graft-versus-host disease in children and adolescents. Biol Blood Marrow Transplant. 2012;18:S74–81.

Lee SJ, Vogelsang G, Flowers MED. Chronic graft-versus-host disease. Biol Blood Marrow Transplant. 2003;9:215–33.

Lee SJ, Flowers MED. Recognizing and managing chronic graft-versus-host disease. In: Gewirtz AM, Muchmore EA, Burns LJ, editors. Haematology 2008: American Society of Haematology Education Program Book. Washington, DC: American Society of Haematology; 2008. p. 134–41.

Magenau J, Reddy P. Next generation treatment of acute graft-versus-host disease. Leukaemia. 2014;28:2283–91.

Martin PJ, Weisdorf D, Przepiorka D, Hirschfeld S, Farrell A, Rizzo JD, Foley R, Socie G, Carter S, Couriel D, Schultz KR, Flowers MED, Filipovich AH, Saliba R, Vogelsang GB, Pavletic SZ, Lee SJ. National Institutes of Health consensus development project on criteria for clinical trials in chronic graft-versus-host disease: VI. Design of clinical trials working group report. Biol Blood Marrow Transplant. 2006;12:491–505.

Meier JKH, Wolff D, Pavletic S, Greinix H, Gosau M, Bertz H, Lee SJ, Lawitschka A, Elad S. Oral chronic graft-versus-host disease: report from the international consensus conference on clinical practice in cGVHD. Clin Oral Invest. 2011;15:127–39.

Olczyk P, Mencner Ł, Komosinska-Vassev K. The role of the extracellular matrix components in cutaneous wound healing. BioMed Res Int. 2014. Published online 2014 Mar 17

Pavletic SZ, Martin P, Lee SJ, Mitchell S, Jacobsohn D, Cowen EW, Turner ML, Akpek G, Gilman A, McDonald G, Schubert M, Berger A, Bross P, Chien JW, Couriel D, Dunn JP, Fall-Dickson J, Farrell A, Flowers MED, Greinix H, Hirschfeld S, Gerber L, Kim S, Knobler R, Lachenbruch PA, Miller FW, Mittleman B, Papadopoulos E, Parsons SK, Przepiorka D, Robinson M, Ward M, Reeve B, Rider LG, Shulman H, Schultz KR, Weisdorf D, Vogelsang GB. Measuring therapeutic response in chronic graft-versus-host disease: National Institutes of Health consensus development project on criteria for clinical trials in chronic graft-versus-host disease: IV. Response criteria working group report. Biol Blood Marrow Transplant. 2006;12:252–66.

Przepiorka D, Weisdorf D, Martin P, Klingemann HG, Beatty P, Hows J, Thomas ED. 1994 consensus conference on AGvHD grading. Bone Marrow Transplant. 1995;15:825–8.

Ringden O, Keating A. Mesenchymal stromal cells as treatment for chronic GVHD. Bone Marrow Transplant. 2011;46:163–64

Rocha V, Wagner JE Jr, Sobocinski KA, et al. Graft-versus-host disease in children who have received a cord-blood or bone marrow transplant from an HLA identical sibling. Eurocord and International Bone Marrow Transplant Registry Working Committee on Alternative Donor and Stem Cell Sources. N Engl J Med. 2000;342:1846–54.

Scarisbrick JJ, Taylor P, Holtick U, Makar Y, Douglas K, Berlin G, Juvonen E, Marshall S, Photopheresis Expert Group. U.K. consensus statement on the use of extracorporeal photopheresis for treatment of cutaneous T-cell lymphoma and chronic graft-versus-host disease. Br J Dermatol. 2008;158:659–78.

Shulman HM, Sullivan KM, Weiden PL, McDonald GB, Striker GE, Sale GE, Hackman R, Tsoi MS, Storb R, Thomas ED. Chronic graft-versus-host syndrome in man. A long-term clinicopathologic study of 20 Seattle patients. Am J Med. 1980;69:204–17.

Treister N, Chai X, Kurland B, Pavletic S, Weisdorf D, Pidala J, Palmer J, Martin P, Inamoto Y, Arora M, Flowers M, Jacobsohn D, Jagasia M, Arai S, Lee SJ, Cutler C. Measurement of oral chronic GVHD: results from the chronic GVHD consortium. Bone Marrow Transplant. 2013;48:1123–8.

Vigorito AC, Campregher PV, Storer BE, Carpenter PA, Moravec CK, Kiem HP, Fero ML, Fero ML, Warren EH, Lee SJ, Applebaum FR, Martin PJ, Flowers MED. Evaluation of NIH consensus criteria for classification of late acute and chronic GvHD. Blood. 2009;114(3):702–8.

Watkins BK, Horan J, Storer B, Martin PJ, Carpenter PA, Flowers MED. Recipient and donor age impact the risk of developing chronic GvHD in children after allogeneic hematopoietic transplant. Bone Marrow Transplant. 2016;52(4):625–626. 1–2 advance online publication 19 December 2016. https://doi.org/10.1038/bmt.2016.328.

Weisdorf D, Haake R, Blazar B, Miller W, McGlave P, Ramsay N, Kersey J, Filipovich A. Treatment of moderate/severe acute graft-versus-host disease after allogeneic bone marrow transplantation: an analysis of clinical risk features and outcome. Blood. 1990;75:1024–30.

Wolf D, von Lilienfeld-Toal M, Wolf AM, Schleuning M, von Bergwelt-Baildon M, Held SEA, Brossart P. Novel treatment concepts for graft-versus-host disease. Blood. 2012;119(1):16–25.

Zecca M, Prete A, Rondelli R, Lanino E, Balduzzi A, Messina C, et al. Chronic graftversus-host disease in children: incidence, risk factors, and impact on outcome. Blood. 2002;100:1192–200.

Graft Versus Tumour Effect

Mairéad NíChonghaile

Abstract

The treatment of relapsed disease remains challenging, and it is well accepted that concept of allogeneic HSCT relies upon both the conditioning or preparative regimen used for the recipient and the graft versus malignancy (GvM) or leukaemia (GvL) effect provided by the donor T cells and NK cells. Strategies which involve harnessing this effect are crucial to success and need to be exploited and refined to improve outcome. Further research is required to identify new strategies and therapies to improve the outlook for patients who relapse post-HSCT.

The nursing challenges following relapse are immense; the psychological support required is complex and largely falls to the nurse to coordinate and deliver regardless of the selected treatment approach.

Keywords

Graft versus malignancy (GvM) or leukaemia (GvL) • Donor lymphocyte infusions (DLI) • Relapse • Chimerism

12.1 Introduction

It is well accepted that concept of allogeneic haematopoetic stem cell transplant (HSCT) relies upon both the conditioning or preparative regimen used for the recipient and the graft versus malignancy (GvM) or leukaemia (GvL) effect provided by the donor T cells and NK cells. The autoimmune attack on the malignancy helps to eradicate the disease in the recipient with the aid of the condition regimen. The susceptibility of a malignant condition being eradicated by GVM of GvL effect varies with the most sensitive conditions being chronic myeloid leukaemia, chronic lymphocytic leukaemia, low-grade B-lymphoproliferative disorders, mantle cell lymphoma and EBV lymphoproliferative conditions. Most other conditions have an intermediate sensitivity to the GvM or GvL effect with conditions that have a special proliferation or that are advanced or chemo-refractory having the least response.

M. NíChonghaile
HOPE Directorate, St James's Hospital,
Dublin, Ireland
e-mail: maireadnichonghaile@eircom.net

M. Kenyon, A. Babic (eds.), *The European Blood and Marrow Transplantation Textbook for Nurses*,
https://doi.org/10.1007/978-3-319-50026-3_12

12.2 Mechanism of GvM/GvL Effect

Both T lymphocytes and NK cells participate in the GvL effect, and it is believed that cytotoxic T cells recognise several classes of antigens on leukaemic cells. The NK cells target MMag self-proteins (present on the tissues of the recipient) which are overexpressed by the leukaemia, e.g. proteinase 3 and elastase tumour-specific antigens, e.g. Wilms tumour 1, and fused proteins, e.g. BCR-ABL, by using the perforin-granzyme pathway to kill their targets. However they are only activated when inhibitory signals from self (recipient) MHC class 1 molecules on the target are missing or overcome by activating signals through the NKG2D receptor. The suppressor of the recipient's immune system allows the donor cells to provoke this effect.

12.3 Minimal Residual Disease (MRD)

The purpose of monitoring MRD in the post-transplant setting is to track disease response or remission or low-level disease recurrence when the quantity of a particular marker starts to increase. This enables a therapeutic intervention to be implemented very early and may optimise the chance of success.

MRD can be monitored using molecular methods – this is where the underlying condition has a specific market or protein that can be monitored by using flow cytometry. Table 12.1 shows the cytogenetic abnormalities that can be targeted in some diseases (page 410 Treleaven and Barrett 2009), and Table 12.2 shows some of the molecular targets (Apperly et al. 2012) if they were present at diagnosis.

12.4 Chimerism

Chimerism analysis is another important tool in the post-HSCT follow-up of the recipient. It demonstrates the degree of engraftment of donor

Table 12.1 Common targets for MRD screening in different malignancies

Disease	MRD target
Myelodysplastic syndromes	Del(5q); monosomy 7, trisomy 8
Chronic myeloid leukaemia	t(9;22)
Acute myeloid leukaemia	t(8;21); inv (16)
Acute lymphoblastic leukaemia	t(9;22) t(4;11); t(8;14)
Follicular lymphoma	t(14;18)
Mantle cell lymphoma	t(11;14)
Chronic lymphocytic leukaemia	del(13q), del(11q); del(17p)
Multiple myeloma	del(13q), del(11q)

Table 12.2 Examples of Molecular targets in different malignacies

Disease	Molecular target
B-ALL	TEL-AML1
	BCR-ABL1
	Ig/TCR gene rearrangements
T-ALL	Ig/TCR gene rearrangements
	Tald1
APML	PML-RARA
AML	AML1-ETO
	CBFb-MYH11
	WT-1
	NPM1 mutated
	FlT3

cells and offers the possibility to identify impending graft rejection and can also be an indicator of disease relapse or recurrence. Chimerism can also be used as a basis for treatment intervention to prevent graft rejection and maintain engraftment and is used as a mechanism to administer pre-emptive immunotherapy to provoke the GvM or GvL effect particularly in high-risk patients.

Chimerism allows the monitoring of the ratio of donor- and recipient-derived cells in non-genetically identical donor and recipient pairs. This allows for timely intervention in the care of the recipient. The term "chimerism" comes from Greek mythology where the chimera was a fire-spitting monster with the head of a lion, body of a goat and the tail of a serpent and is used to describe the fact of two entities – DNA from two people – existing in the one person.

Initially it was felt that in order for all HSCT to be considered successful, an individual would have to be 100% donor chimerism, and this is certainly the case with malignant conditions. However, in non-malignant conditions (e.g. aplastic anaemia or haemoglobinopathies), a mixed chimerism may be enough to restore normal haematopoiesis.

While the total (unfractionated) chimerism result is important, more information can be elicited if lineage-specific chimerism is performed allowing separate tracking of lymphoid and myeloid engraftment and in itself can provide very useful information about possible disease relapse. This should be used in conjunction with other means of MRD analysis and diagnosis.

Schedule and protocols for chimerism analysis are centre, disease and treatment specific, and reference should be made to your institution's policy.

12.5 Management of Relapsed Disease

When a recipient has evidence of MRD or a decrease in chimerism, there are a number of strategies that can be followed. In the case of mixed chimerism, the schema in Fig. 12.1 can be followed.

Relapse usually occurs in the BM but may also be at extramedullary sites, thought to be due to immune escape from patrolling lymphocytes. It is also thought that leukaemia can escape from the immune control provided by the donor's T cells by mutating or becoming a more resistant clone of the original disease. The cause of the relapse may also be different in different haematological malignancies. While relapses can occur many years after HSCT suggesting that perhaps the underlying disease was never eradicated and was held in control by the donor immune system, it is more common with CML, and in this disease, the administration of DLI can often restore remission.

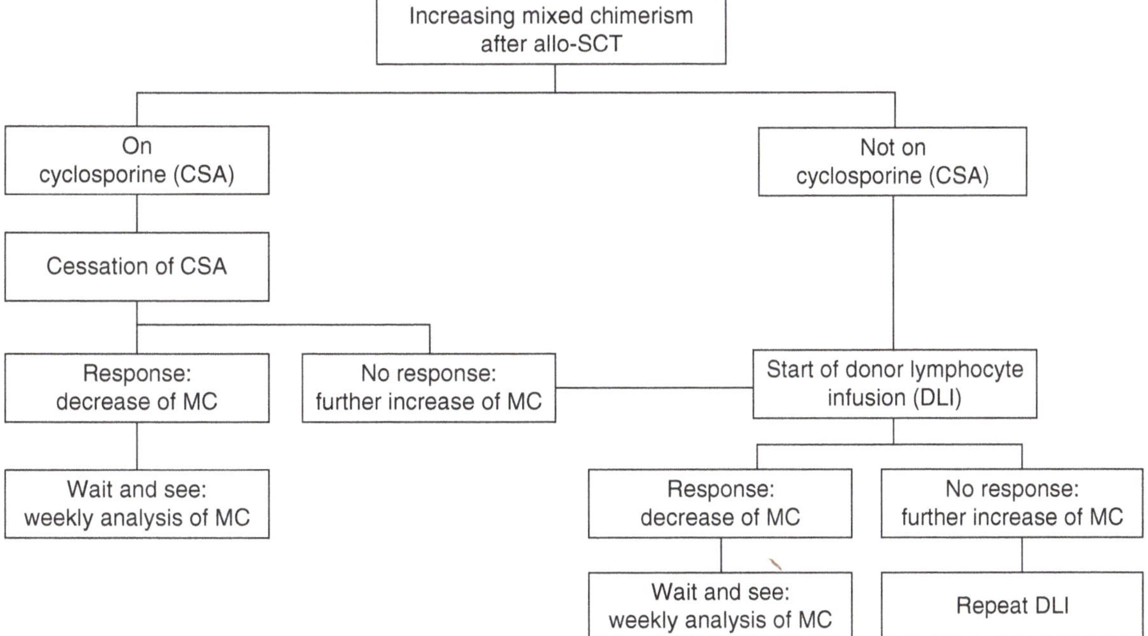

Fig. 12.1 Patients with increasing MC post transplant (5% or more autologous cells) compared to the previous sample are offered further therapy. Immunotherapy for patients receiving CSA consists of immediate discontinuation of the immunosuppressive agent. Chimerism is then assayed weekly until CC status is restored. If MC continues to increase after cessation of CSA, a DLI is given. Immunotherapy for patients not receiving CSA consisted of DLI as frontline treatment. The cell dose administered is based on the number and potential severity of HLA mismatches between the donor and recipient, and starting doses range from 2.5×10^4 to 1×10^6/kg BW. After DLI, chimerism status is assayed weekly until CC status is restored. Patients who show a further increase in MC are given an additional DLI after at least 3 weeks have elapsed. If no GVHD occurs, the dose of DLI is doubled (Bader et al. 2005)

However the outlook for the recipient who relapses post-HSCT is poor and requires frank discussion with the recipient and their family to define the likely outcomes and success. Care for the relapsed patient revolves around five potential strategies:

- Immunotherapy
- Chemotherapy
- Molecular targeting
- Supportive care
- Palliative care

The timing of relapse is extremely important. Early relapses are difficult to treat, and any intervention may be challenging for the patient or precluded due to the proximity to the HSCT and complications experienced by the recipients. Patients who relapse after HSCT may find it extremely difficult to adapt to and accept the fact that further treatment may not be possible or may be ineffective particularly if they have already received intensive treatment prior to HSCT.

However, it is important to provide ongoing support so that patients do not feel abandoned at this stage, and this helps patients to maintain realistic levels of hope and optimism. Palliative and supportive care measures are valid and realistic options to help maintain a good quality of life and should not be ignored. The help and support of the medical team, recipient's local doctor, referring hospital and often primary care services, e.g. GP and hospice, are essential in the management and treatment of the relapsed patient. Referral to psychology, counselling or psychiatric teams may also benefit the patient and their family.

12.6 Treatment Options for Post-allogeneic HSCT Relapse

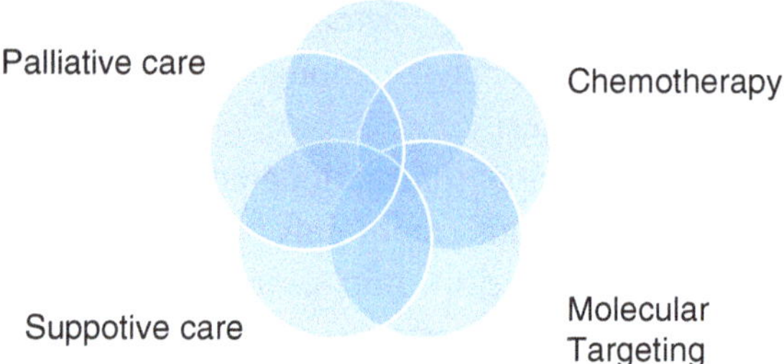

12.7 Management of Relapsed Disease

Immunotherapy This is an important tool in the management of the relapsed patient and can range from withdrawal of immunosuppression (if the patient is still on it) to the administration of donor lymphocyte infusions (DLI) infusions in incremental doses.

12.8 Withdrawal of Immunosuppression

The GvL or GvM effect of HSCT can be enhanced by reducing and stopping the IS (immunosuppressive) agent that the patient may be taking. Nursing care and education is essential in this circumstance as along with GvL the patient needs to be monitored for the development of GVHD which is extensively discussed in another chapter.

12.9 Responsiveness to DLI
(Adapted from Treleaven and Barrett 2009)

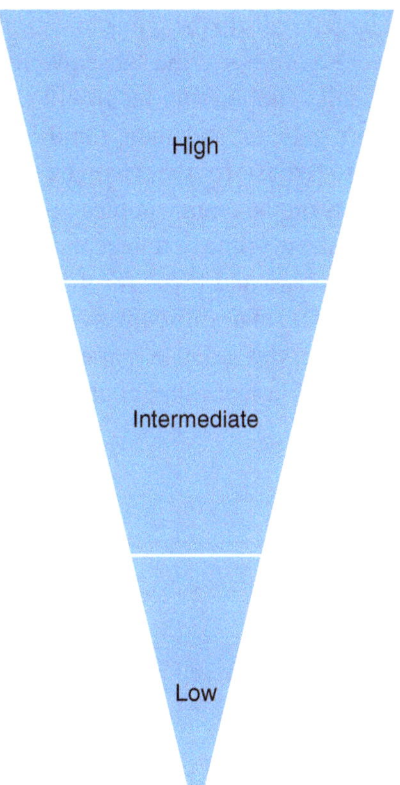

12.9.1 DLI

DLI alone can induce permanent remission of the underlying disease particularly in the case of CML where relapses occur at a molecular level. In other diseases, the response can be varied from effective to ineffective (Fig. 4). Most centres adopt an approach with the administration of graduated doses between 1×10^6 CD3 cells per kg and 1×10^8 per kg recipient body weight depending on time from transplant, patient performance status and type of donor.

DLI may also be administered as an adjuvant therapy to chemotherapy or targeted therapies to augment the effect of that treatment or sustain a remission if achieved.

12.9.2 Chemotherapy

This may be used to palliate the patient, to attempt to reduce the disease burden to facilitate DLI or targeted therapy or to achieve a remission. Patients relapsing within 6 months of HSCT often require reduced or modified dosing due to the toxicity of previous treatment or having reached the dosing limits of particular chemotherapeutic agents. Regimens for relapsed patients tend to be patient specific, and there are currently very few standardised approaches. The nursing care of these patients has been well documented in previous chapters.

12.10 Molecular or Targeted Therapies

Consideration needs to be given to the administration of molecular or targeted therapies to patients who relapse post-HSCT if they are available. Disease-specific monoclonal antibodies, e.g. brentuximab, in some lymphomas; anti-CD33 agents, e.g. gemtuzumab, in myeloid malignancies; and TKIs in BCR-ABL-positive malignancies can have an important role in this setting.

12.11 Second HSCT

If a patient experiences a relapse later post-HSCT, consideration may be given to a second HSCT using stem cells either from the original donor or an alternative donor. In malignant disease, usually a second procedure is only feasible when remission has been achieved following successful administration of chemotherapy, a molecular or targeted therapy. The morbidity and mortality associated with a second HSCT is often significant, and the patient and family should be carefully counselled before such an undertaking.

Conclusion

The treatment of relapsed disease remains challenging, and further research is required to identify new strategies and therapies to improve the outcome for this group of patients.

The nursing challenges are immense, and the psychological support required is complex and largely falls to the nurse to coordinate and deliver regardless of the subseque nt treatment approach. The nursing team will continue to support patients and their families and help them to adjust to the changes ahead. The demands on the team can mean that it is difficult to take the time to reflect and deal with the changing care and focus for the patients. The adjustments and difficulties experienced in caring for the relapse patient need to be matched by a team that continues to support each other.

References

Apperly J, Carreras E, Gluckman E, Masszi T. Haematopoietic stem cell transplantation. 6th revised ed. Genoa: Forum Service; 2012

Bader P, Niethammer D, Willasch A, Kreyenberg H, Klingebiel T. How and when should we monitor chimerism after allogeneic stem cell transplantation. Bone Marrow Transpl. 2005;35:107–19.

Treleaven J & Barrett AJ 2009 Haematopoietic stem cell transplantation in clinical practice. Churchill Livingstone Elsevier; Edinburgh

Engraftment, Graft Failure, and Rejection

Daphna Hutt

Abstract

Engraftment following HSCT is an essential goal for sustained long-term and effective hematopoiesis. It's the most important criteria for a better overall survival. However, stem cell engraftment may be accompanied with a clinical condition known as engraftment syndrome (ES) that could have a devastating outcome. Nurses caring for HSCT recipients must be aware of ES symptoms in order to intervene quickly and appropriately. On the other hand, graft failure (GF) is a major complication and is associated with a dismal prognosis. It is classically divided into primary or secondary graft failure. The risk factors associated with GF may be related to characteristics of the graft, the patient, the donor, or the transplant procedure. The conditions that are associated with an increased occurrence of GF and the available treatment options will be thoroughly discussed in the chapter along with the nursing considerations.

Keywords

Engraftment • Engraftment syndrome • Graft failure • Graft rejection Pediatrics • Nursing

D. Hutt
Department of Paediatric Hematology-Oncology and BMT, Edmond and lily Safra Children Hospital, Sheba Medical Center, Ramat Gan, Israel
e-mail: daphna.hutt@sheba.health.gov.il

13.1 Engraftment

Engraftment is the process by which hematopoietic stem cells (HSC) make their way (homing) to free bone marrow (BM) niches where they can find optimal conditions to survive and proliferate. Once they have reached the BM microenvironment, HSC have to proliferate to generate all hematopoietic cell subsets (Servais et al. 2013). A fundamental goal for successful engraftment is that the transplanted HSC are capable of

© EBMT and the Author(s) 2018
M. Kenyon, A. Babic (eds.), *The European Blood and Marrow Transplantation Textbook for Nurses*,
https://doi.org/10.1007/978-3-319-50026-3_13

sustaining long-term effective hematopoiesis; production of red blood cells, white blood cells, and platelets; and their release to peripheral blood (Locatelli et al. 2014). Engraftment is the most important variable for a better overall survival after stem cell transplant (Cluzeau et al. 2016).

13.2 Engraftment Definition

Various definitions of engraftment exist in the literature. Engraftment is most commonly defined as the first of three consecutive days of achieving a sustained peripheral blood neutrophil count of $>500 \times 10^6$/L (Wolff 2002). Platelet engraftment is usually defined as independence from platelet transfusion for at least 7 days with a platelet count of more than $>20 \times 10^9$/L (Teltschik et al. 2016). The two major factors affecting engraftment are the graft source and the hematopoietic stem cell transplant (HSCT) conditioning regimen. Generally, there are three common sources of HSCT grafts: bone marrow (BM), harvested from the iliac crest; peripheral blood stem cells (PBSC), following G-CSF mobilization of HSC to the peripheral circulation with later collection of these cells by leukapheresis; and cord blood (CB). Champlin et al. (2000) published a large retrospective multivariate analysis which compared results of 288 HLA-identical sibling PBSC transplantations with results of 536 HLA-identical sibling BM transplantations. Patients who received PBSC had significantly faster recovery of neutrophils and platelets compared to BM transplants. Neutrophils exceed the threshold of 500×10^6/L between 2 and 6 days earlier with PBSC than after BM. In an EBMT study, the time interval for engraftment was 12 days for PBSC and 15 days for BM. Platelet recovery is also faster by approximately 6 days, i.e., platelet recovery of 20×10^9/L was reached at day +15 for PBSC patients and day +20 for patients receiving BM (Schmitz et al. 2002). CB transplant is associated with delayed engraftment. A large study of 1268 patients (73% children) with acute leukemia (64% acute lymphoblastic leukemia (ALL), 36% acute myeloid leukemia) in remission analyzed engraftment kinetics and outcomes after a single-unit CB transplantation with

myeloablative conditioning regimen. The median time to neutrophil engraftment was 25 days (range 11–108) for children and 23 days (range 11–116) for adult recipients ($P = 0.6$) (Ruggeri et al. 2014). Furthermore, when comparing intensity of conditioning regimens, Slavin et al. (1998) described for the first time that allogeneic non-myeloablative HSCT was better tolerated than any standard myeloablative conditioning, with a shorter period of neutropenia and a shorter period of platelet dependence.

Methods of determining donor engraftment rely on the assessment of donor and recipient cell components in the recipient BM or PB, termed as chimerism analysis (see Chap. 12).

13.3 Engraftment Syndrome

Engraftment syndrome (ES) is a clinical condition that is characterized by fever, rash, pulmonary edema, weight gain, liver and renal dysfunction, and/or encephalopathy. It occurs at the time of neutrophil recovery after stem cell transplantation (SCT) (Chang et al. 2014). Most data suggest that ES results from a pro-inflammatory state caused by the release of diverse cytokines and other mediators of inflammation. Clinical features of ES are similar in children and adults. Criteria for the diagnosis of ES typically include fever (thought to be not from infection) and features of systemic vascular leak, as ES was previously referred to as capillary leak syndrome. ES can resemble acute or hyperacute GvHD giving rise to the question of whether ES is an early manifestation of GvHD.

13.4 Management of ES

ES may be self-limited and require no therapy. Indications for treatment include a temperature of $>39\,°C$ without an identifiable infectious etiology and clinically significant manifestations of vascular leak, especially pulmonary edema. ES is corticosteroid responsive, and treatment is given only as long as symptoms persist, usually for 1 week (Spitzer 2015).

13.5 Nursing Considerations

Due to the potentially devastating outcomes associated with ES, nurses caring for SCT recipients must be aware of ES and its symptoms in order to intervene quickly and appropriately (Thoele 2014). Nursing assessment, in order to identify changes, should include the assessment of the clinical manifestation of ES, with anticipated presentation 9–13 days posttransplantation:

- Frequent temperature monitoring.
- Routine skin assessment for rashes or abnormalities.
- Respiratory rate, oxygen saturation, and breath sounds (for signs of pulmonary edema).
- Weight changes.
- Appropriate investigations are undertaken to rule out infection such as blood cultures, complete blood count (CBC), and chest X-ray.

Nursing care should include symptom relief by administration of antipyretics; oxygen for hypoxia; diuretics for weight/fluid gain, edema, ascites, and effusions; and a renal dose of dopamine if needed. Nurses should educate patients and caregivers about the signs and symptoms of ES as well as the treatment and management.

13.6 Graft Failure

Although incidence is relatively low, graft failure (GF), when it does occur, is a major complication associated with a dismal prognosis, particularly in recipients of alternative donor HSCT (Ayas et al. 2015). It remains an important contributor to morbidity and mortality after allogeneic SCT. Recent studies indicate that patients experiencing GF have a lower probability of survival in comparison to those with sustained engraftment of donor cells (Olsson et al. 2013; Locatelli et al. 2014).

GF is defined as the lack of hematopoietic cell engraftment following autologous or allogeneic SCT (Lowsky and Messner 2016). It is classically divided into primary or secondary graft failure.

Primary graft failure is defined as no evidence of engraftment or hematological recovery of donor cells, within the first month after transplant, without evidence of disease relapse.

Secondary graft failure refers to the loss of a previously functioning graft, resulting in cytopenia involving at least two blood cell lineages.

Primary graft failure is usually associated with a more significant risk of morbidity and mortality in comparison with secondary graft failure (Olsson et al. 2013; Kato et al. 2013).

13.7 Graft Rejection

The term graft rejection refers to immune-mediated rejection of the donor cells by residual host cells because of genetic disparity between the recipient and the donor. Therefore, this term is only relevant to allogeneic transplants (Lowsky and Messner 2016). Immunological rejection of the hematopoietic stem cell graft is a major cause of graft failure (Olsson et al. 2013). Marrow graft rejection is usually defined by the absence of donor cells in a patient with pancytopenia and reduced marrow cellularity (Martin 2016). Chimerism studies performed by methods of FISH (in sex-mismatched transplant) or by microsatellites enable early diagnosis of GF, and it could be crucial of optimizing the chance of rescuing patients with graft failure (Locatelli et al. 2014). They should be carried out routinely especially in patients who have inadequate marrow function and might be candidates for donor lymphocyte infusion (DLI) or a second transplant (Martin 2016).

The incidence of GF varies between different transplant modalities, studies, and reports. In autologous transplants, a reasonable estimate of GF is between 1 and 3%. The incidence of GF is higher in allogeneic transplant recipients especially if the patient receives an HLA-mismatched or T-cell-depleted graft or a single-unit CB transplant (Lowsky and Messner 2016). Olsson et al. (2013) reported a large retrospective study of 967 transplants performed between 1995 and 2010 and an overall GF rate of 5.6%, with a higher incidence of GF in recipients of SCT for nonmalignant disorders. Analysis of 23,272 patients from the CIBMTR database produced a similar incidence of primary GF (5.5%) in patients with hematological malignancies after myeloablative conditioning (Olsson et al. 2015). Recently, a retrospective study of a large cohort of 4684 unrelated donor HSCT in the period (2006–2012) confirmed a low rate of graft failure (3.8%) (Cluzeau et al. 2016).

13.8 Risk Factors Associated with Graft Failure

Several risk factors that are associated with GF have been identified over the years (Fig. 13.1). They may be related to characteristics of the graft, the patient, the donor, or the transplant procedure (Olsson et al. 2015). The conditions that are associated with an increased occurrence of graft failure include:

1. HLA disparity – Earlier studies reported that an increase in the degree of HLA mismatch was associated with a higher risk for GF for siblings and unrelated grafts (Anasetti et al. 1989). In particular, HLA class I mismatches are important determinants for graft failure (Petersdorf et al. 2001). Donor selection criteria regarding HLA matching have changed over the years, and it is difficult to compare the results of previous to current studies. HLA disparity is not a consistent finding in more recent studies. Passweg et al. (2011) reported

in a study of 709 participants with hematological malignancies who received unrelated donor reduced-intensity conditioning (RIC) transplants that the risk of GF was comparable between the HLA-matched and HLA-mismatched donors. However, immunological T-cell-mediated responses toward HLA contribute to primary GF as seen by the higher risk of primary GF in mismatched compared to both well-matched and partially matched unrelated grafts (Olsson et al. 2015).

2. ABO mismatching in the donor/recipient pair – ABO incompatibility between the donor and the recipient occurs in approximately 25% of HLA-matched transplants. Usually, it has no influence on the neutrophil engraftment, but certain donor/recipient mismatches have been associated with posttransplant pure red cell aplasia (Lowsky and Messner 2016). Olsson et al. (2013) observed that using ABO-incompatible grafts is no longer a risk factor for GF. They assume that removing the red cells from the graft decreases the number of SC by about 30% of the original dose and this might be the reason for GF and not the ABO incompatibility itself, although more recently, in the largest analysis of primary GF (n = 23,272), Olsson et al. (2015) concluded that major ABO incompatibility does in fact still remain a risk factor for primary GF.

3. Reduced-intensity conditioning (RIC) – RIC regimens have lower doses of chemoradiation therapy; the host immune system may persist, resulting with an increased rate of GF (Mattsson et al. 2008; Olsson et al. 2013; Locatelli et al. 2014). Those regimens may result in an intermediate phase, termed mixed chimerism, in which hematopoietic cells are derived from both donor and recipient cells, and thus do not fulfill the traditional definition of GF (Lowsky and Messner 2016).

4. Diagnosis – The primary disease may affect the probability of GF indirectly due to differences in the intensity of pretransplant chemotherapeutic protocols (Olsson et al. 2015).

   Patients with severe aplastic anemia (SAA) have higher incidence of GF due to sensitiza-

- HLA disparity
- ABO-mismatching in the donor/recipient pair
- Reduced-intensity conditioning
- Primary diagnosis
- Graft source
- Cell dose
- Graft manipulation
- Others

Fig. 13.1 Risk factors for graft failure include

tion to components of red blood cell caused by multiple transfusions; therefore, in SAA transfusions should be minimized prior to transplant.

Hemoglobinopathies (thalassemia, sickle-cell disease) – The incidence of GF or rejection remains high probably due to an intact immune system. GF is particularly high in patients who have heavy iron overload and organ damage due to excessive transfusion and inadequate chelation treatment (Gaziev et al. 2008).

Myeloid disorders (myelodysplastic syndrome (MDS) and myelofibrosis (MF)) – These patients, most probably, do not receive prior intensive chemotherapy and might resist donor cell engraftment, due to the presence of residual host cells (Lowsky and Messner 2016). In addition, patients with absence of complete remission (CR) prior to transplant have more GF compared to patients in CR ($P < 0.0001$) (Cluzeau et al. 2016).

5. Graft source – Graft type is the strongest risk factor in the multivariate model for primary GF, with three times higher risk in BM compared to PB grafts (Olsson et al. 2015). Passweg et al. (2011) described that the only characteristic that was associated with GF in that study was the use of BM compared with PB ($P = .002$). Unrelated CB transplants are associated with the highest engraftment failure rate (Kekre and Antin 2014).

6. Cell dose – The higher number of CD3 cells in PB is likely to facilitate engraftment and contributes to the lower incidence of primary GF. BM grafts with low cell dose (TNC doses $\leq 2.4 \times 10^8$/kg) result in a 40% increase in primary GF. PB products per se are associated with cell doses above the threshold that would affect primary GF, or other cell subtypes such as T cells may be equally or more important for engraftment. Nevertheless, while other factors seem more important for primary GF, CD34 cell dose is probably important for subsequent secondary graft failure (Olsson et al. 2015).

7. Graft manipulation – T-cell depletion (TCD) of the graft may cause a potential increased risk for GF (Lowsky and Messner 2016). Various approaches to TCD are used by transplant centers, and they vary in the rates of GF (Kekre and Antin 2014), although Reisner et al. (2011) emphasize in a review of the developments in the last 15 years that haploidentical transplants demonstrate how obstacles to successful transplantation can be overcome making full haplotype-mismatched transplantation a clinical reality that provides similar outcomes to transplantation from matched unrelated donors (MUD). Encouragingly, in recent years, the graft failure rate for haploidentical transplantation has decreased to levels comparable to those of matched unrelated donors (MUD), matched related donors (MRD), and mismatched unrelated donors (MMURD) (Reisner et al. 2011; Kekre and Antin 2014).

8. Other risk factors that have been identified to cause an increased risk of graft failure are infections especially of viral origin, such as cytomegalovirus (CMV), human herpesvirus 6 (HHV-6), and parvovirus, and the use of drugs that may induce myelosuppression, such as ganciclovir (Locatelli et al. 2014).

Identifying and assessing the risk factors for GF, prior to transplant, allow clinicians to make more informed choices for their patients with respect to BM versus PB, donor selection, immunosuppressive regimens, and when to plan for a rescue transplant (Olsson et al. 2015).

13.9 Treatment Options for GF

Whatever the etiology of graft failure or rejection is, it should be identified as early as possible and recognized as a serious and life-threatening issue requiring immediate intervention (Wolff 2002). Routine monitoring of donor cell engraftment is recommended since the evaluation of chimerism status can be crucial for optimizing the chance of rescuing patients from graft failure (Locatelli et al. 2014). No single drug or strategy has incontrovertibly proven to be superior to others for reversing graft failure; current approaches to limit the detrimental impact of this complication are primarily based on its prevention (Locatelli et al. 2014). No standard approach to the management of graft failure exists (Hege et al. 2016), and the rescue strategies are limited (Servais et al. 2013). The common approaches are listed below.

13.9.1 Changes to Immune Suppression

Early detection of decrease in donor chimerism enables to modify the immunosuppressive treatment (Dubovsky et al. 1999). Withdrawal of the immunosuppressive drugs is usually the first measure, which by itself can control leukemia in a limited number of patients (Yoshimi et al. 2005). In case of persistent mixed chimerism after allogeneic transplant, it remains unclear if withdrawal of immunosuppressive drugs will accelerate or prevent GF. The limitation of this method includes an increased risk of graft-versus-host disease.

13.9.2 Donor Lymphocyte Infusion

Donor lymphocyte infusion (DLI) has a potent immunological effect and has been increasingly used to treat relapse, especially molecular relapse, but may also be used to overcome rejection in cases of decreasing donor cell chimerism (Mattsson et al. 2008). Persistent mixed chimerism or declining level of donor cell chimerism is associated with increased risk for GF both in adult and pediatric transplant recipients. A large ($n = 163$) prospective multicenter trial of children with acute lymphoblastic leukemia (ALL) after allogeneic SCT demonstrated that children who developed increased mixed chimerism were at higher risk of developing relapse and can be rescued by preemptive DLI (Bader et al. 2004). Administration of preemptive DLI after day +100 to patients that were withdrawn from immunosuppressive medications enabled 50% of the patients in that study to convert to complete donor type. The majority of the patients required multiple administrations of DLI's. Therefore, DLI may convert mixed donor-host chimerism to full donor chimerism as a surrogate measure to prevent relapse in patients with hematological malignancies (Hale and Petrovic 2014). Frugnoli et al. (2010) reported that escalating doses of DLI is a treatment option for emerging rejection in patients with mixed chimerism following SCT for β-thalassemia. The origin of lymphocytes for DLI could be either frozen aliquots collected from the donor at the time of the original harvest or collected peripherally by leukapheresis or phlebotomy from the donor before DLI (Haines et al. 2015). Side effects of DLI include increased risk of GvHD (Lowsky and Messner 2016) and, in few cases, can lead to marrow aplasia (Mattsson et al. 2008).

13.9.3 CD34+ Boost

Poor graft function is defined by cytopenia of at least two lineages beyond day +28 in patients with complete or near-complete chimerism (Lowsky and Messner 2016). As manifested by the development of a neutrophil count of $<1 \times 10^9/l$ (grade 4) and/or platelet count of $<50 \times 10^9/l$ (grade 3, $25–50 \times 10^9/l$; grade 4, $<25 \times 10^9/l$) (Frugnoli et al. 2010). Cytopenias may be due to viral infection, medication side effect, or GvHD (Lowsky and Messner 2016). In patients with continued poor graft function in the absence of graft rejection, a boost of donor stem cells without additional preparative chemotherapy may improve overall function of the graft. Because this boost may induce GvHD, T-cell depletion of the stem cells can prevent this and improve survival in some patients (Mattsson et al. 2008). CD34+-selected cell boosts without a conditioning regimen prior to infusion can be a valid option in order to improve poor graft function, and fully reverse graft failure, especially in patients with complete donor chimerism or predominance of donor hematopoiesis (Locatelli et al. 2014; Servais et al. 2013).

13.9.4 Autologous Backup

Infusion of autologous hematopoietic stem cells (HSC) that were collected and stored prior to transplant can restore hematopoiesis in case of GF. The collection of autologous backup prior to allogeneic transplant is according to center policy. In patients with hematological malignancies or with marrow failure syndromes, the collection of autologous backup is controversial (Lowsky and Messner 2016).

13.9.5 Growth Factors

Administration of growth factors, after autologous transplant, significantly shortens the time for neutrophil recovery. In case of poor graft function or GF, it is a reasonable approach until a more definitive intervention is decided. Following allogeneic transplants, the role of growth factors for patients with poor graft function or GF is unclear. It is a reasonable approach for the management of low blood counts, and depending on the cause, it may or may not be effective (Lowsky and Messner 2016). Certainly, hematopoietic growth factors should be considered in the management of graft dysfunction, especially with partial donor chimerism (Wolff 2002).

13.9.6 Regrafting

A second allogeneic transplant is the only potential long-term curative option for patients with GF and rejection (Remberger et al. 2011; Servais et al. 2013; Locatelli et al. 2014; Cesaro et al. 2015). There are no conclusive data for supporting the choice of using either the same donor of the first allograft or an alternative donor (Mattsson et al. 2008; Locatelli et al. 2014). Different studies recommend a variety of options depending on the availability of a donor, the patient's clinical condition, and the underlying disease. Gaziev et al. (2008) recommend using the initial donor for second transplant for patients with thalassemia recurrence following the first

graft. The use of the same donor was more frequent in the sibling group compared with the unrelated group, in a report of second transplant in SAA patients. This might be due to the availability of the donor for transplant (Cesaro et al. 2015). However, in patients with an immune-mediated graft rejection, the use of an alternative donor, whenever possible, is recommended (Locatelli et al. 2014). PB might be the best stem cell source for salvage transplantation (Servais et al. 2013) in order to improve engraftment and thus achieve faster hematopoietic recovery (Cesaro et al. 2015).

There are no uniform criteria about the best conditioning approach for a second SCT in patients who have developed GF although it should differ from that used at the first transplant (Mattsson et al. 2008; Cesaro et al. 2015). Many transplant teams favor using an immunosuppressive non-myeloablative, reduced-intensity conditioning (RIC) regimen in order to avoid unacceptable cumulative toxicities of two consecutive high-dose conditionings given in a short interval of time (Remberger et al. 2011; Servais et al. 2013; Ferrà et al. 2015; Cesaro et al. 2015; Cluzeau et al. 2016). The optimal reconditioning regimen after graft failure still needs to be defined, and standardized protocols are lacking (Teltschik et al. 2016).

In general, a second unrelated HSCT is considered a risky procedure with a lower probability of long-term survival on account of a high incidence of GF, noninfectious organ toxicity, and infectious complications. This negative outcome is also influenced by the type of underlying disease. However, second transplant using related and unrelated donors in SAA patients is feasible with a good chance of long-term overall survival in more than 60% of cases (Cesaro et al. 2015). Second transplant should be considered especially for patients with nonmalignant diseases (Remberger et al. 2011).

In conclusion, GF is a rare complication after allogeneic transplant but is associated with poor outcome. Early identification of the patients at risk and aggressive intervention could rescue or prevent some patients from developing GF.

13.10 Pediatric Considerations

The aim of allogeneic transplant in nonmalignant disease is to achieve sustained engraftment in order to improve the hematopoietic function, to correct the immunocompetence, and/or to increase or normalize the respective enzyme shortage (Bader et al. 2005). Children who may have more than 60- to 70-year life expectancy after undergoing allogeneic transplant may benefit from the approach of reduced-intensity conditioning (RIC) or reduced-toxicity conditioning regimens prior to transplant versus myeloablative conditioning. This is especially true in those with nonmalignant diseases and those with malignant diseases that may have a profound graft-versus-tumor effect (Satwani et al. 2013). In the last several years, the use of RIC has expanded from adults with high indices of comorbidity to candidates without comorbidities (Satwani et al. 2013) as well as to the pediatric population. In pediatric nonmalignant diseases, RIC is an attractive alternative with the potential for decreased regimen-related toxicities, lower incidence of long-term complications, as well as preserving fertility. Graft rejection rates are low, especially when stable mixed chimerism is curative if ensured in the lineage that corrects function (Madden et al. 2016). Graft rejection, in children with inborn errors of metabolism undergoing RIC transplants, still remains an obstacle to the success of the transplant since they are immunocompetent (Kato et al. 2016). The incidence of GF in children varies in the different studies. In a large report of 240 classical SCID patients who received allogeneic transplant between 2000 and 2009 by Pai et al. (2014), 18% of the patients received a boost, an additional transplant from the same donor without conditioning (23 children), or a second transplant from a different donor (with or without conditioning) or from the same donor with conditioning (34 children), and 11 children received both a boost and a second transplant at 5 years. A retrospective study by Mitchell et al. (2013) of 135 children with primary immunodeficiency reported that 18 patients (13%) required a second SCT due to

graft failure or rejection. Satwani et al. (2013) reported a large study of reduced-toxicity conditioning allo-SCT, using both related and unrelated allogeneic stem cell sources in pediatric recipients, with both malignant and nonmalignant diseases. Primary GF occurred in 16 patients (16%) all in unrelated CBT recipients and none in MUD/MSD graft recipients. Chemotherapy naivety was the only significant risk factor for primary GF. In a single-center study by Balashov et al. (2015), the incidence of primary and secondary GF in primary immunodeficient patients undergoing MUD and haploidentical transplants was 27% (10 out of 37 patients). This accrued in patients that were initially in high risk for graft failure, such as chronic granulomatous disease (CGD) and congenital neutropenia.

However, as with the adult patients, evidence on the optimal management of GF in children is limited; therefore, analysis of pediatric GF is important in order to establish a standard treatment strategy against this rare event (Kato et al. 2013). The case report (Fig. 13.2) demonstrates the process of graft rejection, its consequences, and treatment options.

13.11 Nursing Considerations

When a patient fails to engraft, he or she faces a life-threatening situation. Patients experiencing disappointment and fear from the failure of the transplant might express feelings of anger, betrayal, grief, depression, and hopelessness. Similarly, healthcare personnel involved in the patient's care may also feel a sense of failure and grief (Wilson and Sylvanus 2005). General nursing care of patients experiencing GF does not differ from the treatment during the neutropenic period of the transplant, as described in Chap. 7, although nurses should routinely monitor the patient engraftment by daily CBC during the engraftment phase, as it enables to assess for signs of GF as well as delayed engraftment. Chimerism analysis should be evaluated frequently as per local policy especially in patients that are at risk for GF (Fig. 13.3).

A 13 month old baby was transferred from another hospital to a specialist unit due to recurrent infections since he was one month old. He initially presented with a necrotic infected wound after a supra pubic aspiration and an extremely swollen belly. Family history: parents are cousins, have 6 children, one died of infection when he was a few months old.

The baby was diagnosed with Leukocyte adhesion deficiency-1 (LAD1), CD11 & CD18 deficiency and he underwent a BM transplant on 13.7.14 from his MRD sister. Conditioning regimen included Fludarabine, Treosulfan and ATG. Stem cell engraftment was on day +17. On day + 24 due to decreased donor chimerism, from 63% to 20%, Cyclosporine was stopped. Three days later on day + 27 he developed skin rash and was diagnosed with acute GvHD. He went on to develop severe acute GvHD (grade III-IV) involving skin, liver and GI tract. GvHD was treated with Solumedrol, CSA, ATG and one dose of mesenchimal stem cells (on day +56). GvHD improved and at discharge, two months post-transplant he had mixed chimerism of 43% donor cells according to XX FISH analysis. Subsequently donor chimerism continued to decrease and at one year post transplant was 3.5% donor cells by XX FISH analysis. CD 11 & CD 18 was measured only on lymphocytes and not on neutrophils (split chimerism). During that year he suffered again from recurrent infections. He underwent a second allogeneic BM transplant on 11.10.15 from another MRD sister. Conditioning therapy included Busulfan & Fludarabine. Engraftment was on day +14 and chimerism was 60% donor cells (XX). Except for CVC sepsis and removal of the central line the transplant went very well and he was discharged home on day +24 in a very good overall condition.

Currently, 11 months post second allogeneic transplant he is in a good general condition. He has stable mixed chimerism of 87% of donor cells (XX). During that period he was at home with no infections, no GvHD and no other complications post-transplant.

This case demonstrates two important points: discontinuation of cyclosporine does not always reverse the situation of increased mixed chimerism and carries the risk of developing severe GvHD. Second allogeneic transplant is feasible with good outcome.

Fig. 13.2 Case report

Routine monitoring of patient engraftment by daily complete blood count

Serial Chimerism testing

Emotional support for patient experiencing graft failure

Fig. 13.3 Be aware of:

Equally important to the physical care is the emotional support for the patient and family experiencing this devastating, disappointing, and life-threatening situation. Nurses can help to reduce patients' fears by providing accurate, timely information about procedures, symptoms, and feelings that the transplant recipient may experience or is experiencing. Nurses should provide support and education on the diagnosis of

GF, treatment options, and decisions regarding the care plan. All information must be individually tailored to the patient and family needs (Wilson and Sylvanus 2005).

Nurses caring for patients who undergo SCT should be aware of the possibility of graft failure following the transplant. They should know the risk factors associated with GF and the treatment options available. This will lead to a better understanding and recognition of this rare but life-threatening situation. The possibility of GF should be discussed with the patient and his family prior to transplant, and they should be counseled with regard to the risk factors for developing GF. The nursing literature regarding graft failure is scarce with no recent study on the implications and the support needed for the patient who develops graft failure.

Bibliography

Anasetti C, Amos D, Beatty PG, et al. Effect of HLA compatibility on engraftment of bone marrow transplants in patients with leukemia or lymphoma. N Engl J Med. 1989;320:197–204.

Ayas M, Eapen M, Le-Rademacher J, et al. Second allogeneic hematopoietic cell transplantation for patients with fanconi anemia and bone marrow failure. Biol Blood Marrow Transplant. 2015;21:1790–5.

Bader P, Kreyenberg H, Hoelle W, et al. Increasing mixed chimerism is an important prognostic factor for unfavorable outcome in children with acute lymphoblastic leukemia after allogeneic stem-cell transplantation: possible role for pre-emptive immunotherapy? J Clin Oncol. 2004;22:1696–706.

Bader P, Niethammer D, Willasch A, Kreyenberg H, Klingebiel T. How and when should we monitor chimerism after allogeneic stem cell transplantation? Bone Marrow Transplant. 2005;35:107–19.

Balashov D, Shcherbina A, Maschan M, et al. Single-center experience of unrelated and haploidentical stem cell transplantation with TCRab and CD19 depletion in children with primary immunodeficiency syndromes. Biol Blood Marrow Transplant. 2015;21:1955–62.

Cesaro S, Peffault de Latour R, Tridello G, et al. Second allogeneic stem cell transplant for aplastic anaemia: a retrospective study by the severe aplastic anaemia working party of the European society for blood and marrow transplantation. Br J Haematol. 2015;171:606–14.

Champlin RE, Schmitz N, Horowitz MM, et al. Blood stem cells compared with bone marrow as a source of hematopoietic cells for allogeneic transplantation. Blood. 2000;95:3702–9.

Chang L, Frame D, Braun T, et al. Engraftment syndrome after allogeneic hematopoietic cell transplantation predicts poor outcomes. Biol Blood Marrow Transplant. 2014;20:1407–17.

Cluzeau T, Lambert J, Raus N, et al. Risk factors and outcome of graft failure after HLA matched and mismatched unrelated donor hematopoietic stem cell transplantation: a study on behalf of SFGM-TC and SFHI. Bone Marrow Transplant. 2016;51:687–91.

Dubovsky J, Daxberger H, Fritsch G, Printz D, Peters C, Matthes S, Gadner H, Lion T. Kinetics of chimerism during the early post-transplant period in pediatric patients with malignant and non-malignant hematologic disorders: implications for timely detection of engraftment, graft failure and rejection. Leukemia. 1999;13:2060–9.

Ferrà C, Sanz J, Díaz-Pérez M-A, et al. Outcome of graft failure after allogeneic stem cell transplant: study of 89 patients. Leuk Lymphoma. 2015;56:656–62.

Frugnoli I, Cappelli B, Chiesa R, et al. Escalating doses of donor lymphocytes for incipient graft rejection following SCT for thalassemia. Bone Marrow Transplant. 2010;45:1047–51.

Gaziev J, Sodani P, Lucarelli G, et al. Second hematopoietic SCT in patients with thalassemia recurrence following rejection of the first graft. Bone Marrow Transplant. 2008;42:397–404.

Haines HL, Bleesing JJ, Davies SM, et al. Outcomes of donor lymphocyte infusion for treatment of mixed donor chimerism after a reduced-intensity preparative regimen for pediatric patients with nonmalignant diseases. Biol Blood Marrow Transplant. 2015;21:288–92.

Hale G, Petrovic A. Clinical options after failure of allogeneic hematopoietic stem cell transplantation in patients with hematologic malignancies. Expert Rev Clin Immunol. 2014;7:515–27.

Hege K, Quigg T, Delgado D. Alemtuzumab, fludarabine, low-dose TBI, and double umbilical cord transplant for primary graft failure in a patient with recurrent HLH. Pediatr Blood Cancer. 2016;63:361–3.

Kato M, Matsumoto K, Suzuki R, et al. Salvage allogeneic hematopoietic SCT for primary graft failure in children. Bone Marrow Transplant. 2013;48:1173–8.

Kato S, Yabe H, Takakura H. Hematopoietic stem cell transplantation for inborn errors of metabolism: a report from the Research Committee on Transplantation for Inborn Errors of Metabolism of the Japanese Ministry of Health, Labour and Welfare and the Working Group of the Japan Soci. Pediatr Transplant. 2016;20:203–14.

Kekre N, Antin JH. Hematopoietic stem cell transplantation donor sources in the 21st century: choosing the ideal donor when a perfect match does not exist. Blood. 2014;124:334–43.

Locatelli F, Lucarelli B, Merli P. Current and future approaches to treat graft failure after allogeneic hematopoietic stem cell transplantation. Expert Opin Pharmacother. 2014;15:23–36.

Lowsky R, Messner H. Mechanisms and treatment of graft failure. In: Negrin RS, Antin JH, Appelbaum FR, Forman SJ, editors. Thomas' hematopoietic cell transplantation. 5th ed, Vol. 2(77). s.l.: Wiley Blackwell; 2016. p. 944–54.

Madden LM, Hayashi RJ, Ka WC, et al. Long-term follow-up after reduced-intensity conditioning and stem cell transplantation for childhood nonmalignant disorders. Biol Blood Marrow Transplant. 2016;22:1467–72.

Martin P. Documentation of engraftment and characterization of chimerism after hematopoietic cell transplantation. In: Negrin RS, Antin JH, Appelbaum FR, Forman SJ, editors. Thomas' hematopoietic cell transplantation. 5th ed, Vol. 1(24). s.l.: Wiley Blackwell; 2016. p. 272–80.

Mattsson J, Ringdén O, Storb R. Graft failure after allogeneic hematopoietic cell transplantation. Biol Blood Marrow Transplant. 2008;14(Suppl 1):165–70.

Mitchell R, Nivison-Smith I, Anazodo A, et al. Outcomes of hematopoietic stem cell transplantation in primary immunodeficiency: a report from the Australian and New Zealand Children's Haematology Oncology Group and the Australasian Bone Marrow Transplant Recipient Registry. Biol Blood Marrow Transplant. 2013;19:338–43.

Olsson R, Remberger M, Schaffer M, et al. Graft failure in the modern era of allogeneic hematopoietic SCT. Bone Marrow Transplant. 2013;48:537–43.

Olsson RF, Logan BR, Chaudhury S, et al. Primary graft failure after myeloablative allogeneic hematopoietic cell transplantation for hematologic malignancies. Leukemia. 2015;29:1754–62.

Pai S-Y, Logan BR, Griffith LM, et al. Transplantation outcomes for severe combined immunodeficiency, 2000–2009. N Engl J Med. 2014;371:434–46.

Passweg JR, Zhang M-J, Rocha V, et al. Donor characteristics affecting graft failure, graft-versus-host disease, and survival after unrelated donor transplantation with reduced-intensity conditioning for hematologic malignancies. Biol Blood Marrow Transplant. 2011;17:1855–77.

Petersdorf EW, Hansen JA, Martin PJ, et al. Major-histocompatibility-complex class I alleles and antigens in hematopoietic-cell transplantation. N Engl J Med. 2001;345:1794–800.

Reisner Y, Hagin D, Martelli MF. Haploidentical hematopoietic transplantation: current status and future perspectives. Blood. 2011;118:6006–17.

Remberger M, Mattsson J, Olsson R, Ringde'n O. Second allogeneic hematopoietic stem cell transplantation: a treatment for graft failure. Clin Transplant. 2011;25:E68–76.

Ruggeri A, Labopin M, Sormani MP, et al. Engraftment kinetics and graft failure after single umbilical cord blood transplantation using a myeloablative conditioning regimen. Haematologica. 2014;99:1509–15.

Satwani P, Jin Z, Duffy D, et al. Transplantation-related mortality, graft failure, and survival after reduced-toxicity conditioning and allogeneic hematopoietic stem cell transplantation in 100 consecutive pediatric recipients. Biol Blood Marrow Transplant. 2013;19:552–61.

Schmitz N, Beksac M, Hasenclever D, et al. Transplantation of mobilized peripheral blood cells to HLA-identical siblings with standard-risk leukemia. Blood. 2002;100:761–7.

Servais S, Beguin Y, Baron F. Emerging drugs for prevention of graft failure after allogeneic hematopoietic stem cell transplantation. Expert Opin Emerg Drugs. 2013;18:173–92.

Slavin S, Nagler A, Naparstek E, et al. Nonmyeloablative stem cell transplantation and cell therapy as an alternative to conventional bone marrow transplantation with lethal cytoreduction for the treatment of malignant and nonmalignant hematologic diseases. Blood. 1998;91:756–63.

Spitzer TR. Engraftment syndrome: double-edged sword of hematopoietic cell transplants. Bone Marrow Transplant. 2015;50:469–75.

Teltschik H-M, Heinzelmann F, Gruhn B, et al. Treatment of graft failure with TNI-based reconditioning and haploidentical stem cells in paediatric patients. Br J Haematol. 2016. https://doi.org/10.1111/bjh.14190.

Thoele K. Engraftment syndrome in hematopoietic stem cell transplantations. Clin J Oncol Nurs. 2014;18:349–54.

Wilson C, Sylvanus T. Graft failure following allogeneic blood and marrow transplant: evidence-based nursing case study review. Clin J Oncol Nurs. 2005;9:151–9.

Wolff SN. Second hematopoietic stem cell transplantation for the treatment of graft failure, graft rejection or relapse after allogeneic transplantation. Bone Marrow Transplant. 2002;29:545–52.

Yoshimi A, Bader P, Matthes-Martin S, et al. Donor leukocyte infusion after hematopoietic stem cell transplantation in patients with juvenile myelomonocytic leukemia. Leukemia. 2005;19:971–7.

Late Effects and Long-Term Follow-Up

Michelle Kenyon, John Murray, Barry Quinn, Diana Greenfield, and Eugenia Trigoso

Abstract

Allogeneic stem cell transplantation was successfully performed in 1968, and its use has grown significantly over the past five decades with the total number now exceeding 1 million patients. HSCT is a curative treatment for many haematological cancers and other disorders. Almost 40,000 HSCT procedures are performed Europe-wide per annum (Passweg et al., Bone Marrow Transplant, 2016), and with a 5-year survival around 50% (Friedrichs, Lancet Oncol 11(4):331–338, 2010), the number of transplant recipients achieving 'long-term survival' and with late effects directly related to their treatment (Majhail et al., Hematol oncol Stem Cell Ther 5(1):1–30, 2012) is increasing. This growth in survivors is the result of improvements in transplant knowledge and expertise, refinements to conditioning regimes, developments in supportive care and increased numbers of procedures due to broadening transplant indications.

The most common cause of death after transplant is relapsed disease. Yet, even without disease relapse, long-term survival is complex for many as other causes of mortality such as graft versus host disease (GvHD), infection, second malignancy, respiratory disease and cardiovascular disease (CVD) (Savani et al., 2011) prove difficult to address.

M. Kenyon (✉)
Department of Haematological Medicine,
King's College Hospital NHS Foundation Trust,
London, UK
e-mail: michelle.kenyon@nhs.net

J. Murray
Haematology and Transplant Unit, The Christie NHS
Foundation Trust, Manchester, UK

B. Quinn
Palliative Care Department, Woking and Sam Beare
Hospices, The Goldsworth Park Centre, Woking,
Surrey, UK

D. Greenfield
Department of Oncology and Metabolism,
Sheffield Teaching Hospital NHS Foundation Trust,
University of Sheffield, Sheffield, UK

E. Trigoso
Paeidatric Transplant Unit, Hospital Universitario
y Politécnico LA FE, Valencia, Spain

© EBMT and the Author(s) 2018
M. Kenyon, A. Babic (eds.), *The European Blood and Marrow Transplantation Textbook for Nurses*,
https://doi.org/10.1007/978-3-319-50026-3_14

Recovery post-HSCT is challenging, lasting several months to years. These individuals are susceptible to the development of post-treatment physical and psychological sequelae years to decades after completion of treatment leading to a reduced life expectancy with greater morbidity when compared to an age-adjusted population (Socié et al., N Engl J Med 341:14–21, 1999). Survivors with late effects experience significantly poorer physical and mental health, report more unmet needs for care and have significantly greater use of health services compared with survivors without late effects (Treanor et al., Psychooncology 22(11):2428–2435, 2013).

Furthermore, as the number of survivors continues to grow, their long-term health problems and subsequent needs demand increasing attention.

The unpredictable, complex and multifactorial nature of these long-term and late effects in HSCT survivors means that patients require regular life-long assessment guided by rigorous protocols. However, it is important to remember that even using standardised protocols, these should be different for adults and children and the resulting care must be tailored to the needs of the individual survivor. And finally, further consideration is needed for the growing number of young people and adult survivors in long-term follow-up who have been treated in childhood and transitioned into adult long-term follow-up care.

Keywords
Late effects • Survivorship • Survivors • Follow-up

14.1 Principles of Care

Protocol-led assessment and treatment is included in the current FACT-JACIE standards (version 6), which has evolved the standard of care recommending the assessment of recipients for evidence of acute and chronic GVHD, need for vaccinations and post-transplant late effects.

There should be policies and procedures in place for monitoring by appropriate specialists of recipients for post-transplant late effects, including at a minimum endocrine and reproductive function, osteoporosis, cardiovascular risk factors, respiratory function, chronic renal impairment, secondary cancers, and the growth and development of pediatric patients. (Standard B7.6.8)

A further benefit of life-long survivorship care is the acquisition of knowledge and understanding through data collection and analysis which in turn facilitates the design and delivery of appropriate services that will better meet the needs of future survivors.

**Late effect: A health problem that occurs months or years after a disease is diagnosed or after treatment has been administered. Late effects may be caused by the primary disease or its treatment and may include physical, mental or social problems and/or secondary cancers.*

14.2 Survivorship and Quality of Life

While there are many definitions of survivorship, it is widely accepted that a survivor is anyone living after a diagnosis of cancer or 'living with and beyond cancer'.

Survivorship includes 'those who are undergoing primary treatment, those who are in remission following treatment, those who are cured and those with active or advanced disease' (DoH 2010).

By developing and implementing strategies to improve the care and support for HSCT survivors, we will also improve their quality of life and experience of care.

There are a broad range of issues experienced by HSCT survivors which are detrimental to overall quality of life (QoL) and have been reported in the literature.

Unmet physical or psychological needs are reported in 60% of cancer survivors. Beyond the first post-HSCT year, a fifth report psychosocial difficulties including fatigue, social reintegration, finance and employment. A third worry about the future and their health (Baker et al. 1999; Andrykowski et al. 2005; Gielissen et al. 2006).

Finance, employment and education are leading survivor concerns. The economic cost of cancer is a substantial personal and societal problem; 92% of sufferers lose income, impacting adversely on QoL for 40% (Bieri et al. 2008). These are among the major challenges that significantly hinder the cancer patient survivorship transition from treatment phase to reintegration phase and limit the post-HSCT potential for personal growth and fulfillment.

Work and education are immensely important to cancer survivors (Snyder 2002) and have health benefits, and interventions addressing return to work are cost-effective (Waddell and Burton 2006). Reintegrated survivors are more likely to self-manage (Richards 2013), make a positive contribution to self and society, depend less on the state financially and potentially reduce healthcare costs.

A range of psychological and psychosocial interventions including education, exercise, counselling, cognitive behavioural therapy (CBT) and psychotherapy have been investigated, aiming to address survivor concerns and improve overall quality of life.

14.2.1 Quality of Life Assessment

There is a new emphasis on understanding and monitoring the concerns and outcomes for cancer survivors through the routine use of patient-reported outcome measures (PROMs) in follow-up services. Quality of life (QoL) is an important outcome measure following HSCT. Treatment-specific QoL tools exist and have been validated in patients receiving haematopoietic stem cell transplant.

Instruments for assessing QoL can be general or specific to a certain disease or treatment. A number of cancer-specific tools (QLQ – LEU, EORTC SF 36, FACT-G/ FACT-BMT) exist and can be seen in publications of large-scale studies. They are often holistic, assessing different dimensions of well-being, such as physical, emotional, social/family and functional. Many of the commonly used scales such as EORTC and FACT are self-complete and produce a numeric score from which an inference on the relative QoL can be drawn.

These holistic assessments can be used to collect information on individuals at set time points during treatment and recovery and also can increase our knowledge of our patients as a group or groups. QoL data can help us to understand the differences between groups, e.g. comparing QoL in male versus female recipients or haplo-identical versus cord recipients.

Standardised assessment tools can reveal information in certain groups or individuals that may not have been previously identified through conventional outpatient consultation alone. This can lead to increases in referrals to other services such as counselling, assisted conception, sexual dysfunction, social work, etc.

At a local level, this increase in referrals can have resource implications, but it can also lead to:

- Formalising referral pathways
- Cultivating interest and expertise in certain areas
- Developing services that meet the unmet holistic needs of the patients

Furthermore, this information can be used to:

- Identify how quality of life can be improved for individuals and to help plan holistic care for individual patients

- Assess quality of care in individual services
- Measure progress on survivorship care across networks or countries

This holistic approach to assessment identifies individual information needs. These needs can be met through a discussion with a healthcare professional, which is supported by written or multimedia materials and offers signposting for individuals to high-quality information and support (Table 14.1). The table below illustrates the most common issues expressed through assessment. They are multidimensional in nature representing psychological, physical and functional concerns.

14.2.2 Common Post-HSCT Concerns

14.2.2.1 Physical Well-Being

Most studies found that survivors report resumption of routine physical activities but describe a greater number of medical problems (Mosher et al. 2009). Fatigue is one of the most commonly reported concerns, and many HSCT patients are dissatisfied with their energy levels many years after treatment. Providing information materials and education on fatigue management is a key area where nurses can positively influence this troubling issue (Anderson et al. 2007; Andorsky et al. 2006).

Table 14.1 Top 10 common concerns (www.eHNA/ Macmillan.org.uk analysis 2015)

1.	Worry, fear or anxiety
2.	Tiredness, exhaustion or fatigue
3.	Sleep problems/ nightmares
4.	Pain
5.	Eating or appetite
6.	Anger or frustration
7.	Getting around (walking)
8.	Memory or concentration
9.	Hot flushes/ sweating
10.	Sore or dry mouth

Accessed Aug 2016

14.2.2.2 Psychological Distress

It is known that 5–19% of HSCT survivors exhibit symptoms that are consistent with post-traumatic stress disorder (PTSD). In those without PTSD, four out of ten report clinically significant psychological distress at an average of 3.4 years post-transplant. The same study found that there was no difference by age, gender, transplant type or time following transplant (Rusiewicz et al. 2008).

14.2.2.3 Return to Work

HSCT survivors return to work despite ongoing physical and psychological symptoms. Younger age and higher levels of education have been linked to a higher probability of post-transplant employment. Those who are unsuccessful in returning to work have poorer physical, cognitive and social functioning and report more pain, sleep disorders and distress (Mosher et al. 2009).

While return to work or education is important to survivors, in guiding our patients, it is essential to consider the following:

- Type of work
  - Physical demand
  - Environment
  - Routine
  - Hours
- Support of employer
  - Phased return is usually the optimal way of enabling people to return to work progressively
- Financial pressure
  - Many people need to return to work due to mounting financial difficulties
- Self-esteem
  - Some people feel 'lost' without their work identity and feel a sense of urgency to return

14.2.2.4 Sexuality

Evidence suggests that sexual function is one of the most prevalent and persistent long-term concerns after HSCT.

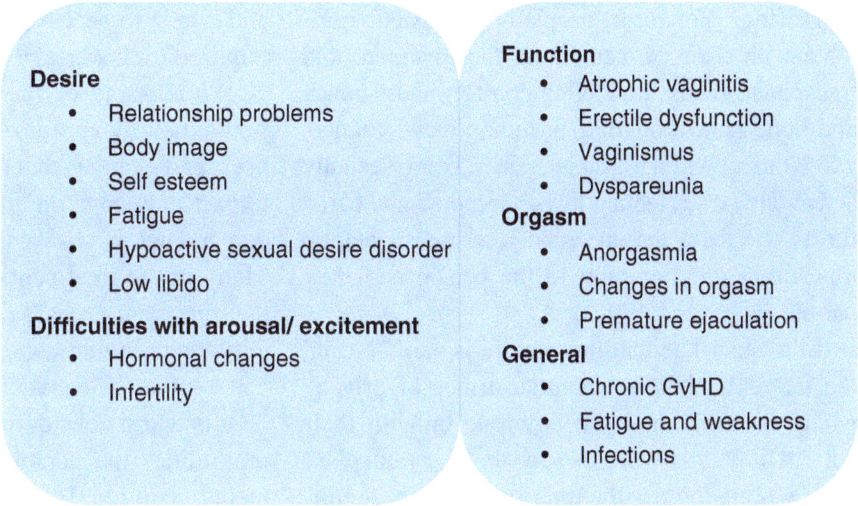

Fig. 14.1 Range of concerns in relation to sexual response cycle (Adapted from Greenfield 2012 www.ebmt.org accessed Sept 2016)

Despite its prevalence and the range of concerns that can be experienced across the entire sexual response cycle (Fig. 14.1), sexual function issues are under-reported. However, a range of sexual concerns have been described with a tendency for women to report more problems than men and women continue to describe more sexual concerns a number of years post-transplant (Mosher et al. 2009). Sexual function is typically multifactorial in origin with endocrine, mechanical and psychological factors. People may benefit from relaxation, massage therapy, aromatherapy or other complementary procedures. Those that resume sexual relations in the first post-transplant year tend to experience fewer long-term issues (Jean and Syrjala 2009).

14.3 Addressing Sexuality

Sexuality is a part of each person's life and identity and is much more than the physical act of sexual intercourse or sexual expression. It is also about less obvious components including how people perceive themselves as sexual beings and the need to be recognised, connected with, loved and cared for by others. Whether the person is in a relationship (gay, lesbian, heterosexual), is single or enjoys sex with one or multiple partners, most people will have sexual needs and desires throughout their life (Osho 2002; Williams 2003; Quinn 2010). There is a danger that in seeing sexuality as merely a physical expression that the haematology and transplant care team may fail to see that sexuality is about the whole person including how they relate to others in an intimate way. Whether the patient is or is not sexually active during the prolonged treatment period before, during and after transplant, patients will need support and advice from the team caring for them, on sexual changes, choices and concerns.

Sex and sexuality are largely seen as a very private matter, and a patient and/or partner may be reluctant to talk about their concerns or unexpected changes to a member of the transplant team who appear busy dealing with other aspects of the treatment process (Schover 1997; Twigg 2000; Mulhall 2008). It is important that the team make it clear that they are there to help with sexual changes and worries and to know what help is available.

There may be a misconception from some members of the transplant team that a person undergoing a stem cell transplant will not have an interest in sex. In reality, whether a person is in a relationship or not, human beings are born as sexual human beings and will die as sexual human beings (Quinn 2010). What that means for each person and how they will express that need throughout periods of their life will change. For some, people being sexually intimate with their partner during the treatment and transplant process may bring comfort, reassurance and hope amidst ongoing uncertainty and change, while others will have no interest in being sexually active. However, feeling loved, accepted and cared for as one faces the uncertainty of transplantation may bring great comfort to the person and their partner (Schover 1997).

In a busy haematology or transplant setting, the team can help to facilitate times of privacy when the individual can be alone or with their partner if this is what they wish. The transplant team who recognise the importance of these intimate moments can often organise treatments and interventions, at less acute points in the transplant process, in order to provide these moments or times of privacy.

The diagnosis of cancer or indeed any illness and the treatments and changes required may have a profound impact on the person and partner, affecting them physically, emotionally, socially and spiritually (Murphy 1990; Brandeburg et al. 2010). For example, facing the reality of temporary or permanent infertility and the multiple body and life changes secondary to disease and treatments can affect a person's sexual identity. The physical and psychological demands of dealing with a serious illness, the transplant demands and setting can interfere with the human sexual response cycle (desire/interest, arousal, readiness (penetration), orgasm and resolution, satisfaction). Any of these points on the response cycle may be affected but can be sensitively addressed (Schover 1997). The team can sensitively support the person and the partner through the transplantation process and treatments mindful of the impact on the person's sexual being. This includes providing accurate information on potential sexual changes that may occur, practical advice on the choice of treatment and interventions and a listening ear. Many sexual concerns arising in the haematology and transplant setting can be resolved or certainly reduced by a member of the team simply listening to the person's concerns and knowing how

and where to access practical and expert help, if required (Schover 1997; Quinn 2010).

While some of the changes to the person's sexuality may appear obvious, many of the more profound changes that a person may face and the impact they have on an individual are often hidden and not so obvious to others (Murphy 1990). Many of the treatments and changes required in the transplant process can affect a person's sexuality including how they relate to their own body and to others (Schover 1997).

It is worth considering the impact of other comorbidities the person may have and the treatments required for these conditions and how these too may affect their sexuality and their ability to have sex. In addressing sexual concerns, the transplant team can be proactive in supporting the person with body changes and psychological concerns that may be interfering with their sexual identity and sexual expression.

Members of the transplant team who are aware of the possible impact that treatments, the transplant protocol and supportive medications may have on a person's sexuality will be better able to speak to the person sensitively, honestly and clearly before the commencement of treatment. These issues should be an important part of the preparation for treatment and transplantation (Quinn 2010). Support may take the form of practical advice, including adjusting to an altered sex life during treatment, adequate pain/symptom control, comfortable positioning during sex, contraception, providing private moments, advice on sexual aids and medical treatments or simply an opportunity to talk about concerns and fears (Table 14.2). Practical support and guidance can help the person returning to sexual activity after transplantation or simply regaining confidence in being sexually expressive again.

Many of the treatment agents (chemotherapy, targeted therapies and radiation) used in the field of haematology and transplantation are known to cause specific problems which can lead to lower sex drive, vaginal dryness (which may cause pain during intercourse), erection concerns, ejaculation and orgasm difficulties (which may lead to loss of con-

Table 14.2 Providing support (Quinn 2010)

Sensitively listening and addressing fears

Creating time and privacy for couples to be alone

Providing adequate symptom relief

Support with body changes

Encouraging couples/sexual partners to talk to one another

Advice on creative foreplay (hugging, stroking, having a shared bath, kissing, mutual masturbation)

Advice on alternative positioning

Alternatives to sexual penetration

Guidance on sexual aids (dilators, vacuum pumps, dildo, toys)

Guidance on medical treatments (oral, injection, pellets)

Counselling

fidence and lack of sexual enjoyment) (Brandenburg et al. 2010). Some drugs including the vinca alkaloids and some targeted therapies may cause nerve damage giving rise to erectile dysfunction and to ejaculation and orgasm difficulties. Following total body irradiation, a small number of patients may experience damage to the nerve, vascular and muscle tissue giving rise to possible erectile difficulties, including the inability to get or maintain an erection suitable for sexual penetration or vaginal changes including stenosis and/or dryness which may cause pain during sexual intercourse.

Women may benefit from the team explaining the use of vaginal lubricants and dilation to prevent vaginal stenosis. Men may require support in exploring treatment options for erectile concerns. These complications may require interventions including advice on oral medications (sildenafil, tadalafil, vardenafil), pellet (intraurethral alprostadil) (MUSE), injection (intracavernosal alprostadil) and appliances (vacuum device) to address erectile dysfunction. Hormone replacement therapy unless contraindicated may have a place, an opportunity to talk through fears and concerns and/or psychosexual therapy support (Brandenburg et al. 2010).

If patients are sexually active during treatment, the team should advise them to use some form of barrier method (condoms, femidoms, dental dams) (Quinn 2010). This is to protect the patient's partner from the minimal risk of irritation caused by a small amount of chemotherapy agents remaining in bodily fluids such as semen, urine and rectal and vaginal secretions. These barrier methods may also reduce the risk of infection especially if the patient is at risk of neutropenia and prolonged immunosuppression. While individuals are advised to take steps to prevent infection, rarely should this prevent the person from enjoying sex with a partner. Occasionally the team may learn of partners no longer sleeping in the same bed for fear of contamination to their partner; the team can reassure the couple that this is not necessary and they can continue with their usual sleeping arrangements. The team can also be sensitive to the demands made and the concerns that arise on the person or couple due to the transplant process.

Other sexual difficulties may arise due to body changes and other symptoms including weight gain or loss, skin changes, graft versus host disease, constipation, diarrhoea, nausea, fatigue, oral complications, depression and anxiety. The person's confidence in being sexual active may be affected by the unwanted body changes that occur. Poorly controlled symptoms, such as nausea, vomiting, constipation, diarrhoea, loss of appetite and extreme tiredness caused by the treatments and the underlying disease, may affect the person physically and psychologically. Carefully assessing and managing these symptoms may enable the person to enjoy the comfort of sexual intimacy with their partner (Schover 1997).

Some of the supportive treatments used in the transplant setting while bringing relief to these unpleasant symptoms can also give rise to sexual difficulties. Pain relief including opiates may give rise to uncomfortable constipation, tiredness, nausea and mucosal dryness leading to painful vagina/anal intercourse and erectile dysfunction. Some anti-sickness medication while providing necessary relief from nausea can effect erectile functioning. While antianxiety and anti-depressant mediations help with stress and anxiety, these medications can lead to a lower sex drive, erectile dysfunction, ejaculatory and orgasm difficulties and vaginal dryness (Quinn 2010).

Many of the chemotherapy agents used in the haematology and transplant setting can affect the person's fertility including alkylating agents which are known to cause most damage, resulting in either temporary or permanent infertility. For many young patients, this may be the first time that they have had to consider the possibility of planning children, and this will require support from the team, family and friends. Facing the possibility of being infertile can have a profound effect on how the person feels about themselves and their place in the world.

Patients will be advised not to plan children during the treatment as the drugs and the demanding treatment requirements will affect the development of the embryo leading to foetal defects and miscarriage. For some people/couples, it may be very painful having to put their plans for a family on hold during the treatment and transplant period. Occasionally a woman may discover a cancer diagnosis during her pregnancy and may be advised to undergo a medical termination because the pregnancy will not be viable and/or in order to proceed with necessary treatment. This can be a very difficult time for the woman and her partner; sometimes the full impact of this loss becomes more apparent following the completion of treatment.

The team can be there to talk about the impact of treatment and to support and advice on the possible options available to support fertility (Schover 1997). For men this may include sperm banking and the possibility of cryopreservation of testicular tissue, generally used for younger patients. For women, this may include cryopreservation of embryos or eggs and ovarian preservation. In some cases, the urgency of treatment may mean that fertility-saving options are not possible. During the transplant process, the focus for everyone including the patient may be on treating the disease, and the reality of being infertile becomes more important in the months and years following transplantation. This can be extremely difficult for patients who are beginning new relationships and have to disclose this to their new partner. This reality can be addressed at follow-up clinics

both in the hospital and community, ensuring the person has support that they can access. Individuals and couples may need support and advice over their concerns of having passed or passing on genes to their children predisposing them to a higher risk of cancer (Quinn 2010).

Some patients will be at risk of bleeding due to thrombocytopenia and should be advised to continue a sex life if they so wish but to be aware of reducing trauma during sex, including vaginal, oral and anal intercourse. Localised trauma may be reduced by using a more gentle thrusting movement during penetration or masturbation.

Many of the drugs used in the transplant setting may bring on the early onset of menopause and the associated symptoms which can cause great distress. Medically induced menopause brings unwanted symptoms including vaginal dryness, mood changes, hot flushes, low confidence and sometimes a lack of interest in sex. Women may find it more difficult to achieve a satisfactory orgasm (Brandenburg et al. 2010). It is important that women and their partners are forewarned about these symptoms but also to ensure these issues are revisited sensitively during and after treatment.

Men and women may need support and advice on finding alternative ways to express themselves sexually both during and after transplant. Although men and women may have a reduced interest in sex for a period of time, their interest in returning to a sexually active relationship may return in weeks and months following the transplant.

Practical measures including the careful positioning of medical devices may enable a person to be held and hugged during prolonged hospitalisation. These measures also include reducing clutter around the persons' bed so that their partner can be closer to them and critically reviewing and removing any unnecessary infection control measures that may act as a barrier to intimacy. Practical advice on how to deal with medical devices including urinary catheters and emptying bowels and/or bladder before having sex can provide greater comfort. While the person may lack the energy to participate in sexual intercourse, they may wish to try alternatives including cuddling, hugging, lying in bed together, increased time for foreplay, sharing a bath or shower together and sharing quiet and private moments together (Schover 1997).

Although the sexual needs of patients in the highly technically setting of transplantation can sometimes be overlooked, the ability to be intimate with a partner might be a welcome relief from some of the demands made on the person by the transplant process.

14.4 Summary

14.4.1 Wider Impact of Survivorship Care

Carers of those with cancer report high levels of emotional distress. The psychological difficulties that carers report can be prolonged. This is exacerbated by their own lifestyle and role disruption; carers report financial difficulties and are often unable to work for periods themselves or have to give up work altogether due to their 'carer role' commitment. It is important to recognise these issues and offer carers support and information.

14.4.2 Models of Long-Term Follow-Up

It is widely recognised that HSCT recipients require structured long-term follow-up and screening to reduce the morbidity and mortality demonstrated in those considered as long-term survivors.

There are clear guidelines around screening requirements (Majhail et al. 2012) but little direction on how these might best be implemented in a late effects (LE) service. A survey of UK transplant centres identified that all had a LE service and most had a standard operating procedure outlining its process but identified wide variability in almost every aspect of the late effects services (Hamblin et al. 2017).

Important components for successful delivery of LE service include:
- Assessment tools incorporating clinical and psychosocial late effects
- Availability of a range of medical and allied health specialists
- Access to psychological services
- Implementation of second malignancy screening, e.g. mammography and PAP smear

14.4.3 Opportunities for Nurses

Nurses have a significant role in delivering and/or coordinating post-HSCT care for patients.

Nurses have an opportunity to:

- Identify useful resources for patients
- Develop post-HSCT services for patients
- Ensure that care meets the needs and concerns of patients
- Develop innovative roles as individual practitioner and as part of a wider multidisciplinary team
- Develop the evidence base by leading/participating in survivorship research
- Develop creative ways of working and providing suitable clinical and supportive care

14.5 Post-transplant Complications and Surveillance

Standardisation of follow-up protocols is important to prevent important tests being overlooked or being duplicated unnecessarily.

14.5.1 Second Malignancies

There is an increased risk of developing a second solid cancer post-transplant in the range of 2–6% at 10 years. Data suggests that second solid cancers occur twice as frequently in the transplant population than in the general public with this increasing to threefold at 15 years. There are several risk factors that may contribute to the development of a second solid cancer (Curtis et al. 1997):

- Total body irradiation
- Primary disease
- Male sex
- Pre-transplant conditioning
- Genetic predisposition contributing to initial cancer and subsequent malignancy

Clinicians have long been aware that radiation leads to second solid cancers with a latent period of approximately 3–5 years before developing a malignancy (Rizzo et al. 2009). The risk for non-squamous cell cancer is higher in younger patients (especially those under 30 years) at ten times that of nonirradiated patients. Other cancers such as breast, thyroid, brain, central nervous system, bone and connective tissue and melanoma are all related to radiation exposure. Screening for some of these cancers is available and aids in early diagnosis (Savani et al., 2011).

All patients should be enrolled into national cancer screening programmes for breast, cervical, colon and skin cancer. Particular attention should be paid to women who receive radiation to their chest >800cGy to ensure they follow guidelines laid down for paediatric survivors. These state that annual mammogram screening should begin at 25 years of age or 8 years after exposure whichever occurs later. Women should have PAP smears annually to three yearly, and those with GvHD should be screened annually. Patients should have at least six monthly dental reviews and an annual thyroid assessment, and if any thyroid nodule is identified, imaging and potential biopsy should be undertaken (Savani et al. 2011).

At the initial consent for transplant consultation, patients should be counselled about the future potential risks of second malignancy. This is an ideal time to engage with the patient and help them make changes to their lifestyle that will have an impact on their lives moving forward. Smoking cessation, a healthy balanced diet, taking regular exercise, reducing alcohol consumption and taking care of their skin in the sun will all have beneficial effects.

14.5.2 Systematic Post-transplant Screening and Investigations

A specific screening plan for transplant patients has been published by Majhail et al. (2012) on behalf of the Center for International Blood and Marrow Transplant Research (DeFilipp et al. 2016), American Society for Blood and Marrow Transplantation (ASBMT), European Group for Blood and Marrow Transplantation (EBMT), Asia-Pacific Blood and Marrow Transplantation Group (APBMT), Bone Marrow Transplant Society of Australia and New Zealand (BMTSANZ), East Mediterranean Blood and Marrow Transplantation Group (EMBMT) and Sociedade Brasileira de Transplante de Medula Ossea (SBTMO).

These comprehensive guidelines written by an expert group in 2006 and updated in 2011 provide a consensus for screening and preventative measures for autologous and allogeneic stem cell transplant patients who have survived for at least 6 months following transplant. There are also patient versions of the guidelines that can be found at www.BeTheMatch.org/Patient (Majhail et al. 2012).

The recommendations take each system and describe the late complication and the general risk factors for developing them. It goes on to suggest the monitoring tests and preventative measures that should be undertaken supported by associated evidence from randomised trials and if none is available from retrospective studies or from expert opinion when no evidence exists at all (Majhail et al. 2012).

Infection and revaccination are described elsewhere in this textbook, but regardless of time since transplant, all presentations of infection should be thoroughly and rigorously investigated and treated aggressively. Revaccination should be initiated as per the widely accepted Tomblyn et al., (2009) guidelines.

Majhail et al. (2012) elegantly describe the general follow-up that a transplant patient should receive in a systematic order and this can be applied fairly easily in the clinic environment. Below is a concise form of the guidance. Please refer to Table 14.3 for the recommended screening guidelines and the full publication for further details.

14.5.3 Ocular Screening

Ocular screening should commence at 6 months and continue on an annual basis for assessment of keratoconjunctivitis sicca syndrome, cataracts and ischaemic microvascular retinopathy. Sicca syndrome (vaginitis, dry skin and xerostomia) occur in 10–40% of patients.

14.5.4 Oral Examination

The oral cavity can be affected with chronic graft versus host disease (cGvHD) and, even in the absence of cGvHD, requires repeated assessment from 6 months especially if there is a sign of xerostomia (dry mouth) as this increases the risk of dental caries. Good oral hygiene and treatment of oral infections should be initiated promptly on recognition. There is an increased risk of secondary oral squamous cell carcinoma in those with oral cGvHD, and patients should be aware to raise concerns.

14.5.5 Pulmonary Screening

Respiratory problems include bronchiolitis obliterans syndrome (BOS), idiopathic pneumonia syndrome (also known as interstitial pneumonitis), cryptogenic organising pneumonia (COP) and sinopulmonary infections. Clinical review at 6 months and annually with physical examination and history should be performed. Counselling with regard to smoking cessation is extremely important. If the patient has GvHD, then it may be appropriate to undertake pulmonary function testing, and if there is evidence of lung involvement, then imaging such as inspiratory and expiratory CT for air trapping to exclude BOS is indicated.

Table 14.3 Recommended screening and prevention (Majhail et al. 2012) printed with permission from Elsevier Inc

Recommended screening/ prevention	6 months	1 year	Annually
Immunity			
Encapsulated organism prophylaxis	2	2	2
PCP prophylaxis	1	2	2
CMV testing	2	2	2
Immunisations	1	1	1
Ocular			
Ocular clinical symptom evaluation	1	1	1
Ocular fundus exam	+	1	+
Oral complications			
Clinical assessment	1	1	1
Dental assessment	+	1	1
Respiratory			
Clinical pulmonary assessment	1	1	1
Smoking tobacco avoidance	1	1	1
Pulmonary function testing	+	+	+
Chest radiography	+	+	+
Cardiovascular			
Cardiovascular risk-factor assessment	+	1	1
Liver			
Liver function testing	1	1	+
Serum ferritin testing		1	+
Kidney			
Blood pressure screening	1	1	1
Urine protein screening	1	1	1
BUN/creatinine testing	1	1	1
Muscle and connective tissue			
Evaluation for muscle weakness	2	2	2
Physical activity counselling	1	1	1
Skeletal			
Bone density testing (adult women, all allogeneic transplantation recipients and patients at high risk for bone loss)		1	+
Nervous system			
Neurologic clinical evaluation	+	1	1
Evaluate for cognitive development		1	1
Endocrine			

(continued)

Table 14.3 (continued)

Recommended screening/prevention	6 months	1 year	Annually
Thyroid function testing		1	1
Growth velocity in children		1	1
Gonadal function assessment (pre-pubertal men and women)	1	1	1
Gonadal function assessment (post-pubertal women)		1	+
Gonadal function assessment (post-pubertal men)		+	+
Mucocutaneous			
Skin self-exam and sun exposure counselling	1	1	1
Gynaecologic exam in women	+	1	1
Second cancers			
Second cancer vigilance counselling		1	1
Screening for second cancers		1	1
Psychosocial			
Psychosocial/QOL clinical assessment	1	1	1
Sexual function assessment	1	1	1

Majhail et al. (2012)

1 recommended for all transplantation recipients, *2* recommended for any patient with ongoing cGvHD or immunosuppression, + reassessment recommended for abnormal testing in a previous time period or for new signs/symptoms

14.5.6 Cardiovascular Tests

Cardiovascular disease is rare in the transplant setting. Clinical review at 6 months and annually with physical examination, blood pressure monitoring and history should be performed. Counselling with regard to a healthy lifestyle, taking regular exercise, maintaining a healthy weight, eating well and not smoking should be reinforced in clinic and be in line with the recommendations for the general public. Risk factors such as diabetes, hypertension and dyslipidaemia can be addressed with non-medication interventions, but some may require treatment if this approach is unsuccessful. If any concerns are raised, investigations with ECG

and ECHO and referral to cardiology may be needed.

14.5.7 Hepatic Complications

Liver function tests are taken at most clinical reviews and aid assessing for the onset of GvHD. Patients with pre-existing liver conditions such as hepatitis B or C should have monitoring of their viral load by polymerase chain reaction (PCR) and referral to a hepatologist or virologist for advice on ongoing antiviral therapy. Serum ferritin levels should be measured at 1 year, and those with elevated levels should be followed more closely and considered for chelation.

14.5.8 Renal Surveillance

Renal injury is common post-transplant as many drugs are nephrotoxic such as ciclosporin, aminoglycosides, acyclovir, etc., and renal function should be checked at 6 months and annually thereafter. In those with chronic kidney disease (CKD), referral to nephrology and assessment with renal ultrasound and/or biopsy should be considered.

14.5.9 Musculoskeletal Assessment

Patients with GvHD and especially those receiving systemic steroids may encounter problems with muscle strength, general weakness and loss of function. All patients should be given advice about regular daily exercise. Those who have developed GvHD should be assessed for range of joint movement to detect sclerotic changes and referred on to physiotherapy for active intervention.

Osteoporosis is common with reports of incidence of 25–50% at 18 months (Majhail et al. 2012). Those with ongoing GvHD requiring long-term use of corticosteroids are at particular risk. DEXA scanning is indicated and advice regarding diet and exercise given to optimise bone mineral density and falls prevention. Supplementation with vitamin D and calcium may be required.

14.5.10 Neurological Assessment

All patients should be assessed annually for signs and symptoms of neurologic deficit such as leukoencephalopathy, cognitive impairment or neurotoxicity as a consequence of long-term use of calcineurin inhibitors. Also any signs or symptoms of peripheral neuropathy should be examined for. If any deficit is found during routine assessment, the patient should be referred for nerve conduction studies or MRI as indicated by the clinical findings. A referral to a neurologist may be appropriate.

14.5.11 Endocrine Surveillance

Endocrine dysfunction is common following stem cell transplant. Thyroid function and gonadal testing are recommended at 1 year and then annually with replacement if needed. Up to 25% of patients who receive total body irradiation will have some thyroid dysfunction (Majhail et al. 2012). Significant gonadal failure requiring hormone replacement is more common in women than men as the ovaries are more sensitive to the effects of chemoradiotherapy than the testes. Sexual dysfunction and assessment of sexual function are described more fully in this chapter. Sexual dysfunction is common although typically under-reported and results in impaired quality of life (QoL) and relationship problems.

14.5.12 Second Malignancy Screening

All patients should be counselled regarding the increased risk of secondary cancers and advised to monitor themselves frequently (breast and testicular examination) and report symptoms promptly. The median time to development is 5–6 years post-therapy although this risk continues to rise with no plateau. Cancers of all organs are well described but the skin, oral cavity, CNS, bone, thyroid and connective tissue are more prevalent. Breast screening should be carried out

for women who receive total body irradiation at age 25 or 8 years following exposure whichever is later but no later than 40 years. Cervical PAP smears should be performed every 1–3 years (yearly if presence of GvHD) in women aged 21 and over or within 3 years of initial sexual activity whichever is earliest. Advice regarding sun exposure, wearing sun screen, loose fitting clothing and a hat and glasses when outside should be given to all patients.

14.5.13 Psychological Screening

Psychological problems may manifest in various ways in the post-transplant setting, and clinicians need to be vigilant for subtle signs and make appropriate referrals for interventions. Depression, anxiety, fatigue and psychosexual dysfunction are frequently observed. This often increases in the transition from early transplant recovery to longer-term follow-up as the patient adjusts to the change in life style, employment and financial independence. Relationships with family and friends may change leading to distressing outcomes. A low level of suspicion should be maintained by the clinician for early signs of psychological distress throughout follow-up.

14.5.14 Fertility Concerns

Fertility is often lost due to high-dose treatments although not in all. Patients should be counselled thoroughly regarding safe sex in those of child-bearing age. Those who are contemplating pregnancy should be referred on to specialist services for advice and monitoring.

14.5.15 Summary

There is no standard instrument guiding post-transplant care that will apply to all patients who have undergone stem cell transplant. Each patient is an individual, and, as such, an individualised plan needs to be generated. Large institutions have published guidelines, such as Fred

Hutchinson Cancer Research Center's LTFU guidelines, the National Marrow Donor Program Be The Match long-term survival guidelines, the Livestrong Care Plan and the Passport for Cure, to name but a few.

The key message is that early screening leads to early detection and treatment, although it is not fully proven that this leads to better outcomes. It is the role of all healthcare providers to raise awareness for the potential for secondary effects of high-dose therapies and to ensure adequate and appropriate survivorship care. Empowering patients to be involved in their own long-term care is paramount. Having 'buy-in' from the patient will help to ensure that they are vigilant for subtle changes and attend screening appointments. They have self-interest at heart and are unlikely to forget that they require certain follow-up tests if they are educated in the late effects clinic. As they enter a passive watchful and waiting period, this is the time when things can be forgotten, so vigilance from the patient and family will help the clinical team avoid errors and omissions.

Having a written care plan or treatment summary detailing the chemotherapies, radiation and side effects suffered with future dates for screening is ideal and can be based on any of the published material listed above. Educate the patient and family on the new normal, what can be expected and when, enable them to become an active participant in their own post-transplant care and help our patients navigate the potentially stormy waters ahead.

14.6 Metabolic Syndrome

In addition to the more familiar post-HSCT sequelae, metabolic syndrome (MetS) is of particular note due to its collection of cardiovascular risk factors that increase the risk of cardiovascular disease, diabetes mellitus and all-cause mortality. Long-term survivors of HSCT have a considerable risk of developing MetS and subsequently cardiovascular disease. The estimated prevalence of MetS is 31–49% among HSCT recipients.

A series of recommendations (Table 14.4) have been developed (DeFilipp et al. 2016) to help clinicians provide screening and preventive care for MetS and cardiovascular disease among HSCT recipients. Furthermore, all HSCT survivors should be advised of the risks of MetS and encouraged to undergo the recommended screening based on their predisposition and ongoing risk factors.

14.7 Compliance and Adherence in the Long-Term Follow-Up Setting

Compliance and adherence issues are common in HSCT survivors. Reasons given in the literature for refusal, noncompliance or abandonment of treatment include the patient's physical discomfort, misunderstanding and uncertainty about the merits of medication, poor communication regarding the diagnosis and treatment regime and inadequate information on illness in general and secondary effects of the disease and its treatment in particular.

Five factors of adherence (WHO 2003):

1. Health system
2. Socio-economic
3. Health or condition
4. Treatment
5. Patient

1. Health System

   A relationship based on a partnership between the patient, relatives and the treating physician improves adherence (Russmann et al. 2010). Insufficient and inadequate doctor/patient/family dialogue, relationship, trust and mutual information are quoted as one of the most important causes of noncompliance.

   Poor attention to patient education with regard to medication benefits and risks, side effects and correct dosing can result in decreased quality of life, more frequent consultations and possible hospital readmissions.

Table 14.4   Screening guidelines for metabolic syndrome (DeFilipp et al. 2016)

Table 2 Screening guidelines for metabolic syndrome and cardiovascular risk factors for adult and pediatric patients among the general population and HCT survivors

	General adult population	Adult long-term HCT survivors	General pediatric population	Pediatric long-term HCT survivors
	(http://www.uspreventiveservicestaskforce.org/)	Majhail et al.[14]	(http://www.nhlbi.nih.gov)	Pulsipher et al.[15]
Weight, height and BMI	Weight height and BMI assessment in all adults (no specific recommendation for screening interval)	No specific recommendations	Weight, height and BMI assessment after 2 years of age (no specified screening interval)	Weight, height and BMI assessment yearly
Dyslipidemia	For persons with increased risk for coronary heart disease, assessments should begin at age 20.	Lipid profile assessment every 5 years in males aged ≥35 years and females aged ≥45 years.	Lipid panel between 9–11 years of age or earlier if family history	Lipid profile at least every 5 years; if abnormal, screen annually
	The interval for screening should be shorter for people who have lipid levels close to those warranting therapy, and longer intervals for those not at increased risk who have had repeatedly normal lipid levels.	Screening should start at age 20 for anyone at increased risk (smokers, DM, HTN, BMI ≥30 kg/m^2 and family history of heart disease before age 50 for male relatives or before age 60 for female relatives).		
Blood pressure	Blood pressure assessment every 3-5 years in adults aged 18-39 years with normal blood pressure (<130/85 mm Hg) who do not have other risk factors	Blood pressure assessment at least every 2 years	Blood pressure assessment yearly after the age of 3 years, interpreted for age/sex/height	Blood pressure assessment at each visit and at least annually
	Blood pressure assessment annually in adults aged ge1;40 years and for those who are at increased risk for high blood pressure (blood pressure 130 to 139/85 to 89 mm Hg, those who are overweight or obese, and African-Americans)			
Hyperglycemia	Screening for abnormal blood glucose (HbA1C, fasting plasma glucose or oral glucose tolerance test) every 3 years in adults aged 40-70 years who are overweight or obese.	Screening for type 2 DM every 3 years in adults aged ≥45 years or in those with sustained higher blood pressure (>135/80 mm Hg)	Fasting glucose every 2 years after the age of 10 years in overweight children with other risk factors	Fasting glucose at least every 5 years; if abnormal, screen annually

Reprinted with permission from Elsevier: Biology of Blood and Marrow Transplantation, 22(8), 1493-1503; doi: 10.1016/j.bbmt.2016.05.007, copyright 2016
Reprinted with permission from Nature Publishing Group: Bone Marrow Transplantation, 52 (2), 173-182; doi: 10.1038/bmt.2016.203, copyright 2016
Abbreviations: *BMI* body mass index, *DM* diabetes mellitus, *HbA1C* hemoglobin A1C, *HCT* hematopoietic cell transplantation, *HTN* hypertension

A whole team approach to education and support facilitates the development of joint strategies that increase likelihood of adherence.

2. Socio-economic

Reasons for noncompliance may revolve around a lack of resources, both in the patient's finances and in the level of clinical expertise and medical facilities available.

The economic cost of cancer plays a significant role in therapy adherence. Many patients need to travel considerable distances to access treatment at substantial personal cost. Furthermore, the majority of patients and many of their carers are unable to work during and for many months following treatment leading to a loss of income and a lack of financial stability.

Availability of social support services is yet another potent factor, especially in patients overwhelmed by multiple pressing needs.

3. Health or Condition

Extensive symptoms such as nausea, vomiting, pain, constipation and fatigue play an important role in a person's ability to manage medication and follow a treatment course with a degree of reliability.

Disease progression and declining health can interfere with the physical ability to manage treatment and also the willingness to continue with treatment.

4. Treatment

Therapy-related factors refer to the treatment regime and the process of taking medication according to the regime. To optimise compliance requires precision and concentration and the ability to follow specific instructions around timing of dosing. Often careful planning around the daily programme of treatment will increase the patient's ability to follow the treatment plan accurately.

Drug frequency, odour, side effects and prior experience of therapy can all impact upon and hinder compliance (Lee et al. 1992).

5. Patient

The patient's attitude towards their illness and treatment are important factors. Their support network, resources, disease knowledge, health beliefs and expectations are central to the degree to which they will be able to follow treatment.

Psychological distress or other psychological factors may also be a cause of poor compliance, often requiring professional intervention and support.

For many patients, a simple lack of understanding of the importance of regular treatment or assessment is the driver for poor adherence or attendance. Others are afraid that annual check-ups may reveal sinister pathology that they would prefer to ignore.

14.8 Immunisations Following Stem Cell Transplantation

Stem cell transplant recipients have a reduction in their antibody levels or titres to vaccine-preventable diseases. This ranges from 50% to 75% loss of cover for tetanus, diphtheria, polio, *S. pneumoniae* and *H. influenzae* at 1 year, rising to 100% loss of protection at 2 years in the non-revaccinated patient Ljungman et al., (2009). This may occur in both autologous and allogeneic stem cell transplant patients having peripheral blood, umbilical cord blood or bone marrow transplantation. Therefore, all stem cell transplant recipients should be routinely revaccinated (Tables 14.5 and 14.6). As limited data exists in alternative donor settings of cord and haplo-identical transplant, the guidelines suggest that for simplicity the same revaccination schedule should be followed for all stem cell transplant patients until further evidence is generated (Ljungman et al. 2009).

There may be some immune function derived from the donated stem cells, but this is unreliable and as such post-transplant vaccine should be used (Johnston and Conly, 2002).

For those patients who develop chronic graft versus host disease (cGvHD), it is likely that all immune function and protection are lost and Ljungman et al. (2009) recommend the same revaccination schedule but advocate measuring antibody levels pre- and post-vaccine to deter-

Table 14.5   Vaccination of haematopoietic cell transplant recipients

Vaccine	Recommended for use after HCT	Time post-HCT to initiate vaccine	No. of doses[a]	Improved by donor vaccination (practicable only in related-donor setting)
Pneumococcal conjugate (PCV)	Yes (BI)	3–6 months	3–4[b]	Yes; may be considered when the recipient is at high risk for chronic GVHD
Tetanus, diphtheria, acellular pertussis[c]	Yes Tetanus–diphtheria (BII) Pertussis (CIII)	6–12 months	3[d]	Tetanus: likely Diphtheria: likely Pertussis: unknown
Haemophilus influenzae conjugate	Yes (BII)	6–12 months	3	Yes
Meningococcal conjugate	Follow country recommendations for general population (BII)	6–12 months	1	Unknown
Inactivated polio	Yes (BII)	6–12 months	3	Unknown
Recombinant hepatitis B	Follow country recommendations for general population (BII)	6–12 months	3	Likely[e]
Inactivated influenza	Yearly (AII)	4–6 months	1–2[f]	Unknown
Measles–Mumps–Rubella[g] (live)	Measles: All children and seronegative adults Measles: BII Mumps: CIII Rubella: BIII EIII (<24 months post-HCT, active GVHD, on immune suppression)	24 months	1–2[h]	Unknown

Ljungman et al., (2009)

Reprinted with permission from Macmillan Publishers Ltd: Bone Marrow Transplantation, 44, 521–526; doi:10.1038/bmt.2009.263, copyright 2009

Vaccinations recommended for both autologous and allogeneic HCT recipients

Abbreviations: *DtaP* diphtheria tetanus pertussis vaccine, *HCT* haematopoietic cell transplant, *PCV* pneumococcal conjugate vaccine, *Tdap* tetanus toxoid-reduced diphtheria toxoid-reduced acellular pertussis vaccine

[a]A uniform-specific interval between doses cannot be recommended, as various intervals have been used in studies. As a general guideline, a minimum of 1 month between doses may be reasonable

[b]Following the primary series of three PCV doses, a dose of the 23-valent polysaccharide pneumococcal vaccine (PPSV23) to broaden the immune response might be given (BII). For patients with chronic GVHD who are likely to respond poorly to PPSV23, a fourth dose of the PCV should be considered instead of PPSV23 (CIII)

[c]DTaP is preferred; however, if only Tdap is available (e.g. because DTaP is not licensed for adults), administer Tdap. Acellular pertussis vaccine is preferred, but the whole-cell pertussis vaccine should be used if it is the only pertussis vaccine available (see text for more information)

[d]See text for consideration of an additional dose(s) of Tdap for older children and adults

[e]Significant improvement of recipient response to hepatitis B vaccine post-transplant can be expected only if the donor receives more than one hepatitis vaccine dose before donation

[f]For children <9 years of age, two doses are recommended yearly between transplant and 9 years of age[306]

[g]Measles, mumps and rubella vaccines are usually given together as a combination vaccine. In females with pregnancy potential, vaccination with rubella vaccine either as a single or a combination vaccine is indicated

[h]In children, two doses are favoured

Table 14.6 Vaccination of haematopoietic cell transplant recipients

Vaccine	Recommendations for use	Rating
Optional		
Hepatitis A	Follow recommendations for general population in each country Ig should be administered to hepatitis A-susceptible HCT recipients who anticipate hepatitis A exposure (for example, during travel to endemic areas) and for post-exposure prophylaxis	CIII
Varicella (Varivax, live)	Limited data regarding safety and efficacy	EIII (<24 months post-HCT, active GVHD or on immunosuppression) CIII (>24 months, without active GVHD or on immunosuppression)
Human papillomavirus	Follow recommendations for general population in each country No data exist regarding the time after HCT when vaccination can be expected to induce an immune response	CIII
Yellow fever (live)	Limited data regarding safety and efficacy The risk–benefit balance may favour the use of the vaccine in patients residing in or travelling to endemic areas	EIII (<24 months, active GVHD or on immunosuppression) CIII (>24 months, without active GVHD or on immunosuppression)
Rabies	Appropriate for use in HCT recipients with potential occupational exposures to rabies Pre-exposure rabies vaccination should probably be delayed until 12–24 months after HCT Postexposure administration of rabies vaccine with human rabies Ig can be administered any time after HCT, as indicated[a]	CIII
Tick-borne encephalitis (TBE)	According to local policy in endemic areas No data exist regarding the time after HCT when vaccination can be expected to induce an immune response	CIII
Japanese B encephalitis	According to local policy when residing in or travelling to endemic areas No data exist regarding the time after HCT when vaccination can be expected to induce an immune response	CIII
Not recommended		
Bacillus Calmette–Guérin (live)	Contraindicated for HCT recipients	EII
Oral poliovirus vaccine (live)	Should not be given to HCT recipients, as an effective, inactivated alternative exist	EIII

Table 14.6 (continued)

Intranasal influenza vaccine (live)	No data regarding safety and immunogenicity Should not be given to HCT recipients, as an effective, inactivated alternative exist	EIII
Cholera	No data were found regarding safety and immunogenicity among HCT recipients	DIII
Typhoid, oral (live)	No data were found regarding safety and immunogenicity among HCT recipients	EIII
Typhoid (i.m.)	No data were found regarding safety, immunogenicity or efficacy among HCT recipients	DIII
Rotavirus	Must be given before 12 weeks of age to be safe	EIII
Zoster vaccine (Zostavax, live)	No data regarding safety among HCT recipients	EIII

Ljungman et al., (2009)
Reprinted withby permission from Macmillan Publishers Ltd: Bone Marrow Transplantation, 44, 521-526; doi:10.1038/bmt.2009.263, copyright 2009
Vaccinations considered optional or not recommended for both autologous and allogeneic HCT recipients
Abbreviation: *HCT* haematopoietic cell transplant
[a]Current Advisory Committee on Immunisation Practices (ACIP) and American Academy of Pediatrics guidelines for post-exposure human rabies Ig and vaccine administration should be followed, which include administering five doses of rabies vaccine administered on days 0, 3, 7, 14 and 28 post-exposure

mine the level of cover that has been achieved and the need for any boosters.

Following transplant, patients will have specific predisposition to some opportunistic or community-acquired infections such as *S. pneumoniae*, *H. influenzae*, measles, varicella or influenza and will have a normal predisposition of contracting regular pathogens such as tetanus, polio or diphtheria. Patients are susceptible to these organisms for a variety of reasons, poor antibody levels, low CD4 and concurrent immunosuppression especially corticosteroid use in the presence of GvHD (Flowers et al., 2015).

There is good evidence that having a low antibody level to vaccine-preventable disease post-transplant and the occurrence of encapsulated bacterial infection such as *S. pneumoniae* and *H. influenzae* are linked which further bolsters the need to have vaccines.

The benefits of revaccination are twofold:

- It directly aids the individual.
- It contributes to a 'herd effect' by maintaining cover within the community.

Live vaccines that are theoretically contraindicated post-transplant are BCG, smallpox, VZV, yellow fever, oral polio and typhoid. Ljungman et al. (1995) published limited data for administration of MMR at 2 years post-transplant in children with no GvHD and who were not on any immunosuppression. They recorded a response rate for those who were seronegative of 65–75%. It is generally accepted that patients who are 2 years post-transplant and at least 1 year from receiving any immunosuppression are able to receive MMR vaccine.

Family members should continue to have all of their routine vaccinations. It is suggested that inactivated polio vaccine is used in family members. If this is not possible, then isolation and avoidance of patient and family member (usually a child) for 4 to 6 weeks are recommended as the live virus may be shed for this time period in body fluids (saliva, vomit, urine, faeces, etc.). If this is not possible, then strict hand hygiene needs to be applied with regard to faeces (nappies or diapers) and avoidance of saliva and shared utensils to reduce risk of transmission (Tomblyn et al. 2009).

Separate guidelines initially existed and were developed by EBMT and the CDC, the IDSA and ASBMT. In order to amalgamate all of the recommendations, an expert group convened in 2009 and produced guidelines for preventing infectious complications among HSCT recipients: a global perspective. From this group, a schedule for revaccination has been agreed as laid out in these two tables and is the adopted practice in most major centres across the world.

14.9 End-of-Life Care in the Haematopoietic Stem Cell Transplant (HSCT) Setting

14.9.1 Background

The famous German philosopher Martin Heidegger once wrote that every human being is a person who is moving towards their own death. Rather than seeing this as something negative, Heidegger suggests that if we truly acknowledge that reality, then it sets us free to live life as we truly want. For many nurses working in the field of HSCT, Heidegger's call to live life to the full is often the driving force in delivering person-centred care and helping people to recover or to live well until they die.

Amidst the great advances in HSCT including increasing cure rates, people living longer and better management of toxicities, the reality still remains that some people will die of their advancing disease and/or treatment-related factors. While the majority of the patients will

return home to continue living their lives, some of the adults and children cared for in this setting may die, while a patient within the hospital or be discharged home to die. In the highly clinical and technical setting of HSCT, this reality can sometimes be overlooked and avoided leaving the patient and family feeling abandoned and alone. In a study exploring the experience of living with advanced cancer, some participants spoke of feeling misunderstood and left alone with their advanced disease, a large part of their suffering and distress arose from the interpretation of their personal pain that was not easily visible to others, and many participants felt that often people did not fully understand what they were going through, leaving them feeling ultimately alone (Quinn 2011).

In reality, the delivery of good end-of-life care can be achieved through each member of the HSCT team (clinical and non-clinical), who have often got to know the patient over a prolonged period of time recognising their important role in supporting patients and their families at this time in their lives. When curative treatment is no longer an option and the focus moves to compassionate care and addressing symptoms, the trusting relationship between the patient, family and the HSCT team is crucial.

14.9.2 End-of-Life Care

End-of-life care and care of the dying have been defined as care that helps all those with advanced, progressive, incurable illness to live as well as possible until the day they die (GMC 2007). Unfortunately, in many parts of the world including some healthcare and HSCT settings, the team may find it difficult to discuss the reality of dying due to a lack of exposure, avoidance, fear of upsetting the patient and sometimes the overmedicalisation and over-specialisation of caring for those who are dying. In reality, care for those moving towards the end of life in the HSCT setting calls for a combination of clinical and human skills, built on sensitivity and humility, coupled with good symptom management – core values of nursing care.

Things have improved, but the challenge remains with some nurses and medical staff in the HSCT setting still reluctant to have a conversation about the reality that the treatment is no longer working and exploring what the patient and family would like as they approach the end of life. This may be a result of living in a society that tends to distance itself from this sensitive subject, coupled with a fear of upsetting people with what is indeed a very sensitive but human subject that, as Heidegger says, touches us all.

The following principles of good end-of-life care or commitments to those moving towards the end of life are worth considering in the HSCT setting:

- When you are moving towards the end of life, we will be honest with you and sensitively support you and your family to ensure your needs and wishes are met, and you are enabled to die in your preferred place of care.
- When you are approaching the end of your life, we will offer you the opportunity to be involved in your care planning. This will include an assessment of your needs and preferences and an agreed set of actions reflecting these choices.
- We will work to ensure that you and your family receive excellent care in accordance with your wishes, at all times of day and night. We will work with our community partners to ensure this happens.
- We will offer you personalised care, based on your wishes and needs. This will include attending to your physical, social, emotional, spiritual and religious needs.
- We recognise the importance of your family, your friends and your support network, and they have the right to have their own needs assessed and reviewed and to have a carer's plan.
- In order to care for you and your family, we will ensure that all staff and volunteers working in our team are aware of the issues surrounding

care at the end of life, in particular the importance of excellence in communicating.
- We will participate in research in order to improve patient and family care at the end of life in the HSCT setting.

This commitment from the HSCT team relies on identifying when a patient may have incurable disease and/or untreatable complications, having the courage to sensitively broach the subject of dying with the patient and family, working with the patient and family to identify and address their physical, social emotional and spiritual needs and planning care together. These core principles will enable nurses, doctors and the HSCT team to support the person to receive, the right care, in the right place, at the right time, every time (GSF 2016).

14.9.3 Caring for Those Who Are Dying

Caring for those who are dying to identify their needs, beliefs and values requires taking the time to hear what they need to say, a process that has been described as an art (Table 14.7).

All nurses and doctors working in HSCT will be required to use the principles of palliative or supportive care in their care of those with

Table 14.7 The art of assessment (Quinn 2014)

Paying attention to the person and hearing their priorities

Thinking beyond the symptom to how it affects the person

Creating time and being present

Cocreating a plan of care with the person and family

Applying 'skilled companionship'[a]

Intervening and reviewing to monitor symptom support and management

[a]Skilled companionship has been described by Alastair Campbell (1984) as the ability to use our clinical skills as nurses and doctors and our humanity to support a person as they strive to cope with the reality of living with advanced disease.

Table 14.8 Principles of palliative/supportive care

Providing relief from pain and other distressing symptoms

Intention not to hasten or postpone death

Integrating the physical, psychosocial and spiritual needs of patients and family

Offering a support system to support the family before and after death

Using a team approach including counselling and chaplaincy

Improving quality of life

Directing treatment, preventing unnecessary and distressing tests or treatments

Supporting the HSCT team

Adapted from Watson et al. (2011)

advanced or incurable disease including the following (Table 14.8):

14.9.4 Managing Pain and Other Symptoms

Mindful that good end-of-life care requires the team to attend to the person and their physical, social, spiritual and emotional needs, some of the common symptoms seen in the end-of-life care setting include those seen in Table 14.9.

Pain continues to be one of the symptoms that people with advanced disease fear and yet research clearly shows that pain management is not always achieved in a consistent and a robust manner. This may be as of a result of a number of reasons including lack of knowledge around – what is meant by pain, which drugs to use, the most therapeutic doses, non-pharmacological approaches and failing to understand what pain means to the individual. While pain is often classified as nociceptive, neuropathic, refractory, breakthrough, chronic or acute and this is important to consider when assessing pain and choosing treatment options, pain can also be understood as a disturbance or a disruption in personal relationships which should be considered (Table 14.4). This approach helps the HSCT team to appreciate some of the more hidden aspects of

Table 14.9 Common symptoms in end-of-life care

Pain (physical, social, emotional, spiritual)[a]

Nausea

Vomiting

Oral problems (dryness, ulcers, mucositis)[a]

Anorexia/cachexia

Agitation/restlessness

Diarrhoea

Excessive secretions[a]

Ascites

Breathlessness[a]

Anxiety/distress[a]

Depression

Confusion

Feelings of loss and grief

Aloneness

Spiritual/religious abandonment[a]

[a]Commonly seen in the last days of life

Table 14.10 Pain as a disturbance or disruptions in key relationships

Physical pain	A disturbance or disruption in the relationship between the person and their body
Social pain	A disturbance or disruption in the relationship between the person and their world including their family, work and society
Emotional pain	A disturbance or a disruption in the relationship between the person and their emotions or how they see themselves
Spiritual pain	A disturbance or disruption in the relationship between the person and their beliefs and values

Managing Advanced Cancer Pain Together – An expert guidance. MACPT (2016) http://www.macpt.eu [Accessed 13 Nov 2016]

pain and how other challenging symptoms can impact on the individual (Tables 14.9 and 14.10).

Rarely will the person's experience of pain happen in isolation from other symptoms/factors including anxiety, fear, loss, fatigue, breathlessness and the inability to sleep or eat. While pain can exacerbate a person's anxiety and their inability to sleep, the inability to sleep and worry can increase the personal experience of pain and make the pain harder to manage; all of these need to be considered. By taking a more person-centred approach (physical, social, emotional and spiritual) to symptom management, better control may be achieved (Fig. 14.2).

Following the principles of the WHO pain ladder (Fig. 14.3), a combination of pharmacological approaches which may include paracetamol, non-steroidal anti-inflammatories, opiates, corticosteroid, anti-depressant, anti-epileptic, anti-muscarinic and benzodiazepine should be considered and reviewed and increased as required. Pain relief should be prescribed on a regular basis and prescribed as needed for 'breakthrough pain'. The HSCT team should also consider the best route of administration (oral transdermal, subcutaneous, sublingual, buccal mucosa, intravenous) for the patient and derived benefit. Pharmacological approaches can be complemented with non-pharmacological interventions including massage, touch, pastoral/spiritual support, hearing the patient's concerns, music and relaxation approaches. A combination of both is often the best approach to managing total pain or indeed any symptom in advanced disease. 'To ignore psychological and spiritual aspects of care may often be the reason for seemingly intractable pain' (Watson et al. 2011. 18)

The following tool (Fig. 14.4) has been designed to encourage patients to talk about their personal experience of pain and what it means to them, but it may also be used to help the patient to talk about their experience of other symptoms. The tool is designed to invite the patient to talk about what is important to them including the reality of their own dying and their fears and concerns.

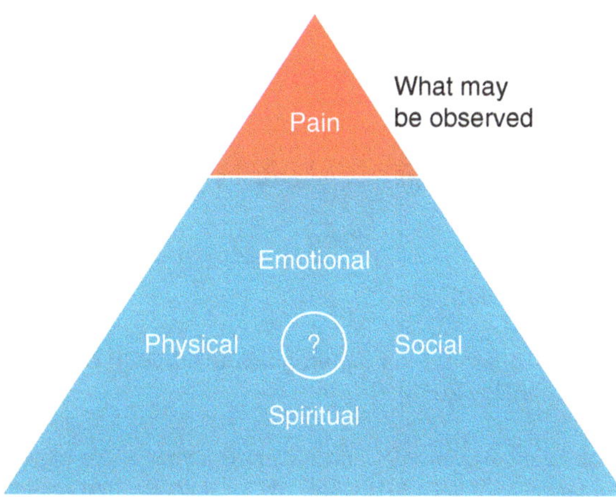

Fig. 14.2 Aspects of pain/other symptoms and what they mean to the individual are often hidden from view and take longer to identify and manage (Managing Advanced Cancer Pain Together – An expert guidance. MACPT (2016) http://www.macpt.eu [Accessed 13 Nov 2016])

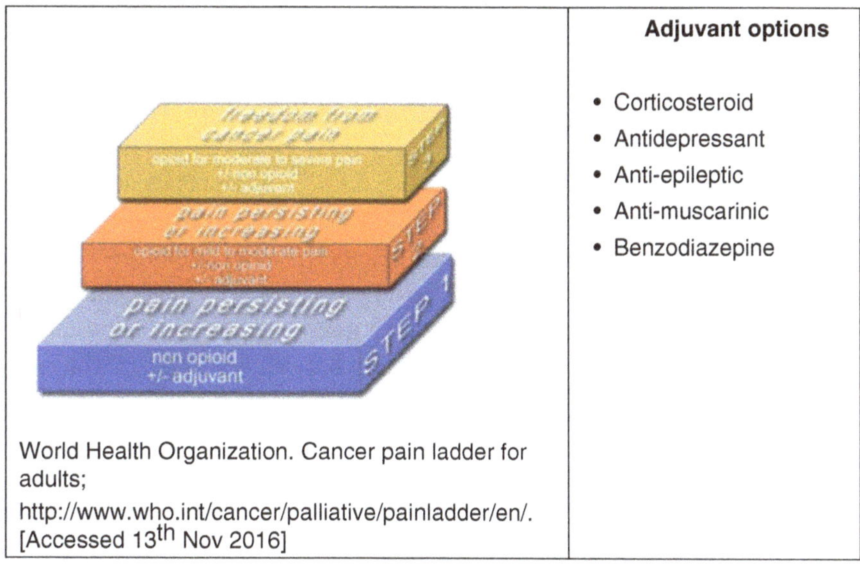

Fig. 14.3 Using the WHO approach to pain management in the HSCT setting

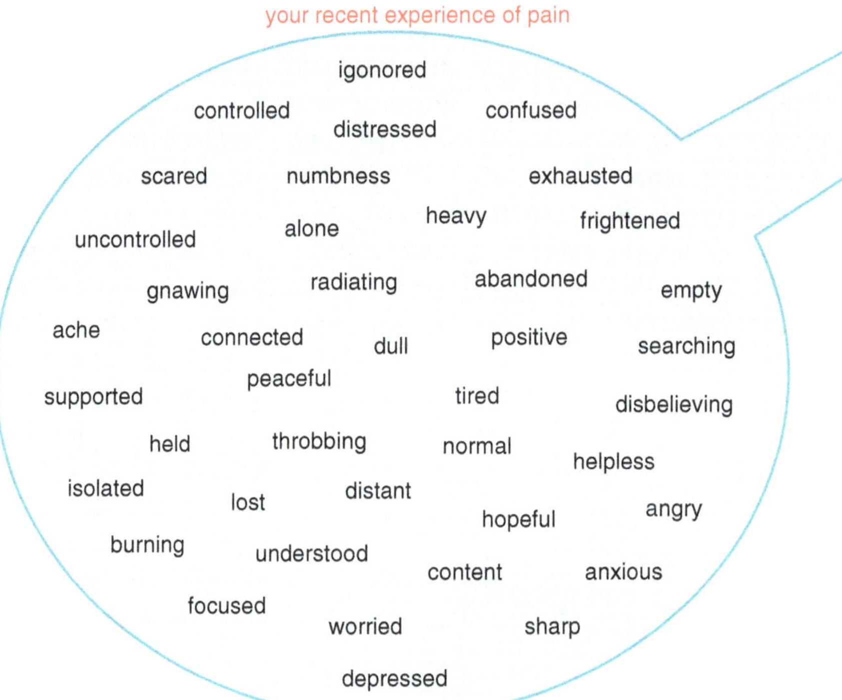

Fig. 14.4 Everyone experiences pain differently – you might find it has an impact on your body, on your sense of well-being and how you feel about yourself, and on your relationships with others and the world around you (Managing Advanced Cancer Pain Together – An expert guidance. MACPT (2016). http://www.macpt.eu [Accessed 13 Nov 2016])

14.9.5 Examples of Drugs Used in the Last Days of Life

Pain: Morphine/diamorphine/oxycodone/alfentanil/fentanyl/Buscopan +/- adjuvant drugs
Excessive secretions: Glycopyrronium
Nausea: Levomepromazine/ondansetron/metoclopramide/cyclizine
Agitation: Midazolam

The management of other symptoms commonly seen in this setting including nausea, agitation and excessive secretions should also take both a pharmacological (Table 14.7) and non-pharmacological approach focussing on what suits the individual patient.

14.9.6 Support

As previously stated, an important aspect of end-of-life care is recognising the HSCT team's role in supporting the patient and their family but also knowing when the person may require more expert help including pastoral care, psychological support and specialist palliative care for challenging aspects of symptom management and/or support/advice for the HSCT team. Pastoral, psychological and palliative/supportive care should be seen as a core part of HSCT care and introduced to the patient earlier so that these approaches are seen as complementing the treatment approach of HSCT. While an individual may not have any religious affiliation or religious needs, many patients will require someone to listen to their hopes and dreams, their concerns and fears. The HSCT team with careful planning, support and working with the patient's community medical and nursing team can in many cases enable patients with advanced disease to be cared for in their own home if that is the patient's wishes. While focussing on the person with advanced disease, the team is well placed to support family members including children and parents.

14.9.7 Conclusion

Although the current public message appears to be one of delivering more care with less resources, this in no way negates the central focus on delivering truly holistic patient-centred care. We can no longer continue to talk about patient-centred care without a willingness to engage with all aspects of the person we support and care for including their physical, emotional, social, existential and spiritual needs. It is time to move away from a medical approach only to care in the HSCT setting to one of attending to the person. With nursing leadership and the reality of dying in the HSCT setting, there is no more urgent time to take forward the reality of person-centred care. Often the greatest gift we can give to those who are dying is our attention and presence. Amidst the uncertainty and the painful realities each person has to face, caring is often perceived as occurring when another person carries out a simple act of kindness with a caring attitude, which requires us to be attentive to them.

14.10 Late Effects and Long-Term Follow-Up in Paediatric Patients

The study of late effects after paediatric haematopoietic stem cell transplantation (HSCT) offers unique opportunities and challenges, magnified by the fact that children going through each developmental stage (infant, toddler, child preadolescent and young adult) have different sensitivities to therapies, resulting in different complications. For instance, infants and toddlers are susceptible to neurocognitive damage with radiation, and adolescents are at high risk of joint/bone issues with steroid therapy (Baker et al. 2011).

Paediatric HSCT survivors have a higher cumulative incidence of late effects compared to the studies of cancer survivors who did not receive HSCT as part of their treatment, with 93% of survivors having at least one late effect with a median follow-up of only 7 years (Bresters et al. 2010).

Children who undergo HSCT with TBI have a significant risk of both growth hormone deficiency (GHD) and the direct effects of radiation on skeletal development. The risk is increased with single-dose TBI as opposed to fractionated TBI, pre-transplant cranial irradiation, female gender and post-treatment complications such as graft versus host disease (GVHD).

Late side effects and complications can include chronic immunosuppression and infections, chronic GvHD, bronchiolitis obliterans, endocrine dysfunction, cataracts, disease recurrence and secondary malignancies (Tomlinson and Kline 2010).

The endocrine system is highly susceptible to damage by high-dose chemotherapy and/or irradiation prior to haematopoietic stem cell transplantation (HSCT) during childhood. Insufficiency of thyroid hormone is one of the most common late sequelae of HSCT and occurs more often in young children. Deficiency in the pituitary's production of growth hormone is a problem of unique concern to the paediatric population (Dvorak et al. 2011).

14.10.1 Specific Late Effects After HSCT in Childhood

14.10.1.1 Growth Impairment

Impaired linear growth after HSCT is multifactorial in origin and can be due to growth hormone deficiency (GHD), hypothyroidism, hypogonadism, corticosteroid treatment as well as poor nutritional status, genetic factors and metabolic status. Because of these confounding factors, the reported prevalence of growth impairment varies widely (9–84%) between studies (Baker et al. 2011).

Treatment includes thyroid replacement therapy and growth hormone therapy, respectively, for thyroid dysfunction and growth delays (Tomlinson and Kline 2010).

Growth hormone deficiency (GHD) replacement therapy provides the benefit of optimising height outcomes among children who have not reached skeletal maturity (Chemaitilly and Robison 2012).

Even though myeloablative conditioning regimens for HSCT are known to affect endocrine function, Myers et al. (2016) recently evidenced that 'poor growth, thyroid dysfunction and vitamin D deficiency remain prevalent despite reduced intensity chemotherapy for haematopoietic stem cell transplantation in children and young adults'.

14.10.1.2 Neurocognitive Impairment

There is limited evidence of neurocognitive and academic outcomes in paediatric HSCT:

- HSCT seems to pose a low risk overall.
- Risk increases for children of age <5years at the time of SCT who received TBI (Phipps et al. 2008).

The procedure of SCT entails probably minimal risk of late cognitive and academic sequelae. Subgroups of patients are at relatively higher risk: patients undergoing unrelated donor transplantation, receiving TBI and those who experience GVHD. No significant changes are seen in global intelligence quotient and academic achievement (Phipps et al. 2008).

Despite substantial exposure to potentially neurotoxic agents, studies have generally shown survivors of paediatric HSCT to be within normal limits in cognitive and academic functioning, and with stable performance over time, although children who are younger at the time of transplantation may be at increased risk for cognitive impairment (Phipps et al. 2008).

Phipps et al. (2008) reported 158 patients who survived and were evaluated at 1, 3 and 5 years' post-transplant and concluded that HSCT, even with TBI, poses low to minimal risk for late cognitive and academic deficits in patients who are at least 6 years old at the time of transplantation. However, socio-economic status was found to be a significant determinant of all cognitive and academic outcomes.

14.10.2 Return to School

A diagnosis of cancer during the teenage years arrives at an important stage of development, where issues of normality, identity and independence are crucial. Education provides opportunity for peer contact, achievement and development for teenagers.

Key areas involved in the impact of a cancer diagnosis on teenagers' educational engagement include school attendance, reintegration and peer relationships. Long-term school absences are a concern for teenagers but do not necessarily lead to a reduction in educational and vocational attainment. It is important to involve healthcare and education professionals, as well as parents and teenagers themselves, in school matters (Pini et al. 2012).

Factors that may place children and teens at increased risk for difficulties in school (Landier et al. 2013) include:

- Diagnosis of cancer at a very young age
- Numerous prolonged school absences
- A history of learning problems before being diagnosed with cancer
- Cancer treatment that results that reduced energy levels
- Cancer treatment that affects hearing or vision
- Cancer treatment that results in physical disabilities
- Cancer treatment that includes treatment to the central nervous system

Collaborative education planning should be initiated on diagnosis and aim to include nonacademic variables, such as peer groups, which can influence successful maintenance of education. Further research is needed to understand the relationship between education engagement and teenagers' cancer experiences as a whole, as well as gaining a more in depth understanding of how teenagers experience their education after a diagnosis of cancer (Pini et al. 2013).

It will therefore be imperative that we continue to follow our HSCT survivors on a long-term basis and continue research efforts to study long-term outcomes (Baker et al. 2011).

References

Anderson KO, Giralt SA, Mendoza TR, Brown JO, Neumann JL, Mobley GM, Wang XS, Cleeland CS. Symptom burden in patients undergoing autologous stem-cell transplantation. Bone Marrow Transplant. 2007;39(12):759–66.

Andorsky DJ, Loberiza FR, Lee SJ. Pre-transplantation physical and mental functioning is strongly associated with self-reported recovery from stem cell transplantation. Bone Marrow Transplant. 2006;37:889–95.

Andrykowski M, Bishop M, Hahn E, Cella D, Beaumont J, Brady M, Horowitz M, Sobocinski K, Rizzo J, Wingard J. Long-term health related quality of life, growth and spiritual well-being after haematopoietic stem cell transplantation. J Clin Oncol. 2005;23:599–08.

Baker F, Zahora J, Polland A, Wingard J. Reintegration after bone marrow transplantation. Cancer Pract. 1999;7:190–7.

Baker S, Bhatia S, Bunin N, Nieder M, Dvorak C, Sung L, Sander J, Kurtzberg J, Pulsiphe M. NCI, NHLBI first international consensus conference on late effects after pediatric hematopoietic cell transplantation: state of the science, future directions. Biol Blood Marrow Transplant. 2011;17(10):1424–7.

Bhatia S, Francisco L, Carter A, Sun CL, Baker KS, Gurney JG, McGlave PB, Nademanee A, O'Donnell M, Ramsay NK, Robison LL, Snyder D, Stein A, Forman SJ, Weisdorf DJ. Late mortality after allogeneic hematopoietic cell transplantation and functional status of long-term survivors: report from the bone marrow transplant survivor study. Blood. 2009;110(10):3784–92.

Bieri S, Roosneck E, Helg C, Verholen F, Robert D, Chapius B, Passweg J, Miralbell R, Chalandon Y. Quality of life and social integration after allogeneic hematopoietic SCT. Bone Marrow Transplant. 2008;42:819–27.

Brandenburg D, Grover L, Quinn B. Intimacy and sexuality for cancer patients and their partners: Pan-Birmingham Cancer Psychology Services; 2010.

Bresters D, van Gils IC, Kollen WJ, Ball LM, Oostdijk W, van der Bom JG, Egeler RM. High burden of late effects after haematopoietic stem cell transplantation in childhood: a single-centre study. Bone Marrow Transplant. 2010;45(1):79–85.

Chemaitilly W, Robison LL. Safety of growth hormone treatment in patients previously treated for cancer. Endocrinol Metab Clin North Am. 2012;41(4):785–92.

Curtis RE, Rowlings PA, Deeg J, Shriner DA, Socié G, Travis LB, Horowitz MM, Witherspoon RP, Hoover RN, Sobocinski KA, Fraumeni JF, Boice JD, Gary Schoch G, Sale GE, Storb R, Travis WD, Kolb H-J, Gale RP, Passweg JR. Solid cancers after bone marrow transplantation. N Engl J Med. 1997;336:897–904.

DeFilipp Z, Duarte RF, Snowden JA, Majhail NS, Greenfield DM, Miranda JL, Arat M, Baker KS, Burns LJ, Duncan CN, Gilleece M, Hale GA, Hamadani M, Hamilton BK, Hogan WJ, Hsu JW, Inamoto Y, Kamble RT, Lup-Stanghellini MT, Malon AK, McCarthy P, Mohty M, Norkin M, Paplham P, Ramanathan M, Richart JM, Salooja N, Schouten HC, Seber A, Steinberg A, Wirk BM, Wood WA, Battiwala M, Flowers MED, Savani BN, Shaw BE; on behalf of the CIBMTR Late Effects and Quality of Life Working Committee and the EBMT Complications and Quality of Life Working Party. Metabolic syndrome and cardiovascular disease following hematopoietic cell transplantation: screening and preventive practice recommendations from CIBMTR and EBMT. Bone Marrow Transplant. 2016:1–10.

DoH. National cancer survivorship initiative – vision. London: Crown; 2010.

Dvorak CC, Gracia CR, Sanders JE, Cheng EY, Baker KS, Pulsipher MA, Petryk A. NCI, NHLBI/PBMTC first international conference on late effects after pediatric hematopoietic cell transplantation: endocrine challenges-thyroid dysfunction, growth impairment, bone health, & reproductive risks. Biol Blood Marrow Transplant. 2011;17(12):1725–38.

Flowers M, et al. 2015. https://www.fredhutch.org/content/dam/public/Treatment-Suport/Long-Term-Follow-Up/LTFU_HSCT_guidelines_physicians.pdf. version June 03, 2015. Accessed 22 Sept 2016.

Freidrichs B, Tichelli A, Bacigalupo A, Russell N, Ruutu T, Shapira M, Beksac M, Hasenclever D, Socie G, Schmitz N. Long-term outcome and late effects in patients transplanted with mobilised blood or bone marrow: a randomised trial. Lancet Oncol. 2010;11(4):331–8.

Gielissen M, Verhagen S, Witjes F, Bleijenberg G. Effects of cognitive behaviour therapy in severely fatigued disease-free cancer patients compared with patients waiting for cognitive behaviour therapy: a randomized controlled trial. J Clin Oncol. 2006;24:4882–8.

Hamblin A, Greenfield DM, Gilleece M, Salooja N, Kenyon M, Morris E, Glover N, Miller P, Braund H, Peniket A, Shaw BE, Snowden JA, on behalf of the British Society of Blood and Marrow Transplantation (BSBMT). Provision of long-term monitoring and late effects services following adult allogeneic haematopoietic stem cell transplant: a survey of UK NHS-based programmes. Bone Marrow Transplant. 2017;52:889–894. (June 2017). https://doi.org/10.1038/bmt.2017.67.

International Standards for Hematopoietic Cellular Therapy Product Collection, Processing, and Administration. Sixth Edition (2015) from the Federation for Accreditation of Cell Therapy (FACT) and the Joint Accreditation Committee of ISCT-Europe and EBMT (JACiE). Available from: http://www.jacie.org.

Jean CY, Syrjala KL. Sexuality after hematopoietic stem cell transplantation. Cancer J (Sudbury, Mass). 2009;15(1):57.

Johnston BL, Conly JM. Immunization for bone marrow transplant recipients. Can J Infect Dis. 2002;13(6):353–7.

Landier W, Leonard M, Ruccione KS. Children's Oncology Group's 2013 blueprint for research: nursing discipline. Pediatr Blood Cancer. 2013;60:1031–6. https://doi.org/10.1002/pbc.24415.

Lee CR, Nicholson PW, Souhami RL, Deshmukh AA. Patient compliance with oral chemotherapy as assessed by a novel electronic technique. J Clin Oncol. 1992;10(6):1007–13.

Ljungman P, Cordonnier C, de Bock R, Einsele H, Engelhard D, Grundy J, Link H, Locasciulli A, Prentice HG, Reusser P, Ribaud P. Immunisations after bone marrow transplantation: results of a European survey and recommendations from the infectious diseases working party of the European Group for Blood and Marrow Transplantation. Bone Marrow Transplant. 1995;15:455–60.

Ljungman P, Cordonnier C, Einsele H, Englund J, Machado CM, Storek J, Small T. Vaccination of hematopoietic cell transplant recipients. Bone Marrow Transplant. 2009;44:521–6.

Majhail NS, Rizzo JD, Lee SJ, Aijurf M, Atsuta Y, Bonfim C, Burns LJ, Chaudhri N, Davies S, Okamoto S, Seber A, Socie G, Szer J, Van Lint MT, Wingard JR, Tichelli A. Recommended screening and preventive practices for long-term survivors after hematopoietic cell transplantation. Hematol Oncol Stem Cell Ther. 2012;5(1):1–30.

Mosher CE, Redd WH, Rini CM, Burkhalter JE, DuHamel KN. Physical, psychological, and social sequelae following hematopoietic stem cell transplantation: a review of the literature. Psychooncology. 2009;18(2):113–27.

Mulhall J. Saving your sex life. Munster: Saving your Sex Life. Münster, Germany: Hilton Publication; 2008.

Murphy RF. The body silent. New York: W.W. Norton; 1990.

Myers KC, Howell JC, Wallace G, Dandoy C, El-Bietar J, Lane A, Davies SM, Jodele S, Rose SR. Poor growth, thyroid dysfunction and vitamin D deficiency remain prevalent despite reduced intensity chemotherapy for hematopoietic stem cell transplantation in children and young adults. Bone Marrow Transplant. 2016;51:980–4.

Osho L. Sex matters: from sex to superconsciousness. New York: St Martin's Griffin; 2002.

Passweg JR, Baldomero H, Bader P, Bonini C, Cesaro S, Dreger P, Duarte RF, Dufour C, Kuball J, Farge-Bancel D, Gennery A, Kröger N, Lanza F, Nagler A, Sureda A, Mohty M. Hematopoietic stem cell transplantation in Europe 2014: more than 40000 transplants annually. Bone Marrow Transplant. 2016. Advance online publication 22 Feb 2016. doi:10.1038/bmt.2016.20.

Phipps S, Rai SN, Leung WH, Lensing S, Dunavant M. Cognitive and academic consequences of stem-cell transplantation in children. J Clin Oncol. 2008;26(12):2027–33.

Pini S, Hugh-Jones S, Gardner PH. What effect does a cancer diagnosis have on the educational engagement and school life of teenagers? A systematic review. Psychooncology. 2012;21(7):685–94.

Pini S, Gardner P, Hugh-Jones S. The impact of a cancer diagnosis on the education engagement of teenagers – patient and staff perspective. Eur J Oncol Nurs. 2013;17(3):317–23.

Quinn B. Sexual side effects of cancer treatments and the person living with cancer. In: Brandenburg D, Grover L, Quinn B, editors. Intimacy and sexuality for cancer patients and their partners: Pan Birmingham Cancer Psychology Services; 2010. p. 22–32.

Richards M, Corner J, Maher J. The National Cancer Survivorship Initiative: new and emerging evidence on the ongoing needs of cancer survivors. British Journal of Cancer. 2013;105:S1–4.

Rizzo DJ, Curtis RE, Socié G, Sobocinski KA, Gilbert E, Landgren O, Travis LB, Travis WD, Flowers MED, Friedman DL, Horowitz MM, Wingard JR, Deeg JH. Solid cancers after allogeneic hematopoietic cell transplantation. Blood. 2009;113:1175–83.

Rusiewicz A, DuHamel KN, Burkhalter J, Ostroff J, Winkel G, Scigliano E, Papadopoulos E, Moskowitz C, Redd W. Psychological distress in long-term survivors of hematopoietic stem cell transplantation. Psychooncology. 2008;17(4):329–37.

Russmann S, Curkovic I, Huber M. Adverse reactions and risks associated with non-compliance. Ther Umsch. 2010;67(6):303–7.

Savani B, Griffith M, Jagasia S, Lee SJ. How i treat late effects in adults after allogeneic stem cell transplantation. Blood. 2011;117:3002–9.

Schover LR. Sexuality and fertility after cancer. New York: John Wiley & Sons; 1997.

Snyder C, Harris C, Anderson J, Holleran S, Irving L, Sigmon S, Yoshinobu L, Gibb J, Langelle C, Spelten E, Spragers M, Verbeek J. Factors reported to influence the return to work of cancer survivors: a literature review. Psycho-Oncology. 2002;11:124–31.

Socié G, Stone JV, Wingard JR, Weisdorf D, Henslee-Downey J, Bredeson C, Cahn J-Y, Passweg JR, Rowlings PA, Schouten HC, Kolb H-J, Bender-Götze C, Camitta BM, Godder K, Horowitz MM, Wayne AS, Klein JP, for the Late Effects Working Committee of the International Bone Marrow Transplant Registry. Long-term survival and late deaths after allogeneic bone marrow transplantation. N Engl J Med. 1999;341:14–21.

Tomblyn M, Chiller T, Einsele H, Gress R, Sepkowitz K, Storek J, Wingard JR, Young JH, Boeckh MA. Guidelines for preventing infectious complications among hematopoietic cell transplantation recipients: a global perspective. Biol Blood Marrow Transplant. 2009;15:1143–238.

Tomlinson D, Kline N. In: Tomlinson D, Kline N, editors. Pediatric oncology nursing advanced clinical handbook. Berlin Heidelberg: Springer-Verlag; 2010.

Treanor C, Santin O, Mills M, Donnelly M. Cancer survivors with self-reported late effects: their health status, care needs and service utilisation. Psychooncology. 2013;22(11):2428–35. https://doi.org/10.1002/pon.3304. Epub 2013 May 16

Twigg J. Bathing: the body and community care. London: Routledge; 2000.

Waddell G, Burton A. Is work good for your health and wellbeing? London: The Stationary Office; 2006.

Wells M, Williams B, Firnigl D, Lang H, Coyle J, Kroll T, MacGillivray S. Supporting 'work-related goals' rather than 'return to work' after cancer? A systematic review and meta-synthesis of 25 qualitative studies. Psycho-Oncology. 2013;22:1208–19. https://doi.org/10.1002/pon.3148.

Williams SJ. Medicine and the body. London: Sage Publications; 2003.

World Health Organisation. Adherence to long-term therapies, evidence for action. Geneva: World Health Organization; 2003.

Useful Resources

EBMT Swiss Nurses Group. Adherence to oral anti-tumour therapies. 2011.

Nursing Research and Audit in the Transplant Setting

Corien Eeltink, Sarah Liptrott, and Jacqui Stringer

Abstract

Nursing research is a systematic inquiry that uses disciplined methods to answer questions or solve problems in order to expand the knowledge base within a given field. There are various issues to address in order to complete a successful study. The aim of this chapter is to provide the reader with an overview of the key topics for consideration and give guidance as to where to go for further information. Providing best care to patients undergoing HSCT is the moral and ethical duty of all nurses. As a consequence, awareness of, and involvement in, research as the vehicle to ensuring best practice is also our moral duty.

Keywords

Nursing research · Audit · Methodology · Quantitative · Qualitative
Mixed methods · Cross-sectional · Longitudinal · Prospective
Retrospective

C. Eeltink
Department of Hematology, Cancer Center
Amsterdam/ VU University Medical Center,
Amsterdam, The Netherlands
e-mail: c.eeltink@vumc.nl

S. Liptrott
Division of Haemato-oncology,
European Institute of Oncology, Milan, Italy
e-mail: sarah.liptrott@ieo.it

J. Stringer (✉)
Clinical Lead Complementary Health and Wellbeing,
The Christie NHS Foundation Trust, Manchester, UK
e-mail: Jacqui.Stringer@christie.nhs.uk

15.1 Introduction/Background

Nursing research is a systematic inquiry that uses disciplined methods to answer questions or solve problems. It has only been in the last four decades that nurses have had access to knowledge from nursing research to inform their practice. Nowadays nurses are expected to use the best type of evidence to base their nursing care on, so-called evidence-based practice (EBP).

In 1859, Florence Nightingale's book *Notes on Nursing* was first published, with the aim of providing guidance to women who have personal charge of the health of others. At this time, there

© EBMT and the Author(s) 2018
M. Kenyon, A. Babic (eds.), *The European Blood and Marrow Transplantation Textbook for Nurses*,
https://doi.org/10.1007/978-3-319-50026-3_15

were no nursing schools and no trained nurses. She was the pioneer of modern nursing. She combined knowledge, her systematic approach, developing instruments, and statistics into an early form of evidence-based practice. Based on her analysis and presentations, she was able to make changes in nursing care with the effect of reducing mortality and morbidity.

In 1997, Molassiotis reported the lack of nursing training in research techniques, problems with funding nursing research, staff shortages, and language barriers as the reasons for the limited contribution of nursing research and the utilization of research findings to the field of bone marrow transplantation (BMT) in Europe. However, he also reported that nursing research was moving forward and starting to be integrated into many European BMT centers.

Currently, huge progress is being made. JACIE accreditation, demonstrating excellence of practice, is a legal requirement for transplant centers in many countries (more information about JACIE in Chap. 1), and as a consequence, nurses have an important role in validating protocols of care. The EBMT nurses group is making it possible to form multi-institutional collaborative models of research. An example of this is the many surveys our nurses have developed looking at current practice in relation to, for example, mouth care, CVCs, isolation, low bacterial diet, nutrition, medication adherence, and patient information. Such surveys are the ideal baseline from which to explore where there is inconsistency in nursing practice across Europe and whether further work is required to clarify what can be seen as best practice. Patient-focused research looking at mouth care, sexuality, and quality of life has been extensively explored and indicates an increasing use of evidence-based practice. Finally, the number of PhDs among registered nurses is growing, which is increasing the capacity of the nursing community to carry out independent research. Nursing research is moving in the right direction.

However, we have been undertaking hematopoietic transplantation for over 60 years with increasing success, and the longer HSCT survivors live, the more long-term effects they report. Much remains to be done. This chapter aims to provide

guidance on carrying out research and information about the types of methodology, which can be used in nursing research and what support may be required to complete a successful project.

15.2 Service Evaluation: Audit or Research?

Before focusing on research as a topic, it is worth first clarifying the differences between service evaluation, audit, and research. These are all valid methods nurses can use to review, benchmark, or enhance their practice, but there are differences in the way they are performed, and these differences have resource implications (financial, staff, and time). Probably the key difference between the three strategies is the overall aim of the work. Both service evaluation and audit are looking at assessing or confirming the quality of the care being provided to patients, whereas research aims to add new information to the field. It is often the case that a service evaluation or audit will trigger questions, which become the basis of a research study.

> **Box 15.1 Definitions of Service Evaluation, Audit and Research**
>
> *Service evaluation*: service evaluation seeks to assess how well a service is achieving its intended aims. It is undertaken to benefit the people using a particular healthcare service and is designed and conducted with the sole purpose of defining or judging the current service. The results of service evaluations are mostly used to generate information that can be used to inform local decision-making
>
> *Audit (clinical)*: the English Department of Health states that clinical audit involves systematically looking at the procedures used for diagnosis, care, and treatment, examining how associated resources are used and investigating the effect care has on the outcome and quality of life for the patient. Audit usually involves a quality improvement cycle that measures care against predetermined standards (benchmarking), takes specific actions to improve care, and monitors ongoing sustained improvements to quality against agreed standards or benchmarks
>
> *Research*: research involves the attempt to extend the available knowledge by means of a systematically defensible process of enquiry
>
> Adapted from Twycross and Shorten (2014)

Table 15.1 Key criteria to consider when deciding whether your project is service evaluation, audit, or research

Criteria	Service evaluation	Audit	Research
Overall aim (intent)	To judge the quality of the current service	To measure clinical practice against a standard	To generate new knowledge/add to the body of knowledge
Initiated by	Service providers	Service providers	Researchers
Involves a new treatment	No	No	Sometimes
Randomization	No	No	Sometimes
Allocates patients to treatment groups	No	No	Sometimes

Adapted from Twycross and Shorten (2014)

Because research may change the care that a patient is currently receiving, there is a significant amount of preparation required and mandatory approvals from statutory bodies (e.g., ethics committee) to be obtained prior to starting a study. This is to ensure the patient is protected from poor study design and unethical research practice. The situation can become confusing as research methodologies are often used for both service evaluation and audit. Equally, there may not always be clear standards available against which to audit practice. However, there are papers offering guidance on how to confidently decide which category a specific project falls into. The following table provides a succinct set of criteria for assessing any new project (Table 15.1):

It is beyond the remit of this chapter to go further into the issue. However, there are resources available to support nurses to make decisions regarding what classification their work falls into, which is not always obvious. The Health Research Authority (HRA) in the UK, for example, has an online tool which has been designed to help clinicians with exactly this challenge: http://www.hra.nhs.uk/research-community/before-youapply/determine-whether-your-study-is-research/.

15.3 Performing/Undertaking Research

Few people are born as researchers. The majority become researchers through education and training, practical experience, and always hard work. Research is demanding yet rewarding – even when results are not what were expected, as the aim is to learn and increase knowledge in a particular field. When initiating research, it can be challenging to know where to begin. Planning and organization are key concepts in research performance, in order get started and keep focus with the project. For novice researchers, those looking to undertake research in a new field or using a methodology that they may not be familiar with, there is usually help at hand. It is important to build a team to undertake the research, which may begin within the local organization itself; many hospitals have research and development departments (particularly those with links to academic institutions) and/or access to statisticians and support for analysis where necessary. Often difficulties arise when there is a lack of resources or time to undertake research. Getting support from management and senior clinical staff to undertake research can aid in getting some protected time.

Financial support for undertaking research is an important consideration and may be available from a variety of sources. Registration for a personal postgraduate degree (either a master's or a doctorate) is supported by some institutions and has the added benefit of ongoing training and supervision. Nursing associations/organizations – both national and international such as the European Oncology Nursing Society – provide the possibility of applying for research grants. Information on other available resources can be obtained from, for example, national departments of health and health research boards; however, this will vary from country to country and will need investigation.

Issues of interest for investigation through research and development of the research question can be the work of a team. All healthcare professionals will have their own views of what is important and potentially how it can be investigated. By involving other members of staff in the research process, there is a "buy-in" where the project becomes the property and interest of all rather than just one individual. This is important when thinking about the practicalities of undertaking research as it is particularly challenging if one person has to do everything. Research planning can also benefit from user (e.g., patient) involvement in terms of advising on, for example, study design, strategies for recruitment, and data collection methods that may or may not work.

Support can also be sought from a wider field such as via local academic institutions, universities, or other centers for multicenter studies. Knowledge of the literature and contacting those who are the experts in the field can be useful when questions or ideas are unclear. Other professional groups that may be disease or intervention focused such as the EBMT Nurses Group can also be a useful resource. The EBMT NG Research Committee is one such group that promotes collaboration with researchers in order to encourage presentation of ideas and aspirations for research within a wider setting. Please see the website for more details: http://www.ebmt.org/Contents/Nursing/WhoWeAre/NursingCommittes/Pages/default.aspx.

15.4 Interpreting Nursing Research

In order to complete a successful project, regardless of which criteria it comes under (audit, service evaluation, or research), it is important to identify any work that has already been performed within the field of interest. A scoping exercise to identify key relevant research and a critical appraisal of existing literature will facilitate the identification of current knowledge and as such, which studies can be used as a baseline for further work (e.g., to audit against as best practice). It will also identify where gaps in knowledge exist

and provide a focus for where research can aid in developing our understanding.

To interpret and evaluate the significance of nursing research, knowledge of the various methodologies is required. This will provide the potential researcher with confidence to know whether the methodology and study design selected were appropriate to answer the research question and, as a consequence, will provide an indicator as to the quality and reliability of the results presented.

Evaluating the quality of existing literature can be complex and time-consuming, but a thorough review can inform future research direction and methodological choices. There are a variety of appraisal checklists available that can facilitate evaluation of research such as the CONSORT statement for randomized controlled trial (RCT) reporting, Critical Appraisal Skills Programme (CASP) tools, and PRISMA Statement. A published paper will usually have a title, abstract, introduction (including study aims), methods (including statement of ethical approval), results, discussion, acknowledgment of funding sources, and a reference section. The abstract is concise while communicating key information and will give the reader an indication of whether the paper is relevant to their field of interest. The main article will provide a more detailed description. The introduction, for example, should provide an overview of previous literature to "set the scene" and state the study rationale and consequent aims/objectives. The methodology and results sections require the reader to undertake a critical appraisal of sampling and recruitment strategies. This includes where appropriate, whether the correct calculation has been made to ensure sufficient subjects were entered, the "power calculation," to provide meaningful results and data collection methods and analysis of results to inform them of the overall methodological quality and therefore reliability of the study results. The discussion section will provide a summary of the results and their interpretation, often comparing with other pertinent research. It should also describe the limitations of the research and implications for both future research and clinical practice.

It is difficult for a research study to be conducted perfectly; an open and critical reflection of limitations will assist in judging the impact on quality and perhaps generalizability of the results. Equally, suggestions of future studies which may be required and implications for clinical practice can be used as validation of a proposed piece of research. A review of the references may identify recent work and prevent repetition as well as older studies, which are still relevant and can provide a lot of information. If the reference list consists mainly of old or outdated sources, it may be an indicator that the research is based on outdated information or that there is the necessity for more work to be done on the issue in question. Similarly noting the presence of peer-reviewed journals will support evidence of reading around the topic.

15.5 Nursing Research

15.5.1 The Research Question

Once the general topic has been identified, it is important to refine this further to a more specific area of interest. Asking a librarian to assist with finding the appropriate literature as a background reading exercise allows for a greater understanding of the topic. Narrowing the focus may be helped by talking with colleagues about the topic and by working with a team and using sources of support as described earlier. Formulating the research question is about restating your topic as a question. The research question needs to be clear, focused, and ethical – and obviously something that can be researched. The acronym "PICO" is a reminder used to help clarify the clinical question (Box 15.2). It acts as a framework, requiring reflection about different aspects of interest to investigate. Building the PICO requires clarity and specificity, which helps in targeting the right evidence to use in practice. The question must be specific. What type of patient group is of interest? Is there a specific test as an intervention or a broad group? If looking for better outcomes, what are examples of those outcomes?

Box 15.2 PICO: Worked Example, Aslam and Emmanuel (2010)

P: patient, problem, or population	P: allogeneic HSCT recipients
I: intervention	I: psychologist
C: comparison	C: no psychologist
O: outcome	O: effect on psychological distress

Sample question using PICO:
In allogeneic hematopoietic stem cell recipients (P), what is the effect of a psychologist in the multidisciplinary team (I) on psychological distress (O) compared to no psychologist (C)?

15.5.2 Designs for Nursing Research

Once the question has been clearly defined, identifying the appropriate methodology to answer the question most effectively is the next step. The research design has to be pertinent to the question itself, with the nature of the question guiding the choice of approach. Research questions may be exploratory (i.e., with no a priori theory of outcome), wanting to investigate a phenomenon that we know little about and how it is perceived by a group of individuals. This type of question lends itself to in-depth interviews and a qualitative research approach. If a research question is, for example, interested in the efficacy of a novel intervention, perhaps in comparison with to standard care, then a randomized controlled trial may be more appropriate.

Two overarching categories of research are basic research, used to obtain empirical data (e.g., laboratory-based studies), which is unlikely to be immediately translatable to clinical practice, and applied research, which is usually directly relevant to the clinical setting. Nursing research tends to be applied research.

Research can also be categorized into experimental or non-experimental. Although the suggested gold standard of evidence is the experimental approach of an RCT, it is not always possible or appropriate to use this approach, for example, where randomization may be unethical. This does not mean research other than that of an

RCT is not of value; on the contrary, well-conducted research will always add to the knowledge base, and studies using more exploratory methodologies often provide a foundation for clinical trials. Common approaches for nursing research include descriptive or explorative research (e.g., using questionnaires), correlational studies, and both experimental and quasi-experimental approaches.

15.5.3 Literature Reviews

With the ever-increasing amount of research being produced and published, it is possible that answers to research questions already exist, but they sometimes lack the culmination, critical appraisal, and interpretation of individual studies together in one single document. This is where reviews of the literature to identify the evidence base are sources of research in themselves. Systematic reviews have increased in number within the field of nursing care. They use strategies in order to limit bias and systematically critically appraise and synthesize pertinent studies of interest (Greener and Grimshaw 1996). This means having defined objectives for the review, criteria for study inclusion, an organized approach to searching databases, and a clearly defined method for critical appraisal, analysis, and subsequent synthesis of data. Systematic reviews can potentially combine research findings from smaller individual studies, in order to provide a broader overview of findings in which detection of "minor" findings may be amplified or discredited. Box 15.3 describes two examples of systematic reviews within the HSCT setting.

> **Box 15.3 Systematic Reviews Within the HSCT Setting**
> In the review by Chaudhry et al. (2016), the incidence and outcomes of oral mucositis (OM) in allogeneic HSCT patients and its association with conditioning regimens were analyzed, reviewing 395 patients in 8 eligible myeloablative regimen studies and 245 patients in 6 eligible reduced-intensity conditioning (RIC) regimen studies. Severe mucositis (defined as either grades 2 to 4 or grades 3 and 4, depending on the studies' definition of severity) occurred among 79.7% patients treated with myeloablative regimen studies and 71.5% patients treated with reduced-intensity conditioning regimen studies. RIC regimens led to a high incidence of OM similar to that of MA regimens.
> Riley et al. (2015) reviewed the effects of oral cryotherapy in patients with cancer receiving treatment. For this they included 14 RCTs analyzing 1280 participants. After high-dose melphalan before HSCT, cryotherapy reduces considerable oral mucositis. However, the size of the reduction could not be detected.

15.5.4 Quantitative, Qualitative, and Mixed Method Research

Research is generally divided into three groups – quantitative, qualitative, and mixed method approaches. Quantitative research is particularly focused on theory testing and relationships between variables (factors which are either changed within an experimental design, such as mouth wash in oral care, or influenced by such changes, e.g., level of oral pain/mucositis), where measurement instruments (e.g., pain scale) provide numerical data which can be subjected to statistical analysis (Creswell 2014). Examples of quantitative designs include those producing numerical data such as experiments or clinical trials (often sponsored by pharmaceutical companies or academic groups that coordinate research projects), observations (looking at frequencies), and surveys with closed questions (using questionnaires, in person, online, or by phone). At the other end of the spectrum, qualitative research is focused on understanding meanings and experiences of human beings, also within a given context (Kielmann et al. 2011). Researchers using these methods do not have any theory on which to base their work; rather they may use their results to develop a theory. Examples of qualitative data include interviews, focus groups, and secondary data (such as written accounts or reports). Both quantitative and qualitative approaches have positive and negative aspects, and a more recent "mixed method" approach to research lies somewhere between these two ends. A combination of qualitative and quantitative data collection methods is aimed to benefit from the advantages of each approach, in order to provide a robust method of validating and investigating findings. Mixed methods may be used within a study or over a program of research, and an example of such is provided in Box 15.4.

Box 15.4 Mixed Method Research in the HSCT Setting

Niederbacher et al. (2012) investigated quality of life (QoL) following allogeneic hematopoietic stem cell transplantation (HSCT). Forty-four patients were monitored and followed up for at least 3-month posttransplant. Quality of life was evaluated via the Functional Assessment of Chronic Illness Therapy–Bone Marrow Transplantation (version 4) questionnaire with all patients and semi-structured, problem-oriented interviews with seven subjects. The authors compared results from the quantitative and qualitative parts based on triangulation – a method aimed to increase confidence in findings by use of two or more independent measures (Bryman 2008). Findings suggested <25% were highly satisfied with their QoL, with women scoring lower than men. The results revealed a positive correlation between the post-HSCT period and QOL ($r_s = 0.338$, $P = 0.025$), especially regarding the social/family ($r_s = 0.411$, $P = 0.006$) and emotional well-being ($r_s = 0.306$, $P = 0.043$) aspects. Interviews, however, revealed

dependence and inability to work while also acknowledging support from family and healthcare professionals and a shift in priorities. By using mixed method approach, authors were able to say that the comparative quantitative and qualitative parts of the study demonstrated corresponding results.

15.5.5 Classifications of Research by Time

Research can also be categorized according to the time in/over which it is conducted. This can include retrospective studies, prospective studies, and cross-sectional and longitudinal research.

15.5.6 Cross-Sectional Study Design

A cross-sectional study is an observational study that collects data from a group of similar individuals (cohort) or a representative population at one specific point in time or over a period of time. It may be descriptive and used to assess certain distress of a disease or treatment in a defined population. A cross-sectional study is quick and easy to conduct and good for generating hypotheses, and an example of such is provided in Box 15.5. A weakness is that the onset of the outcome is difficult to determine and that associations may be difficult to interpret.

Box 15.5 Cross-Sectional Studies in the HSCT Setting

Dyer et al. (2016) assessed 421 Australian survivors (57% male, 43% female) of HSCT sexuality and reported sexual inactivity in 12% of both male and female survivors and sexual difficulties in 51% of sexually active male survivors and 66% of sexually active female survivors. Men reported erectile dysfunction (80%) and decreased libido (62%), and female survivors reported loss of libido (83%), painful intercourse (73%), vaginal dryness (73%), less enjoyment of sex (68%), vaginal narrowing (34%), and vaginal irritation (26%). They also studied associations and found age and cGVHD significantly associated with sexual dysfunction. However, this study is the largest up till now; a weakness of this study is that it is not prospectively examined. After all, how sexual function evolves over time cannot be concluded. For some outcomes, a prospective design is better.

15.5.7 Longitudinal Study Design

A longitudinal study is alternative to a cross-sectional study in that data is gathered for the *same* subjects repeatedly over the study period. As a consequence, longitudinal research can extend over many years or even decades depending on the aims of the study.

> **Box 15.6 Longitudinal Study in the HSCT Setting**
>
> Kupst et al. (2002) undertook a prospective longitudinal study of cognitive and psychosocial functioning in pediatric HSCT patients. They assessed the children on three occasions: pre-HSCT, 1 year post-HSCT, and 2 years post-HSCT. 153 children and adolescents were evaluated pre-HSCT and at 1 year, with 2-year data available for 74 children. Longitudinal analyses of Wechsler IQ data were completed on 100 children (longitudinal exact test) and 52 children (repeated measures analysis of variance). Results of cognitive assessment indicated (1) stability of IQ scores over time and (2) that the strongest predictor was pre-HSCT cognitive functioning. Psychosocial assessment results indicated (1) a low prevalence of behavioral and social problems, (2) stability in functioning over time, and (3) pre-HSCT functioning strongly predictive of later functioning.

15.5.8 Prospective Study Design

A prospective study design is a specific type of observational study that follows a group of similar individuals (cohort) over time and ideally begins enrolling before exposure (baseline) and then follows over a period of time (longitudinally), to determine if and when exposure (e.g., HSCT) changes outcomes. In this way, more associations can be identified between "risk factors" and outcomes – examples of prospective studies are provided in Box 15.6.

> **Box 15.7 Prospective Studies in the HSCT Setting**
>
> Syrjala et al. (2008) reported the most extended longitudinal study in relation to sexual function changes during 5 years after HSCT report that 46% of males and 80% of the female patients have sexual problems 5 years posttransplant. Both men and women declined in average sexual function from before transplantation to 6 months after transplantation. Women did not improve from 6-month posttransplantation levels by 5 years. Men improved significantly by 2 years. A weakness of this study is that the baseline measurement is before transplantation, ideally the baseline measurement would be carried out before induction chemotherapy.
>
> Crooks et al. (2014) determined whether the use of a single-item screening tool and a problem list could monitor patients' distress and the relations. All consecutive

patients scheduled for an allogeneic transplant between January 15, 2012, and December 17, 2012, who gave informed consent after being informed were handed a packet that included a short demographic sheet, distress thermometer, and problem list. The final sample included 37 patients; they were approximately 54 years of age, range 32–66 years, and had more males (62%) than females (38%). Distress was measured at the transplant talk, discharge, and 3 and 6 months post-discharge. Using the distress cutoff score of 4 as the criterion, 59% had clinically significant distress at time point 1, 58% at discharge, 43% at 3 months, and 19% at 6 months. The results show the use of a one-item screening tool and problem list to monitor psychosocial distress over time as a potential method to coordinate the care to address problems.

15.5.9 Retrospective Study Design

A retrospective study is one which looks backward, often by looking through patients' notes or registries. It will collate information and examine variables in relation to an outcome (e.g., survival) that is established when the protocol is written at the start of the study. This methodology is useful if the outcome of interest is uncommon, and a prospective investigation would have to be too large to be feasible. Retrospective studies may be carried out prior to commencement of a more targeted prospective study to validate the field of study.

Box 15.8 Retrospective Study in the HSCT Setting

Aoudjhane et al., on behalf of the Acute Leukemia Working Party of EBMT (2005), compared the results of patients who underwent a reduced intensity conditioning regimen (RIC) prior to HLA identical HSCT, to those after myeloablative (MA) regimen HSCT, in patients with acute myeloblastic leukemia (AML) over 50 years of age. Outcomes of 315 RIC were retrospectively compared with 407 MA HSCT recipients. In multivariate analysis, acute GVHD (II–IV) and transplant-related mortality were significantly decreased ($P = 0.01$ and $P < 10\text{–}4$, respectively), and relapse incidence was significantly higher ($P = 0.003$) after RIC transplantation. Leukemia-free survival was not statistically different between the two groups. These results may set the grounds for prospective trials comparing RIC with other strategies of treatment in elderly AML.

15.6 Ethical Issues in Nursing Research

Throughout the research process, the protection of those participating is paramount. Guidance on the ethical conduct of clinical trials is provided both locally within institutions and nationally and internationally and is based on key documents such as the Nuremberg Code (1947) and the Declaration of Helsinki (2002). Methods to protect human rights include the process of gaining informed consent from each potential subject to participate in a trial, as well as the review of any study and its documentation, by an independent ethics committee.

The process of informed consent is more than a signature on a document. Participants must be aware of the implications of participating in the study, the potential risks and benefits, anonymity and protection of privacy, the voluntariness of their participation, and right to withdraw consent to participate at any time without suffering negative consequences. This information tends to be within a participant information sheet (PIS) and related consent form (CF). These are documents that will also be revised by the independent ethics committee. Potential participants should be provided with these documents and have time to both read and assimilate the information, with opportunity to discuss and ask questions so that there is a clear and complete understanding of all aspects of the study. The purpose of ethics committees, however, is to ensure the interests of the participant are accounted for when evaluating studies for approval. This includes evaluating whether the study is ethical, the completeness and appropriateness of documents such as the PIS and CF, and reviewing aspects of the design to ensure its correct conduct.

Ethical considerations in nursing research are sometimes rather complex, and just a simplified overview has been described in this chapter. The requirement for approval to conduct research should be discussed at a local level with research and development units or with the local ethics committee secretary, who will usually be able to provide guidance on the types of approval for the type of research being undertaken. This may also include approval from the national regulatory bodies in some cases. Research should not be undertaken until all necessary approvals have been received and documented. The process of approval may be lengthy if amendments to documents or even research protocols are required in order to address concerns raised by one or more of the approval bodies. This potential for delay should be considered when research is being planned.

Conclusion

One of the key factors for nursing research is that we are aiming to produce results and increase our knowledge base in a way that is quickly translatable into clinical practice. In a rapidly developing field such as HSCT, research helps to provide evidence on which to base standards for care, thus helping to ensure the safety and efficacy of our practice with a very vulnerable patient population. Planning a potential study is often the aspect of work which is most time-consuming. It is, however, imperative to get this right to prevent delays further down the line (e.g., with the ethical approval process). For that reason,

teamwork is highly recommended as is support from experts/experienced researchers. It is beyond the scope of this chapter to provide specific details for all aspects of the research process, but rather the aim was to provide guidance on the main concepts, which require thought in order to complete a successful project. Research is an integral part of the future of HSCT, and as qualified nurses, we have a duty of care to our patients to become involved in whatever way we can. Finally, it is important to remember that negative results can be just as useful as positive ones, if not more so; please do not let such an outcome, if it should occur, put you off publishing.

References

Aoudjhane M, Labopin M, Gorin NC, Shimoni A, Ruutu T, Kolb H-J, Frassoni F, Boiron JM, Yin JL, Finke J, Shouten H, Blaise D, Falda M, Fauser AA, Esteve J, Polge E, Slavin S, Niederwieser D, Nagler A, Rocha V. Comparative outcome of reduced intensity and myeloablative conditioning regimen in HLA identical sibling allogeneic haematopoietic stem cell transplantation for patients older than 50 years of age with acute myeloblastic leukaemia: a retrospective survey from the Acute Leukemia Working Party (ALWP) of the European group for Blood and Marrow Transplantation (EBMT). Leukemia. 2005;19:2304–12.

Aslam S, Emmanuel P. Formulating a researchable question: a critical step for facilitating good clinical research. Indian J Sex Transm Dis. 2010;31(1):47–50.

Bryman A. Social research methods. 3rd ed. Oxford: Oxford University Press; 2008.

Chaudhry HM, Bruce AJ, Wolf RC, Litzow MR, Hogan WJ, Patnaik MS, Kremers WK, Phillips GL, Hashmi SK. The incidence and severity of oral mucositis among allogeneic hematopoietic stem cell transplantation patients: a systematic review. Biol Blood Marrow Transplant. 2016;22(4):605–16.

Creswell JW. Research design: qualitative, quantitative and mixed methods approaches. 4th ed. London: Sage; 2014.

Crooks M, Seropian S, Bai M, McCorkle R. Monitoring patient distress and related problems before and after hematopoietic stem cell transplantation. Palliat Support Care. 2014;12(1):53–61.

Declaration of Helsinki. (As amended in Tokyo, Venice, Hong Kong and Somerset West and Edinburgh) October 2000; 2002.

Dyer G, Gilroy N, Bradford J, Brice L, Kabir M, Greenwood M, Larsen SR, Moore J, Hertzberg M,

Kwan J, Brown L, Hogg M, Huang G, Tan J, Ward C, Kerridge I. A survey of fertility and sexual health following allogeneic haematopoietic stem cell transplantation in New South Wales, Australia. Br J Haematol. 2016;172(4):592–601.

Greener J, Grimshaw J. Using meta-analysis to summarise evidence within systematic reviews. Nurse Res. 1996;4:27–38.

Kielmann K, Cataldo F, Seely J. Introduction to qualitative research methodology. Manual, UK.Gov website; department for international deveolment 2011.

Kupst MJ, Penati B, Debban B, Camitta B, Pietryga D, Margolis D, Murray K, Casper J. Cognitive and psychosocial functioning of pediatric hematopoietic stem cell transplant patients: a prospective longitudinal study. Bone Marrow Transplant. 2002;30:609–17.

Molassiotis A. Nursing research within bone marrow transplantation in Europe: an evaluation. Eur J Cancer Care (Engl). 1997;6(4):257–61.

Niederbacher S, Them C, Pinna A, Vittadello F, Mantovan F. Patients' quality of life after allogeneic haematopoietic stem cell transplantation: mixed-methods study. Eur J Cancer Care. 2012;21(4):548–59.

The Nuremberg Code. Br Med J (1996). 1947;313:1448.

Riley P, Glenny AM, Worthington HV, Littlewood A, Clarkson JE, McCabe MG. Interventions for preventing oral mucositis in patients with cancer receiving treatment: oral cryotherapy. Cochrane Database Syst Rev. 2015;12:CD011552. https://doi.org/10.1002/14651858.CD011552.pub2.

Syrjala KL, Kurland BF, Abrams JR, Sanders JE, Heiman JR. Sexual function changes during the 5 years after high-dose treatment and hematopoietic cell transplantation for malignancy, with case-matched controls at 5 years. Blood. 2008;111(3):989–96.

Twycross A, Shorten A. Service evaluation, audit and research: what is the difference? Evid Based Nurs. 2014;17(1):65–6.

www.ingramcontent.com/pod-product-compliance
Lightning Source LLC
Chambersburg PA
CBHW080251030726
47593CB00009B/2440